Diagnostic Controversy

T0229713

This collection is dedicated to the diagnostic moment and its unrivaled influence on encompassment and exclusion in health care. Diagnosis is seen as both an expression and a vehicle of biomedical hegemony, yet it is also a necessary and speculative tool for the identification of and response to suffering in any healing system. Social scientific studies of medicalization and the production of medical knowledge have revealed tremendous controversy within, and factitiousness at the outer parameters of, diagnosable conditions. Yet the ethnographically rich and theoretically complex history of such studies has not yet congealed into a coherent, structured critique of the process and broader implications of diagnosis. This volume meets that challenge, directing attention to three distinctive realms of diagnostic conflict: in the role of diagnosis to grant access to care, in processes of medicalization and resistance, and in the transforming and transformative position of diagnosis for 21st century global health. Smith-Morris's framework repositions diagnosis as central to critical global health inquiry. The collected authors question specific diagnoses (e.g., Lyme disease, Parkinson's, andropause, psychosis) as well as the structural and epistemological factors behind a disease's naming and experience.

Carolyn Smith-Morris is a medical anthropologist and Associate Professor at Southern Methodist University.

Routledge Studies in Anthropology

Diagnostic Controversy

Cultural Perspectives on Competing
Knowledge in Healthcare

Edited by Carolyn Smith-Morris

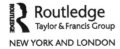

Routledge
Taylor & Francis Group

NEW YORK AND LONDON

First published 2016
by Routledge
605 Third Avenue, New York, NY 10017

and by Routledge
4 Park Square, Milton Park, Abingdon, Oxon OX14 4RN

First issued in paperback 2017

*Routledge is an imprint of the Taylor & Francis Group,
an informa business*

Library of Congress Cataloging-in-Publication Data
Diagnostic controversy : cultural perspectives on competing knowledge in
    healthcare / edited by Carolyn Smith-Morris.
        pages cm. — (Routledge studies in anthropology ; 25)
    Includes bibliographical references and index.
    1. Diagnosis—Cross-cultural studies.   2. Decision making—Cross-cultural
studies.   I. Smith-Morris, Carolyn, 1966–
    RC71.D523 2016
    616.07'5—dc23   2015015188

Typeset in Sabon
by Apex CoVantage, LLC

ISBN 13: 978-0-8153-4655-5 (pbk)
ISBN 13: 978-1-138-93825-0 (hbk)

Contents

PART III
Diagnosis in a Global Community

Figures

1 Introduction

Diagnosis as the Threshold to 21st Century Health

Carolyn Smith-Morris

The diagnostic moment has an unrivaled capacity for encompassment and exclusion, both as an expression and as a vehicle of authoritative medical reference. Inside this moment, when an illness is named, there exists a cascade of response and resistance through which relationships of power are negotiated. Social scientists have long recognized that governmental funding patterns, private market investment, and social responses ranging from care to stigma cohere around and respond to these diagnostic moments, and to the nosological categories that hold sway over them, while unrecognized and unnamed suffering remains invisible.

Although the authoritative nature of a diagnostician's pronouncement leads us to believe otherwise, diagnosis hovers at the edge of scientific certainty, in the epistemological battlegrounds of professionalized and bureaucratized practice. Diagnosis also lives in the resistance of those disenfranchised actors whose diagnosis—or failure to receive a diagnosis—spells certain social, economic, or political demise. The undiagnosed, HIV-positive seasonal farm laborer, soon to return to his village to marry; a business executive suffering from intermittent and unexplained abdominal pain, visiting his fifth doctor in as many months; and the hallucinating woman whose healing treatments include beatings and prayer, but not the expensive and inaccessible medication that wealthier others might receive—these are but a few reminders of the controversial role and socially debated space of diagnosis. These men and women do not share a diagnosis, but they do share its transubstantiating impact. And it is the shared impact of a diagnostic event, and not a particular disease state, that unifies our discussion in this volume. By questioning the diagnostic act, this collection not only removes the pronouncement of an authoritative agent from its otherwise sturdy moorings in objectivity and immutability; it also mobilizes a vocabulary of competition, resistance, and positionality. This vocabulary can unmoor diagnosis and allow an alternative focus, if not framework, for critical studies of biomedical praxis to emerge.

Why should just one subject, one moment within the expansive theme of illness and healing, carry such weight? One reason may be because diagnosis is among the first responses to suffering, the one that initiates and organizes all others. Even more importantly, there is perhaps nothing more unifying in all of healing's endless activities, nothing more consistent across all recognized illnesses and the efforts to ameliorate them, than this sentinel act. If diagnosis is correct and successful, it conveys not just meaning, but *shared* meaning. When diagnosis is successful, it is not only because it leads to efficacious care, but also because it affirms a set of relations and response behaviors. The authors in this volume exploit the unifying moment of diagnosis to consider how disease states are fashioned in professional nomenclature, and from there are molded into action and policy within professional and clinical spaces. These actions manage and manipulate vast populations—even all of humankind—through increasingly biologized and racialized language (Hunt and Kreiner 2013; Petryna 2009; Smedley and Smedley 2005).

Social theorists have been irresistibly drawn to diagnosis for millennia. Ours is therefore an ancient problem, as old as the practice of diagnosis itself. So while we are certainly not the first to focus attention on diagnostic nosology and processes, we offer the first ethnographic and deeply contextualized collection into this subject. We look beyond social issues and clinical challenges to frame diagnosis as a broadly constructed, and constructive, process. These insights into the designs, influence, and impacts of diagnosis are a timely meta-analysis into the structures of authoritative—and now global—power differentials in health. The complexity, regulation, and regimes of diagnosis have expansive capacity for shaping medicine as a whole. And as global healing is made evermore interdependent through internationally coordinated campaigns and capitalist expansion, there is cause to view diagnosis as a doorway guarded not by the beneficent hand of an omniscient science, but as one contested by self-interested, incompletely informed, and ethically divergent powers.

To be sure, an inquisition into the parameters and meaning of a diagnosis attends every illness ethnography and many clinical texts. Anthropological and sociological examinations of stigma and the social negotiation of diagnosis have been robust since the 1980s (Good and Good 1986; Young 1981). But there are few volumes dedicated to the analysis of the patterned, speculative, and proliferating acts of diagnosis *per se* (exceptions include: Hunt and Kreiner 2013; Smith-Morris 2005). A recent and important exception is the edited volume by Jutel and Dew (2014). This is a textbook that lays out many of the complex topics that both clinicians and their patients face in arriving at a diagnosis. It is a unique resource for clinicians in training. A second important exception is in mental health diagnoses, for which early and critical perspectives probed the social meaning and clinical ambiguity of not only certain mental disorders, but of the process of labeling behaviors and ways of thinking as "disordered" (Fabrega 1987; Gaines 1982, 1986, 1992; Summerfield 1998). Atwood Gaines's Afterword to this collection suggests the pioneering work in the arena of mental health diagnosis, of which his own contributions to the diagnoses of Alzheimer's, depression, and ethnopsychiatry are influential. Mental health is particularly fraught for diagnosis because, as Summerfield wrote, "the 'nature of reality' is bound up with local forms of knowledge and philosophy. . . . To assume that the contemporary Western way of being a person . . . is good for mental health in Africa or Asia. . . is medical imperialism" and risks "pseudodiagnosis" (Summerfield 1998: 336).

The unique offering of this collection is to capture some of the diagnostic complexity and controversy of real-world settings. We consider those patterned aspects of diagnosis that operate across disease and illness categories, as well as the multiple and competing ways that social factors in diagnosis interact, compete, and conflate with each other. Therefore, we are distrustful of the performed certainties of healing praxis. Through detailed and contextually rich case studies, we probe the deep and local detail of medical ambiguities, particularly the multi-layered and situational production of a diagnosis.

The clinical context of diagnosis presents both epistemological and nosological challenges across both infectious and non-infectious, chronic and acute conditions, high-income and low-income communities. But only social scientists of health may be convinced, at the outset, that a critique of this process is worth making. Clinicians, after all, must arrive at a diagnosis before they can proceed to the more iconic aspects of their work: treatment and healing. To entangle oneself in epistemological arguments at all, much less at the very outset of patient contact, is a treacherous business that only the philosophically inclined physicians may be willing to take on. But in exposing this important process to such scrutiny, I am questioning not *whether* to diagnose, but how, when, and why a particular diagnosis yields certain results.

I will use this Introduction to review the fundamental purpose of diagnosis: to identify and sort a group of symptoms into the uniform, taxonomic categories of known diseases. I devote some attention to the issue of uniformity so that the readers of this conversation have the same starting place: that is, we recognize diagnosis as part of a healing strategy, one that simultaneously indexes and deploys the disease lexicon and instructions of a particular healing system. The uniformity and distinctiveness of these categories help justify one diagnosis over another, but it is also a particular strategy of knowing, of carving up the world of experience into bytes and bits of "evidence," some to be taken seriously, others to be discarded. So uniformity's great benefits do have an epistemic price.

DIAGNOSTIC UNIFORMITY

In biomedical dictionaries, diagnosis is typically given a two-part definition: (1) it is the determination of the nature of a case of a disease; and (2) it is the art of distinguishing one disease from another (Dorland's Illustrated

Medical Dictionary, 28th edition, 1994). Sydenham's early writings on the subject explained that "[i]n the first place, it is necessary that all disease be reduced to definite and certain *species*, and that, with the same care which we see exhibited by botanists in their phytologies"(1858; quoted in Engle and Davis 1963). Each category must be both uniform in character and clearly bounded from other categories. Medical anthropologists have shown that every ethnomedical system is structured around a limited set of diagnostic categories in order to set limits on its illness lexicon. This need is perfectly sound. To be effective, diagnosis must, therefore, be taxonomic. For the clinician, good diagnosis yields a single lexicon, a dictionary of known maladies. It is from this lexicon that diagnosticians learn how to identify a disorder, when to diagnose, and what a given diagnosis implies and connotes.

The theme of uniformity is a good place to start because it lends at least an illusion of clarity, boundaries, and regularity to diagnosis. Where the boundary line between positive diagnosis and non-diagnosis is clear, clinical debate is minimal and the focus can turn to the next phase, be it treatment or monitoring or prayer. But when differential diagnosis is more difficult or contested, the peculiar requirements and thresholds for a diagnosis will receive more debate. Several cases in this volume are concerned with this pattern of diagnostic debate and negotiation, the recognition and weighing of evidence within a scientific arena (Crane or Myers, this volume). Several others draw attention to cases in which a diagnosis is not about certainty or truth so much as it is about a social and professional negotiation (Rohden, Potter, this volume); over what signs are deemed relevant, what counts as evidence, and how to interpret whatever evidence is available (Sachs, Warren and Manderson, and Davis and Nichter, this volume). All recognize that there is more to diagnosis than its taxonomic function: its most stark and homogenizing purpose.

Diagnosis in reality attempts to map an irregular human experience onto a landscape of uniformity. The fit is often imperfect. As anyone who has ever had acne, or pink eye, or a UTI will know, superimposed over this diagnostic label are other layers of interpretation, meaning, and social experience. In the deep topography of social and human space, things like race, gender, technology, politics, economies, and cultural hierarchies complicate both disease and illness. At its full, globally scaled dynamic, diagnosis exists within the broadest context of science, where the politics and power struggle of specific actors create medical definitions that are refined and deployed to achieve certain goals. This space is inhabited by both professionals and patients, both experts and laypersons, consumers and producers. So, to arrive at a diagnostic decision depends on the evidentiary technologies available, the authority of both patient and healer, and the ability of patient and healer to communicate effectively. Work toward a diagnosis is uncertain, an approximation. Burnam (1993) offered this:

More often [as physicians,] we proximate meaning: rather than certitude, we deal with what is most likely. Inferring from the signs what might be wrong, we test for truth and discriminate among competing diagnostic possibilities by examining for the presence of a mosaic of harmonious signs that we might expect to find if our conjecture (or one of them) was tenable. (1993: 941)

These uncertainties, approximations, and conjectures in diagnosis abrade the ideal and empirical within biomedicine. More than the stages of decision-making prior to a correct diagnosis, they are fundamental to the process and do not necessarily lead to clear and "harmonious" signs. The presence of a virus, for example, may be relatively plain through contemporary visualization technologies. So too might the fracture of a bone or the impairment of one's ability to maintain the vertical line of gravity. But for other conditions, diagnosis involves more guesswork about invisible processes and events, or about potential *future* events. A conservative approach in predictive diagnoses—e.g., diabetes, heart disease, hypertension—leaves the diagnostic moment until late in the disease course, when certainty is at a maximum. A more aggressive approach pushes the diagnostic moment earlier in time, through a lower threshold, to capture more of those at risk for complications (Rapp 1999; Smith-Morris 2006b). A few patients who would not have developed the harmful conditions will be captured, diagnosed, and possibly treated, and some of those may suffer because of the false positive prediction. But by definition, those people will inhabit a predetermined, tolerable margin of error (tolerable, at least, to the diagnosticians).

We can therefore enumerate a few aspects of the diagnostic enterprise that belie its underlying uncertainty and mutability. Engle and Davis (1963) pointed to a continuing truth that not only do we not have universally accepted definitions for all disease, but our ability to confidently diagnose a condition varies considerably across disease states. Further:

[O]ur definitions of some diseases are continually changing, with the result that there is no fixed number of disease. Finally, the manifestations of some well-delineated diseases are also changing. (1963: 113)

In other words, even if diagnostic clarity is achieved, that clarity may not last. Diagnoses will always be modified to better capture those at risk, and wholly new diagnoses will arise as organisms evolve and environments change. The pressure toward uniformity and clarity, then, is met with constant resistance, while diagnostic controversy can be seen as a valuable mechanism in the advance of both the medical sciences and the healing arts.

Scientific advance engenders new ways of seeing and conceptualizing events in the human organism. Here, I suspect, most readers will have an example or two in mind of relatively recently medicalized human events; trends in the diagnosis and treatment of "excessive" skin after weight loss or pregnancy, for instance; of "dysfunctional" or "reduced" sexual appetite after a threshold age; even male pattern baldness. But rather than address these favorites of medical sociological analysis, let us consider the example of a new diagnosis built not on previous diagnostic categories, but wrought out of trends in health data.

The example comes from obstetrical medicine, in which the concept of "term" is carved out of the temporal continuum, forming a new diagnostic category where none seemed necessary before. Gestation in human single-ton pregnancies lasts an average of 40 weeks from the first day of the last menstrual period to the estimated day of delivery. In the past, the period from three weeks before until two weeks after the estimated date of delivery was considered "term," with the expectation that neonatal outcomes from deliveries in this interval were uniform and good. Increasingly however, new technologies and research have identified *unsatisfactory* neonatal outcomes, especially respiratory morbidity, *within* this five-week gestational age range. In other words, the formerly normal and good "term" was deemed to *lack uniformity*, and was subsequently carved into smaller, more precise units between 37 0/7 weeks of gestation and 42 0/7 weeks of gestation. A work group was convened in late 2012 that included representatives from the Eunice Kennedy Shriver National Institute of Child Health and Human Development, the American College of Obstetricians and Gynecologists, and the Society for Maternal-Fetal Medicine. It was driven by a desire for "uniform definitions of term predicated on a uniform method of determin-ing gestational age" (Medicine 2013). The participants created four new classifications of pregnancy outcome (early term, full term, late term, and post-term).

In the construction of "term" as a new diagnostic category, taxonomic uni-formity was deployed where simple temporal information was not enough. The distinction is both ephemeral and epidemiological, because the need for these ~13-day distinctions derives from predictive and population-based science, prior to (and possibly in the absence of) any actually distress or problem in the patient at hand. What's more, the demand for uniformity in diagnosis is a productive epidemiological priority, both responding to but also *creating* assumptions about the need to track those distinctions. In this case, time is diagnostically reimagined, given a nominal firmness, as if "37 weeks' gestation" was somehow different from "early term." The conse-quent centrality of diagnostic testing to this process, and particularly the exactness of risk categorization and monitoring, are presumed and inscru-table. This becomes problematic only with the corresponding expectations for maternal follow-through (which occurs, by the way, through equally standardized, population-based modes of treatment). This is just one of many examples that illustrate the epidemiological imperative: where the tracking of vast, if not all, human populations is needed, those populations must also be visualized, made "legible" (Biehl 2004), in more uniform, less diverse ways. Time becomes pathological, and uniformity is deployed (or overlain) where human experience was once chaotic. Finally, the example suggests not positive, negative, or neutral outcomes to diagnosis, but a new way of creating uniformity and order. It is meant to contrast the diagnosis of symptoms with the diagnosis of statistics, and to raise a first question about the role of diagnosis in practice.

How does a drive toward uniformity—whether informed by biology or by statistics—shape the practice of healing? Despite structuralist attention to the teaching hospital and university research institute, these are not the most influential institutions of diagnostic authority. Instead, the most influential structures are those unquestioned forms of naming: the taxonomies from which and through which dominant relationships are built and institutionalized. Members of a medical profession embrace this disease taxonomy and its uniformity for important and practical reasons. It can be known by experts in the field, and deployed for broad use. It is reliable, stable, and referential, not just signal. And in the taxonomy of diagnoses, the chaotic details of human experience, in theory, fall into beautiful, uniform order.

DIAGNOSTIC CONTROVERSY

Diagnostic controversies are more widespread in some areas of medicine than others. My own interest in the impact of diagnosis emerged from my work on metabolic syndrome, a single diagnosis that integrates several risk factors for future coronary heart disease and/or diabetes (Aguilar-Salinas et al. 2005). Confusion and resistance to a diagnosis of diabetes, for which professional controversy is both regular and unlikely to be resolved soon (Pettitt 2001), was the subject of my first inquiry into this topic (Smith-Morris 2005). Type 2 diabetes is a condition in which the body's production or use of insulin is impaired, leading to harmful, elevated glucose levels in the blood. The medical marketplace surrounding this diagnosis could not be more complex. It represents around 4 million deaths per year, most of them premature deaths among working adults, direct costs of 2.5–15 percent percent of national health care budgets, and indirect costs stemming from lost production, which are as high as five times the direct costs (World Health Organization 2015). Yet, despite a near global omnipresence, the diagnosis of diabetes is still actively debated and researched.

Gestational diabetes is particularly vexing because of the vulnerability of pregnant women to moralizing interventions, debates over the primary patient (mother or fetus), and the many cultural tropes surrounding reproduction. At the center of the diagnostic controversy are concerns about macrosomia (high birth weight) and other birth outcomes, as well as the potential need for different diagnostic criteria for some ethnic groups. Aspects of the controversy have included: the appropriateness of testing; the methods by which testing should be done; the cutoff values for diagnosis; the costs of various methods; the need for different cutoff values for different ethnic groups; and the implications of fetal origin research for public health interventions in high diabetes risk populations.

As with a variety of metabolic and chronic conditions, a diagnosis of diabetes is based on more than current biological complications. Late in the last century, diabetes was typically diagnosed late in its destructive processes, after the body had been battling vascular complications for a long time. Increasingly, diagnostic thresholds have been lowered to catch the disease early and prevent its worst effects. But this means that the lived experience of diagnosis is substantially different and opaque. Only through biotechnological intervention has early diagnosis been possible. Pregnant women who are susceptible to Gestational Diabetes Mellitus (GDM) or the form of diabetes that occurs and is diagnosed in pregnancy, but which disappears after the birth of the child, may have expectations about diabetes that contradict their symptomless experience (Smith-Morris 2005 2006a). This means that reaction to an early diagnosis would be very different from reaction to a late diagnosis. As a result, the social and emotional impact of a diagnosis may be incorporated into the diagnostic algorithm itself. If it were not already obvious, we are now well outside the clear and concise boundaries of some easier diagnoses.

Lay controversies in diagnosis include resistance to diagnostic practice (Dew 2014; Trundle et al. 2014), activism and advocacy for diagnostic legitimacy (Nguyen 2010; Davis and Nichter, this volume; Petryna 2009), and communicative and power struggles between patients and healers. These are particularly true for GDM, which is often symptomless and which disappears after the birth of the child. That is, the patient cannot keep a diagnosis of GDM after birth; any subsequent disease would therefore have to be re-diagnosed. This feature of GDM is a profound complication in the diagnostic process for Pima women. In many cases among Pima Indians, early diagnosis (technically, a diagnosis of GDM is considered to be a precursor to but not the same disease as type 2 diabetes) was not helpful for prevention, and instead was understood as a doctor's error.

The case of Pima diabetes also reveals the problem of what might be called "correlate prevention;" that is, the manipulation of diagnostic thresholds to compensate for social determinants of health. Correlate prevention (also taken up later in this volume by Hardon and by Koch) includes the targeted amplification of diagnostic practice in an area for a variety of purposes. For example, the capture of poor and marginalized new patients with early diagnosis is justified, epidemiologically, by their greater statistical risk for disease; but is there not a corresponding ethical obligation of treatment being made available to those patients? Diabetes diagnosis in indigenous communities has undergone such a strategy, through not only additional screening efforts but also the creation of lower diagnostic thresholds just for these ethnic groups. In sum, whereas early prevention may be beneficial in terms of morbidity, there are moral and social burdens to diagnosis that should impact diagnostic practice.

The relationship between epidemiological targeting and diagnostic practice is heavily charged. As Hardon, with HIV surveillance, and Koch, with TB detection, will discuss, the ethical implications of these epidemiological regimes can be dangerously over-simplified. Farmer's (1992) study of the early HIV targeting of Haitians showed how epidemiological error led to a costly stigmatization of an entire nation's population. But in addition to the problem of epidemiological overreach, early prevention assumes several things about the target population's understanding of and willingness to engage with a preventative intervention plan. In the case of Pima diabetes, whether women complete and respond to prenatal diabetes education is "contingent upon their interpretation of the diagnostic process that, for Gestational Diabetes, seems to contradict subsequent normal blood glucose levels" (Smith-Morris 2005: 166). Some women resisted testing and diagnosis as an unjustified (or unhelpful) policing of pregnant women and their prenatal behaviors and health. The slippery slope of medico-epidemiological logic must be counter-balanced by patient interpretations and experience, and by recognizing that patients can "question the same vagaries of the . . . diagnostic process that are questioned by professionals themselves" (ibid.: 169–170).

The cases I've discussed thus far—"term" pregnancy and gestational diabetes in Pima Indians—help illustrate the poles of the uniformity/complexity continuum. At one end, new diagnostic categories are carved using clean, precise temporal units; at the other, social and economic factors complicate statistical prognostication, making diagnosis a variable and irregular target. Diagnosis seeks to create or identify order from chaos, whether for symptom alleviation or for more numerical, epidemiological goals. And so certain diagnoses, like gestational diabetes, must constantly grapple with fluid contexts, differences in appearance and presentation, and sincere disagreement from the highest scientific levels to the everyday encounters between patients and their healers.

Finally, we cannot question the uniformity of diagnosis without recognizing some of the many possibilities for honest error, misdiagnosis, or simple uncertainty. The credible diagnostician needs some discursive tools for dealing with uncertainty, for managing disagreement and controversy, and for the periods of time during which a diagnosis is ambiguous. This vocabulary does exist. It is a crucial aspect of clinical practice because it makes possible a very wide margin of exploration of those things that *might* be incorporated later into the diagnostic lexicon. One of the most salient examples of this language is the biomedical category of "syndrome." For Whitmarsh, the syndrome is:

> [A]nother way of saying symptom ambiguity, a moment where medicine appears to return to its preclinical gaze, to the disease as a collection of symptoms, not having a fixed origin" (2013: 320).

There is a danger that such a category will be overly large, that it will collect too many unrelated conditions in its conceptual net, and that it will slip too great a variety of conditions into its net of costly diagnosis and treatment. Such broad and irregular diagnostic categories are, therefore, not well tolerated in biomedicine. A complete, framed differential diagnosis—arrived at through probabilistic, prognostic, or pragmatic approaches—is ranked and tested until a diagnosis can be confirmed and treated (Stern et al. 2010). And once the etiology of a syndrome has been determined, that nomenclature should then be removed and a new name (e.g, "disorder" or "disease") assigned.

And so, in certain respects, it seems that uniformity and controversy can be contained reasonably well within the diagnostic lexicon. A few terms are needed to deal with controversy and uncertainty, but ultimately, the system remains functional. But in the remaining space of this Introduction, I move beyond the nosological tasks of diagnostic practice and into the cultural and embodied perspectives that will be the priority of this collection. These variables take our conversation into much greater depths of complexity than the diagnostic lexicon can tolerate. Indeed, these complexities are often more than even the best diagnosticians can account for (although the volume by Jutel and Dew is a hopeful exception).

⌗

In the pages ahead, I lay the framework on which the rest of this volume, including the organization of the chapters, is built. This framework involves three fundamental questions: First, what does a diagnosis mean, not just in terms of nosological categories, but in terms of access to treatment, a good prognosis, and healing resources for any given context? Second, how do the twin forces of medicalization and resistance to medicalization influence the shape, content, and impact of a given diagnosis? And third, what are the dynamics of post-modernity that create 21st century diagnostic communities?

DIAGNOSIS AS ACCESS

The diagnostic doorway allegedly grants access to whatever resources of treatment, validation of suffering, or social support may exist. Returning to the term "syndrome," we have a useful historical vantage point from which to consider how passage through this diagnosis doorway impacts patients' lives. As I have mentioned, the vast majority of named "syndromes" are genetic conditions. But prior to the discovery of DNA's double helix structure and the opening of our current molecular era, the term "syndrome" was used to allow diagnosticians to communicate about unexplained patterns of symptoms or illness. There were relatively few syndromes then, corresponding with the less precise and more laborious methods for data collection on new conditions. But since methods of genetic mapping and cytogenetics have been refined and expanded, there has been an explosion in diagnostic activity for genetic disorders (Gilbert 2000). The vast majority of named syndromes today are conditions for which an inheritance mechanism is either known or partially known. But we also continue to use the term "syndrome" to describe non-genetic conditions (e.g., AIDS) and for collections of symptoms whose etiology is not clear, or even genetic conditions whose manifestation is irregular (e.g., CHARGE syndrome for the highly complex and variable pattern of birth defects that include: coloboma of the eye; heart defects; atresia of the choanae; significant delays of growth and development; genital or urinary abnormalities; and ear abnormalities and deafness).

Another diagnostic transformation over time has occurred for Marfan syndrome, a connective tissues disorder (Faivre et al. 2012: 434). Marfan syndrome is a dominant genetic trait, meaning that people who inherit only one copy of the Marfan *FBN1* gene from either parent will develop the syndrome and be able to transmit it to their children. People with Marfan—Abraham Lincoln, for example—tend to be unusually tall, with long limbs and long, thin fingers. Their symptoms can range from mild to severe, the most serious being defects of the heart valves and aorta, but also possibly of the lungs, the eyes, the dural sac surrounding the spinal cord, the skeleton, and the hard palate. The history of this condition's named existence is both long and dynamic. First named in 1896, its diagnosis was based primarily on phenotypic presentations and late-stage complications and symptoms. Marfan syndrome's nosology has undergone several changes, updates, and modifications since then, in parallel with evolving technology over this time span. By 1988, the first international symposium established a nosology based on molecular evidence. Further revisions in 1992, 1994, and 1996 addressed several more of the former diagnostic problems: the age-dependent nature of some clinical manifestations (making diagnosis in children difficult); the potential diversity of clinical presentations; and several unclear and vague thresholds (e.g., flat feet and pulmonary artery dilatation).

Also noteworthy is the 1996 revision the specifically addressed patients' access to treatment resulting from these proposed diagnostic changes. Consulting diagnosticians expressed concern over the social and economic impacts of diagnosis, and not just the biology of the disease, raising specific concerns about limiting patients' access to insurance benefits or career opportunities (Faivre et al. 2012). Experts therefore modified the definition not only because of the changes in the known aspects of the condition, but also because of the changing societal attitudes about the economic and interpersonal impacts of the diagnosis itself.

Contemporary health care legislation in the U.S. now precludes restrictive access due to pre-existing conditions, reducing one of the risks of diagnosis. The long and evolving diagnostic history of conditions like Marfan syndrome helps make visible the human hands at work in the evolution of science, and the growing relevance of social and economic access issues to diagnostic practice. Such policies also de-link some of the damaging consequences of diagnosis from the naming of disease. But other relevant access issues may surface relating to the diagnosis of chronic and genetic conditions. In the next section, I take up these issues and the broader social context of diagnosis.

MEDICALIZATION & RESISTANCE

Medicalization is the process by which either new or ambiguous symptoms enter into professional medical awareness, and is fundamental to diagnostic debate and medical discovery. The process can be initiated by scientists, practitioners, or lay people, and occurs both inside and outside of the laboratory and clinic. Medicalization has a long history of its own, tied to politics, marketplaces, and embodied human experience.

The naming of a set of symptoms is a landmark event in the process of medicalization. The degree to which that name is agreed upon and the breadth of its use are indicative of the term's incorporation into medical status and the privileges that status conveys. But in the process of medicalization, the tension between disease and not-disease is yet unresolved. When we use terms like "syndrome" and other diagnostic categories that are either new or ambiguous, we embrace both the drive to medicalize and the need to resist it. All possibilities remain open, real and unreal, legitimized and illegitimate. So when de Figueiredo coined the term "medically unexplained symptoms" in 1980 to describe a set of symptoms known simultaneously as Briquet *syndrome*, or a somatization *disorder* (APA 2000: #300.81), or a psychiatric *disease*, the diagnostic controversies were unresolved and the process of medicalization unfinished. The multiple terms in use is indicative of the uncertainty attached to the diagnosis and to de Figueiredo's reluctance to offer a more definitive name.

These types of struggle toward medical legitimacy have been an anthropological concern since the origins of the discipline, but we have succeeded not so much in resolving the tension as in ethnographically describing the process of medicalization. Physician Muhammad Yunus argues the inadequacy of this resolution more forcefully. He says that ambiguous terms like "syndrome" are a product of "the single most destructive force in the practice of medicine today. . . the drumbeat dichotomization between disease and illness" (2008: 348). The disease/illness distinction has been both friend and foe to medical anthropology: friend, because anthropologists like George Foster, Arthur Kleinman, and Allan Young could lean on this dualism in promoting the relevance of our field (and cross-cultural research generally) to clinical audiences; and foe, for the inevitable ranking and prioritizing that categorical reasoning provokes. The term "syndrome" binds together certain symptoms and experiences, moving them one step closer to the legitimacy of diagnosis, while sloughing off some of the surrounding occurrences or feelings deemed unworthy. Yunus argues that the disease/illness dichotomy creates a "fallacious dogma. . . a 2-class classification of patients: those with structural pathology are the 'real' patients who deserve real care, and those without . . . are second-class patients (analogous to second-class citizens) not worthy of serious physician attention" (2008: 348).

To avoid such fallaciousness, those psychosocial and politico-economic factors typically relegated to "illness" and irrelevance in diagnostic terms must be brought further into the language of researchers and patient care providers. Kleinman, Good, Young, and a generation of their students have labored to make visible those social, economic, and cultural factors of illness and particularly, of diagnosis (Good and Good 1986; Kleinman 1981; Young 1981). These are the variables that transform certain events or experiences into what we recognize as a problem, a symptom, or a dysfunction, and the chapters ahead illustrate how they find their way into the diagnostic lexicon.

But medicalization in the 21st century is increasingly sophisticated. There is pressure for biomedical practitioners to attend to social and human factors in the diagnostic process (Jenkins 2014; Mezzich and Caracci 2008; Prior 2014), to diagnosis-related social costs and stigma (Dew 2014; Jutel 2014), or to diagnose with sensitivity to the impacts of follow-up care or the long-term management of a condition (Faivre et al. 2012). Diagnosticians must address marital or reproductive decisions relevant to genetic diagnoses, and the worsening of mental health symptoms following a depression diagnosis (Horwitz 2011). They must even consider a delay in diagnosis due to social attitudes that under-recognize or under-value certain symptoms (Hudelist et al. 2012). In short, the social impacts of a diagnostic label are a major responsibility in ethical diagnostic practice (Estroff 1981; Scott and Leboyer 2011). Medicalization can been seen as the social and economic marketplace in which some of these factors are debated, a space available to patients and laypeople.

DIAGNOSIS IN A GLOBAL COMMUNITY

The positional superiority conveyed by the diagnostic act, no matter how speculative or incomplete, is profound. It is also profoundly profitable. Within biomedicine, the diagnostic pronouncement mobilizes vast resources across a global context. This is true not only for vectors of infection that terrorize us by making irrelevant the vaporous borders of nation-states; it is also true for chronic and metabolic disorders that are transmitted by "free" markets, aggressive advertising, and a healthy demand for the cheapest possible food. The profit-seeking agenda can create demand where none existed before, and can crowd the exam room with commercial interests (Ebeling 2014). Now as much a marketplace as a population of people, the "global public" is a health industry and an ingredient to international politics in ways never before imagined. Pharmaceuticalization (Biehl 2004; Petryna et al. 2006; Whyte et al. 2002) judicialization (Biehl 2013), and projectification (Whyte et al. 2013) now join commodification and standardization (Adams 2002; Adams et al. 2005; Brody 2010; Hunt and Kreiner 2013) as "schemes" that evaluate, verify, and falsify the human experience (Biehl and Petryna 2013: 8). Humans are twisted and contorted into the ledgers of accountants, many of them at work in health corporations.

Because of the incredible fertility and productivity of this health market, diagnosis is an essential instrument for expanding the biomedical system's authority as well as for the growth of its profits. Indeed, prescribing medication to an ever-expanding set of diagnostic categories is tied to what Whitmarsh calls "the public health necessity of diagnosing the pre-ill" (Whitmarsh 2013: 316). As with GDM, contemporary biotechnological healing means that a diagnosis is made long prior to the appearance of any experienced symptom, when future disease is only a statistical probability and not a current reality. For these illnesses, diagnosable evidence is likely to come from our revolutionary new biotechnologies.

In other words, diagnosis is sometimes about naming what is *present*, and at other times about the naming of what we *expect* to see in the future. This dual, context-dependent character of diagnosis contributes to its reputation as a chaotic and mutable process. Were diagnosis to hinge on a process of deduction from an encyclopedic knowledge of existing categories of disease, then physicians would need only be taxonomists. Diagnostic skill would be no more than a mathematical one, based not in perception or even necessarily in the diagnostician's experience, but in the robustness of the statistical model for predicting future distress. Parson's version of this *gen d'armes* of diagnosis deals in stark categories and clear boundaries, rather than the shifting and vague realities of many illness experiences.

But diagnosis is neither so formulaic nor so immune to the social world in which it operates. Just as experts modified and updated the definition of Marfan syndrome, first in response to changing technologies and medical knowledge, and later in recognition of the social stigmas and barriers associated with the diagnosis, experts are increasingly scrutinized for having been influenced by factors unrelated to biological events. This has good and bad consequences.

To illustrate the point, we need only consider the basic process by which diagnoses respond to changes in technologies, treatments, medical knowledge, and cultural norms. These changes cause experts to review and modify disease definitions and diagnostic thresholds. This task is commonly undertaken by expert panels, consensus meetings, or influential workgroups who publish findings as statements, special reports, or as part of clinical practice guidelines. While such changes can be beneficial, there is an increasing recognition that the widening of disease definitions may contribute to over-diagnosis occurring across a range of conditions. The concern expressed by some researchers is that for some people with milder symptoms, at lower risks, or in earlier stages of possible disease, the harms of a diagnostic label and treatment may outweigh the benefits. At the same time, there is accumulating evidence about the pervasive financial ties between pharmaceutical companies and health professionals, including those who are writing the guidelines and disease definitions (Cosgrove and Krimsky 2012; Moynihan et al. 2013; Perlis et al. 2005; Roseman et al. 2012).

One illustration of this process comes from a study by Moynihan et al. (2013), who selected a sample of the most costly conditions and most prescribed medications, then evaluated the most recent publications from panels that made these disease definitions. Finally, the researchers evaluated the industry ties of the panel members. Among the panels that disclosed ties, almost all chairs had financial ties to industry, and an average of three-quarters of the members had ties to a median of seven companies, commonly working as consultants, advisers, and/or speakers, as well as receiving research support. Companies with financial relationships with the greatest proportion of panel members were marketing or developing drugs for the same conditions about which those members were making critical judgments. GlaxoSmithKline, for example, which was marketing top-selling products for asthma, had financial ties to 20 of the 24 members of the 2009 asthma panel, and all 20 were consultant/advisers and/or had declared speaker/honoraria ties to the company (ibid.).

There is no firewall between for-profit medical companies and purportedly neutral expert panels on clinical practice and diagnostics. Of course, this unscrupulous affair between diagnosis and capitalism is not new. Colonial and post-colonial governments, international agencies, and local catalysts have improved the catch of Western ideology using biomedicine's panacea as bait. Critical studies of health began with the realization that indigenous and subaltern bodies were medicalized, and eventually controlled, through their diagnosis as flawed, dangerous, or weak. Colonial medicine, for example, was primarily concerned with maintaining the health of Europeans in colonial settings rather than the indigenous people, and only insofar as was a pre-requisite for sustaining the colonies and for making them productive. Randall Packard described the era of tropical medicine as narrowly technical in focus, "driven by a faith in the ability of Western science to overcome the health problems of colonized subjects" and pleasing to colonial administrators, since a strictly technical or chemical arsenal for combatting infectious disease released government authorities from learning more, diagnostically or otherwise, about the colonized population (Packard 2000: 98–99).

Social scientists of medicine are now vigilant to the colonizing effects and dependency fostered by market-driven health care. Packard blames the "the internationalization of health," through which international health agencies become central in defining all levels of health intervention (2000). This means that a limited number of international organizations control health funding, the production and distribution of expert knowledge, and new systems of agencies that separate health from broader social and economic development initiatives (Erikson 2012; Litsios 1997; Ong and Collier 2004). Biehl's work on bureaucratization, Petryna's on pharmaceuticalization, and Adams (2005) or Landsman (2006) on the politics of evidence in medicine are built upon and contribute to several goals of broader post-colonialism. These include the de-centering of European notions of modernity (Chakrabarty 1992), particularly as they are tied to technology, science, and biomedicine; the problematizing of the trope of territoriality and geopolitical boundaries (King 2002), because these physical demarcations are increasingly irrelevant in the mobility of infectious people (Farmer 1999); and treating local (and translocal, Anderson 2002) knowledge without essentializing it, and without mapping a false diversity onto underlying hegemony (see work by Jeffrey Cohen, for example 1999). One of Adrianna Petryna's informants, Krol, sums it up well: that diagnosis is about "drumming up business" (2009: 125). That business is the engineered window through which pre- and newly diagnosed patients can be turned into a placebo subjects for study trials and lifelong consumers of health goods.

⌗

Up to this point, I have introduced three organizing themes for an investigation into diagnostic practice. They include the position of diagnosis as threshold to treatment resources and support, the process of medicalization, and the contemporary particularities for diagnosis given the global scale and impact of economic marketplaces on health care and healing. These same themes organize the rest of the volume, which I now summarize: (1) Diagnostic Access; (2) Medicalization & Resistance to Diagnosis; and (3) Diagnosis in a Global Community.

Part I: Diagnostic Access

The use of diagnosis as a framework—something that structures and shapes other things—is the common thread in Part I: Diagnostic Access. The first chapters look at diagnosis as a threshold, the doorway to the resources promised. This strategic position makes diagnosis a valuable and sought-after nosological event, but one that is not uniformly reliable for delivering relief from suffering.

Anita Hardon discusses the use of HIV diagnosis in pregnant women as a global surveillance strategy aimed at preventing mother-to-child transmission of HIV. This strategy exposes how diagnosis—historically a threshold to care—is de-linked from treatment, and care for identified patients left undone. In the case of PMTCT, diagnosis is a development tactic: a clinical strategy employed without adequate resources for the ethical care of and engagement with diagnosed women. Hardon suggests how diagnosis may be used in ethically questionable ways, creating gateways for some but not others, and justifying (or sustaining) some governmental and non-governmental investments in some countries, but not others.

In "Resisting Tuberculosis or TB Resistance: Enacting Diagnosis in Georgian Labs and Prison," **Erin Koch** reveals another way in which diagnosis is used strategically for something other than—or in addition to—treatment.

In this case of tuberculosis in post-Soviet Georgian prisons, the strategizers are not just clinicians or development agents, but lab technicians and even the prisoners themselves. Koch investigates standardization as a fundamental element of the diagnostic enterprise. She shows how standardized diagnostic regimens become "situated within and informed by a moral economy that is inseparable from political economy." Like Hardon, Koch points to how diagnostics are decoupled from treatment and become a tool for the management of people rather than a fixed nosological threshold.

Part II: Medicalization & Resistance to Diagnosis

Patients and healers are experiencing diagnosis in some surprising new ways in the 21st century. While struggling to make sense out of suffering and/or to treat it effectively, the actors in the diagnostic process fill multiple roles simultaneously. In Part II, the moral, embodied, and epistemological aspects of diagnosis are the focus.

The section begins with **Fabiola Rohden** and a diagnosis in development. Her chapter, "Promotion of Andropause in Brazil: A Case of Male Medicalization," views this diagnosis as neither clear nor agreed upon across professional and lay groups. Here, at the edge of diagnostic certainty, different actors compete to be heard and influential. Rohden examines the role of the popular, news, and clinical media and campaigns to establish those boundaries for andropause. She redraws the parameters of medicalization in a highly technical and strategically marketed arena. The case of andropause shows how processes of commercialization, social movements, and the popularization of health ideas come together in new ways, and on larger scales than ever before, to impact medical debates and pharmaceutical science.

In "Making Sense of Unmeasurable Suffering: The Recontextualization of Debut Stories to a Diagnosis of Chronic Fatigue Syndrome," **Lisbeth Sachs** considers the modes of interpretation through which bodily experience becomes "symptoms" and narratives of suffering are transformed into "relevant" medical histories. Chronic fatigue syndrome (CFS), Sachs relates, is a "diagnostic success story"—a tale of the achieved diagnosis for decades of formerly marginalized and ignored sufferers. Yet even while CFS is now a better-recognized syndrome, it remains a "negatively determined diagnosis," with substantial work remaining for the doctor and patient to do. In the crafting of Debut Narratives, patients portray their own reliability as informants, nourish hope for healing, and struggle with the ambiguity of this diagnosis.

Narelle Warren and Lenore Manderson take up the challenge of patient credibility in a case study of Parkinson's disease. "Credibility and the Inexplicable: Parkinson's Disease and Assumed Diagnosis in Contemporary Australia" is a study of the diagnostic negotiation that occurs over time, between patients, selves, and others. Parkinson's disease has multiple "pathways to diagnosis" and is a condition that contests the very nature of medical authority for its many uncertainties. Warren and Manderson argue that whereas the moment of diagnosis may resolves professional ambiguities, the personal uncertainties—of future decline, of medication, of eventual death—remain. The treatment of diagnosis as process suggests a more flexible and responsive strategy for this and similar conditions.

Philosopher **Nancy Nyquist Potter** introduces a concept from critical race theory called "epistemologies of ignorance." In applying this concept to psychiatric diagnosis, Potter wants to give uptake to deviant behavior as an important element in diagnostic negotiations. Building on Part II's themes of medicalization and negotiation, Potter asks, "What are we doing to not-know, to maintain ignorance of structures of oppressive, systemic harms?" She examines the *DSM*, the nosological dictionary of psychiatric illness, as an organizing epistemology; and its application, through diagnosis, as an authoritative strategy for maintaining ignorance of certain meanings and experiences. In response, Potter suggests that defiance of such authoritative epistemes is a virtue and may help correct some of the harms done to people living with a mental illness, or who are at risk of earning a mental illness label.

Part III: Diagnosis in a Global Community

In Part III, we turn to the implications that globalization, social networking, and transnational mobility have for diagnosis. From activist communities constructed around a diagnostic category, to epidemiologically drawn communities of risk, to a push for diagnostic uniformity for psychosis, this section recognizes global connections in, and the global scale of 21st century diagnosis.

For patients who become suspect in the panic about globally mobile infections, diagnosis is a moral burden. **Johanna Crane**'s chapter "Supervirus: The Framing of a Doomsday Diagnosis" reveals how diagnostic authority is being harnessed in new ways this century. Speaking to the issue of drug resistance, rather than disease *per se*, this case reveals the semiotic and materials impacts of a diagnosis that is simultaneously a moral burden, a paradox, and a contested event. Using ethnographic research, Crane explores the framing of HIV drug resistance as a stand-alone diagnosis. The case reveals the gap between the science in the laboratory and patient experience in the real world, where patients with near-perfect adherence to medications were more likely to develop this "supervirus."

Global psychiatric diagnosis may be facing a revolutionary moment in the new focus on dysregulated neural circuits, as examined by **Neely Myers** in "Diagnosing Psychosis: Scientific Uncertainty, Locally and Globally." Responding to the leadership in this arena expressed by the Director of the National Institute of Mental Health, Myers explains how genetic biomarkers and psycho-neural structures have been posited as the future of psychiatric diagnosis. She then offers two striking case studies—one in a high-income country, another in a low-income country—to illustrate such dangers as diagnostic rigidity, the label of a "brain disorder," and the erroneous assumption that a proper diagnosis would indicate the best treatment.

Georgia Davis and Mark Nichter show how media and technological advances have changed the way patients learn about and communicate with each other about their experiences. In "The Lyme Wars: The Effects of Biocommunicability, Gender, & Epistemic Politics on Health Activation and Lyme Science," we have a vibrant example of 21st century diagnostic negotiation. In a deeply contextualized and ethnographically rich discussion, they explore three controversies in this diagnosis: the signs of Lyme disease; post-treatment Lyme disease syndrome; tests; and geography. Exposing the vulnerability and responsibility of individuals in contemporary health care decision-making, this chapter reviews the privilege and influence of clinical evidence, and the role of activated Lyme patients in improving diagnostic guidelines.

And in his Afterword, **Atwood Gaines** considers the relational qualities of diagnosis and its multi-vocal meanings. Drawing particularly on long diagnostic debates and controversies from psychiatry, to which he has added not only ethnographic detail but also a policy-oriented critique, Gaines ends the volume with a forward-looking comment. He challenges us to critique medicine's "move to deeper and deeper levels of biology" which "remove the often obvious cultural involvement with diagnosis," and he urges to engage with both the theory of diagnosis and in its particulars.

꤇

It has been almost a decade since I began my work on the critique of diagnosis and started paying closer attention to its treatment in both anthropological and culturally sensitive clinical literatures. Because there have been some excellent articles on this in that time, my goal in this collection is not to promote new attention, but to refocus the attention paid to this moment in healing. The message of the collection is that diagnosis is a tipping point in the processes of encompassment and exclusion in health care. By directing a critical ethnographic inquiry to these moments, and by then engaging in community activation around these moments, culture advocates of any discipline might intensify the impact of anthropological sensibilities in health care.

Diagnosis is a necessary and speculative tool for the identification of and response to suffering in any healing system. But it is also an expression and a vehicle of bio-medico-capitalist power. Social scientific studies of medicalization and the production of medical knowledge have revealed tremendous controversy within, and factitiousness at the outer parameters of, diagnosable conditions. This collection offers an ethnographically rich and structural critique of this process more generally than has been available before.

I have spent most of my Introduction offering a map to the complex layers of diagnosis and diagnostic activity. But the simple concept of uniformity remains instructive and essential, not only to the diagnostic enterprise, but to our critique of it. Were it not for the goal of an effective healing system, diagnosticians would be a chaotic and disorganized, if not a dangerous, mob. Culture advocates, and medical anthropologists specifically, share the goal of effective healing, although they work from different points on the stream bank. Indeed, diagnostic consensus may be the one shared purpose that unites social, laboratory, *and* clinical scientists. We vary in our tolerance for chaos and uncertainty, and in our interest in and willingness to take up the social, political, and capitalist variables that create and influence bodily suffering. But we agree that our efforts hinge on a common language for diagnosis and on the fact that, to be effective, diagnosis must be the gateway to an organized system of treatment.

The cases in this collection speak to social, laboratory, and clinical conundrums. We bring gripping and sometimes painful accounts to light, while acknowledging both the demand for uniformity and clarity and the undeniable irregularity of the human experience. Because the healing arts can now be ruinously expensive, healers and scientists must examine anew the process of medicalization, and of diagnostic incorporation into what is now a techno-capitalist iron cage. We must make more, and make more of, diagnostic controversies. For it is in this space of debate, where the questioning of scientific advancement and knowledge production are made public, that the impact of the marketplace, social norms, and profit-seeking biases are laid bare.

SOURCES

Adams, Vincanne. "Randomized Controlled Crime: Postcolonial Sciences in Alternative Medicine Research." *Social Studies of Science* 32, no. 5/6 (2002): 659–90.

Adams, Vincanne, Suellen Miller, Sienna Craig, Arlene Samen, Nyima, Sonam, Droyoung, Lhakpen, and Michael Varner. "The Challenge of Cross-cultural Clinical Trials Research: Case Report from the Tibetan Autonomous Region, People's Republic of China." *Medical Anthropology Quarterly* 19, no. 3 (2005): 267–89.

Aguilar-Salinas, Carlos A., R. Rojas, F. J. Gómez-Pérez, R. Mehta, A. Franco, G. Olaiz, and J. A. Rull. "The Metabolic Syndrome: A Concept Hard to Define." *Archives of Medical Research* 36 (2005): 223–31.

The American College of Obstetricians and Gynecologists Committee on Obstetric Practice Society for Maternal-Fetal Medicine. *Definition of Term Pregnancy*. Washington, DC: American College of Obstetricians and Gynecologists, 2013.

Anderson, Warwick. "Postcolonial Technoscience." *Social Studies of Science* 32, no. 5–6 (2002): 643–58.

Biehl, João. "Global Pharmaceuticals, AIDS, and Citizenship in Brazil." *Social Text* 22, no. 3 (2004): 105–32.

———. "The Judicialization of Biopolitics: Claiming the Right to Pharmaceuticals in Brazilian Courts." *American Ethnologist* 40.3 (2013): 419–36.

Biehl, João, and Adriana Petryna. *When People Come First: Critical Studies in Global Health*. Princeton, NJ: Princeton University Press, 2013.

Brody, Howard. "The Commercialization of Medical Risks: Physicians and Patients at Risk." In *The Risks of Prescription Drugs*, edited by D. W. Light, 70–91. New York: Columbia University Press, 2010.

Burnum, John F. "Medical Diagnosis through Semiotics." *Annals of Internal Medicine* 119, no. 9 (1993): 939–43, 1993.

Chakrabarty, Dipesh. "Postcoloniality and the Artifice of History: Who Speaks for "Indian" Pasts?" *Representations* 37 (1992): 1–26.

Cohen, Jeffrey H. *Cooperation and Community: Economy and Society in Oaxaca.* Austin: University of Texas Press, 1999.

Cosgrove, Lisa, and Sheldon Krimsky. "A Comparison of DSM-IV and DSM-5 Panel Members' Financial Associations with Industry: A Pernicious Problem Persists." *PLoS Medicine* 9, no. 3 (2012): e1001190.

Dew, Kevin. "Patient-Centered Care or Discrimination? Diagnosis among Diverse Populations." In *Social Issues in Diagnosis: An Introduction for Students and Clinicians*, edited by A. G. Jutel and K. Dew, 93–104. Baltimore, MD: Johns Hopkins University Press, 2014.

Ebeling, Mary. "The Promotion of Marketing-Mediated Diagnosis: Turning Patients into Consumers." In *Social Issues in Diagnosis: An Introduction for Students and Clinicians*, edited by A. G. Jutel and K. Dew, 134–50. Baltimore, MD: Johns Hopkins University Press, 2014.

Engle, Ralph L., and B. J. Davis. "Medical Diagnosis: Present, Past, and Future." *Archives of Internal Medicine* 112(October 1963): 108–15.

Erikson, Susan L. "Global Health Business: The Production and Performativity of Statistic in Sierra Leone and Germany." *Medical Anthropology* 31, no. 4 (2012): 367–84.

Estroff, Sue. *Making It Crazy: An Ethnography of Psychiatric Clients in an American Community.* Berkeley, CA: University of California Press, 1981.

Fabrega, H. "Psychiatric Diagnosis: A Cultural Perspective." *The Journal of Nervous and Mental Disease* 175 (1987): 383–94.

Faivre, L., G. Collod-Beroud, L. Adès, E. Arbustini, A. Child, B. L. Callewaert, B. Loeys, C. Binquet, E. Gautier, K. Mayer, M. Arslan-Kirchner, M. Grasso, C. Beroud, D. Hamroun, C. Bonithon-Kopp, H. Plauchu, P. N. Robinson, J. De Backer, P. Coucke, U. Francke, O. Bouchot, J. E. Wolf, C. Stheneur, N. Hanna N, Detaint D, A. De Paepe, C. Boileau, G. Jondeau. "The New Ghent Criteria for Marfan Syndrome: What Do They Change?" *Clinical Genetics* 81 (2012): 433–42.

Farmer, Paul.*Infections and Inequalities: The Modern Plagues.* Berkeley, CA: University of California Press, 1999.

———. *AIDS and Accusation: Haiti and the Geography of Blame.* Berkeley, CA: University of California Press, 1992.

Gaines, Atwood. "From DSM-I to III-R; Voices of Self, Mastery and the Other: A Cultural Constructivist Reading of U.S. Psychiatric Classification." *Social Science & Medicine* 35, no. 1 (1992): 3–24.

———. "Definitions and Diagnoses: Cultural Implications of Psychiatric Help-Seeking and Psychiatrists' Definitions of the Situation in Psychiatric Emergencies." *Culture, Medicine & Psychiatry* 3 (1986): 381–418.

———. "Cultural Definitions, Behavior and the Person in American Psychiatry." In *Cultural Conceptions of Mental Health and Theory*, edited by A. J. Marsella and G. M. White, 167–192. Dordrecht, Netherlands: Reidel Publishing Company, 1982.

Gilbert, Patricia, ed. *Dictionary of Syndromes and Inherited Disorders.* 3rd ed. Chicago: Fitzroy Dearborn Publishers, 2000.

Good, B. J., and M-J. Good. "Cultural Context of Diagnosis and Therapy: A View from Medical Anthropology." *Mental Health Resource & Practice in Minority Communities* (1986): 1–27.

Horwitz, Allan V. "Creating an Age of Depression: The Social Construction and Consequences of the Major Depression Diagnosis." *Society and Mental Health* 1, no. 1 (2011): 41–54.

Hudelist, G., N. Fritzer, A. Thomas, C. Niehues, P. Oppelt, D. Haas, A. Tammaa, and H. Salzer. "Diagnostic Delay for Endometriosis in Austria and Germany: Causes and Possible Consequences." *Human Reproduction* 27, no. 12 (2012): 3412–416.

Hunt, Linda M., and Meta J. Kreiner "Pharmacogenetics in Primary Care: The Promise of Personalized Medicine and the Reality of Racial Profiling." *Culture, Medicine and Psychiatry* 37, no. 1 (2013): 226–35.

Hunt, Linda M., Meta J. Kreiner, and Fredy Ridriguez-Mejia. "Changing Diagnostic and Treatment Criteria for Chronic Illness: A Critical Consideration of Their Impact on Low-Income Hispanic Patients." *Human Organization* 72, no. 3 (2013): 242–53.

Hunt, Linda M., Nicole Truesdell, and Meta J. Kreiner. "Race, Genes, and Culture in Primary Care: Racial Profiling in the Management of Chronic Illness." *Medical Anthropology Quarterly* 27, no. 2 (2013): 253–71.

Jenkins, Tania M. "Who's the Boss? Diagnosis and Medical Authority." In *Social Issues in Diagnosis: An Introduction for Students and Clinicians*, edited by A. G. Jutel and K. Dew, 105–19. Baltimore, MD: Johns Hopkins University Press, 2014.

Jutel, Annemarie Goldstein. "When the Penny Drops: Diagnosis and the Transformative Moment. *In* Social Issues in Diagnosis: An Introduction for Students and Clinicians, edited by A. G. Jutel and K. Dew, 78–92. Baltimore, MD: Johns Hopkins University Press, 2014.

Jutel, Annemarie Goldstein, and Kevin Dew, eds. *Social Issues in Diagnosis: An Introduction for Students and Clinicians*. Baltimore, MD: Johns Hopkins University Press, 2014.

King, Nicholas B. "Security, Disease, Commerce: Ideologies of Postcolonial Global Health." *Social Studies of Science* 32, no. 5–6 (2002): 763–89.

Kleinman, A. "On Illness Meaning and Clinical Interpretation." *Culture, Medicine and Psychiatry* 5 (1981): 373–77.

Landsman, Gail H. "What Evidence, Whose Evidence? Physical Therapy in New York State's Clinical Practice Guideline and in the Lives of Mothers of Disabled Children." *Social Science & Medicine* 62 (2006): 2670–80.

Litsios, Socrates. "Malaria Control, Rural Development and the Post-War Re-ordering of International Organizations." *Medical Anthropology* 14, no. 2 (1997): 255–78.

Mezzich, Juan E., and Giovanni Caracci, eds. *Cultural Formulation: A Reader for Psychiatric Diagnosis*. Lanham, MD: Rowman & Littlefield Publishing, 2008.

Moynihan, Raymond N., Georga P. E. Cooke, Jenny A. Doust, Lisa Bero, Suzanne Hill, and Paul P. Glasziou. "Expanding Disease Definitions in Guidelines and Expert Panel Ties to Industry: A Cross-sectional Study of Common Conditions in the United States." *PLoS Medicine* 10, no. 8 (2013): e1001500.

Nguyen, Vinh-Kim. *The Republic of Therapy: Triage and Sovereignty in West Africa's Time of AIDS*. Durham, NC: Duke University Press, 2010.

Ong, Aihwa, and Stephen J. Collier. *Global Assemblages: Technology, Politics, and Ethics as Anthropological Problems*. Oxford: Wiley-Blackwell, 2004.

Packard, Randall M. Post-Colonial Medicine. In *Companion to Medicine in the Twentieth Century*, edited by R. Cooter and J. Pickstone, 97–112. London: Routledge, 2000.

Perlis, Roy H., C. S. Perlis, Y. Wu, C. Hwang, M. Joseph, and A. A. Nierenberg. "Industry Sponsorship and Financial Conflict of Interest in the Reporting of Clinical Trials in Psychiatry." *American Journal of Psychiatry* 162, no. 10 (2005): 1957–60.

Petryna, Adriana. *When Experiments Travel: Clinical Trials and the Global Search for Human Subjects*. Princeton, NJ: Princeton University Press, 2009.

Petryna, Adriana, Andrew Lakoff, and Arthur Kleinman, eds. *Global Pharmaceuticals: Ethics, Markets, Practices.* Durham, NC: Duke University Press, 2006.

Pettitt, D. J. "The 75-g Oral Glucose Tolerance Test in Pregnancy." *Diabetes Care* 24, no. 7 (2001): 1129.

Prior, Lindsay. "Lay Diagnosis: An Oxymoron?" In *Social Issues in Diagnosis: An Introduction for Students and Clinicians*, edited by A. G. Jutel and K. Dew, 183–97. Baltimore, MD: Johns Hopkins University Press, 2014.

Rapp, Rayna. *Testing Women, Testing the Fetus: The Social Impact of Amniocentesis in America.* Hove, UK: Psychology Press.

Roseman, Michelle, Erick H. Turner, Joel Lexchin, James C. Coyne, Lisa A. Bero, Brett D. Thombs. "Reporting of Conflicts of Interest from Drug Trials in Cochrane Reviews: Cross Sectional Study." *BMJ* 345 (2012): e5155.

Scott, J., and M. Leboyer. "Consequences of Delayed Diagnosis of Bipolar Disorders." *L'Encephale* 37, no. S3: S173–S175.

Smedley, Audrey, and Brian D. Smedley. "Race as Biology Is Fiction, Racism as a Social Problem Is Real: Anthropological and Historical Perspectives on the Social Construction of Race." *American Psychologist* 60, no. 1 (2005): 16–26.

Smith-Morris, Carolyn. *Diabetes among the Pima: Stories of Survival.* Tucson: University of Arizona Press, 2006a.

———. "Prenatal Mysteries of Symptomless Diabetes in the Gila River Indian Community." In *Diabetes Around the World: Critical Perspectives, Creative Solutions*, edited by M. F. a. G. Lang, 187–202. Durham, NC: Carolina Academic Press, 2006b.

———. "Diagnostic Controversy: Gestational Diabetes and the Meaning of Risk for Pima Indian Women." *Medical Anthropology* 24, no. 2 (2005): 145–77.

Stern, Scott D. C., Adam S. Cifu, and Diane Altkorn. *Symptom to Diagnosis: An Evidence-Based Guide.* 2nd ed. New York: McGraw-Hill, 2010.

Summerfield, Derek. "The Invention of Post-Traumatic Stress Disorder and the Social Usefulness of a Psychiatric Category." *British Medical Journal* 322 (1998): 95–98.

Trundle, Catherine, Ilina Singh, and Christian Broer. "Fighting to be Heard: Contested Diagnosis." In *Social Issues in Diagnosis: An Introduction for Students and Clinicians*, edited by A. G. Jutel and K. Dew, 165–182. Baltimore, MD: Johns Hopkins University Press, 2014.

Whitmarsh, Ian. "The Ascetic Subject of Compliance: The Turn to Chronic Diseases in Global Health." In *When People Come First: Critical Studies in Global Health*, edited by J. Biehl and A. Petryna, 302–24. Princeton, NJ: Princeton University Press, 2013.

Whyte, Susan Reynolds, Sjaak van der Geest, and Anita Hardon, eds. *Social Lives of Medicines.* Cambridge, UK: Cambridge University Press, 2002.

Whyte, Susan Reynolds, Michael A. Whyte, and Lotte Meinert. "Therapeutic Clientship: Belonging in Uganda's Projectified Landscape of AIDS Care." In *When People Come First: Critical Studies in Global Health*, edited by J. Biehl and A. Petryna, 140–165. Princeton, NJ: Princeton University Press, 2013.

World Health Organization. *Diabetes: The Cost of Diabetes.* Geneva: World Health Organization, 2015.

Young, Allan. "The Creation of Medical Knowledge: Some Problems in Interpretation." *Social Science & Medicine* 15, no. 3 (1981): 379–86.

Yunus, Muhammad B. "Central Sensitivity Syndromes: A New Paradigm and Group Nosology for Fibromyalgia and Overlapping Conditions, and the Related Issue of Disease Versus Illness." *Semin. Arthritis Rheum* 37 (2008): 339–52.

Part I

Diagnostic Access

2 Testing Pregnant Women for HIV
Contestations in the Global Effort to Reduce the Spread of AIDS

Anita Hardon

Globally orchestrated programs for the prevention of mother-to-child transmission (PMTCT) of HIV emerged in the late 1990s, when public health policy makers were at a loss over how to control the epidemic, and when providing universal access to AIDS therapies was not yet seen as a feasible option (Hardon 2012). This chapter focuses on the ways in which HIV testing has been pursued in these programs, and shows how procedures in some settings and historical moments only screened women for HIV, whereas in other settings, the tests were gateways to further clinical diagnoses and life-saving treatment.

Programs to prevent the spread of HIV see pregnant women as an easy target. Whereas reducing the mother-to-child transmission of HIV is an unquestioned good, specifically targeting pregnant women in the battle against HIV has ethically questionable implications. Without access to further diagnostics and treatment for the women themselves, routine testing for HIV introduces the psychological burden of diagnosis without adequate health care, and also increases the potential of women being stigmatized as vectors of HIV. It also casts into doubt the quality of life for their HIV-negative children, who may well find themselves orphaned in the foreseeable future.

Antiretroviral medicines grew more accessible worldwide following the United Nations's endorsement of PMTCT and the entry of generic drugs manufacturers on the market (Hardon 2012). Thereafter, PMTCT programs expanded their aims to the treatment of HIV-positive pregnant women (UNFPA 2005). Note that the availability of follow-up care for the mother became a *possible* outcome of diagnosis, not an assured one. Diagnosis remained de-linked from treatment, which is already controversial. But a second controversy arose over the appropriate pre-test counseling to offer pregnant women. Each site and context produces different pre-test concerns, including the likely social stigma attached to taking an HIV test or to the illness itself; the likely availability of follow-up treatment should a diagnosis be positive; and the ability of women to positively apply the knowledge gained from the diagnosis to their lives.

This article first provides a brief history of PMTCT. How have its programs and technologies evolved over time? What kinds of assumptions inform its diagnostic practices? Here, I describe the contrasting views in the controversy over pre-diagnostic counseling. The ethnographic vignettes that follow reveal how pregnant women and frontline antenatal care workers in four developing countries—Indonesia, Vietnam, Kenya, and Uganda—implement and experience PMTCT programs. While many global health advocates expected women to value comprehensive pre-test counseling, our research suggests that pregnant women in most settings are satisfied with routine screening for HIV. The key issue, as it turned out, was not whether testing should be routine or not, but whether social support, treatment, and care were available when pregnant women are identified as HIV positive.

PMTCT: A BRIEF HISTORY

Preventing the mother-to-child transmission of HIV emerged as a global strategy in the late 1990s (WHO/UNAIDS 1998). It entailed using antiretroviral medications (ARVs) to prevent the transmission of the virus during childbirth. At the time, ARV prophylaxis for HIV-positive pregnant women had been used in Europe and North America for half a decade. But treatment regimes were expensive and complicated—involving long-term treatment during pregnancy, delivery, and postpartum—and were considered inappropriate for developing countries (Dabis et al. 2000). PMTCT was not yet feasible in resource-poor settings.

A trial completed in Thailand in 1998—which found a 28-day course of twice-daily oral Zidovudine (AZT) to be safe, well tolerated, and, in the absence of breast-feeding, to lessen the risk of mother-to-child transmission of HIV1 from 18.9 percent to 9.4 percent (Shaffer et al. 1999)—prompted the World Health Organization (WHO) to publish guidelines on the use of AZT to prevent the mother-to-child transmission of HIV (WHO/UNAIDS 1998). The use of AZT required testing pregnant women for HIV. By 2000, UNICEF and the WHO had set up a pilot project in 11 resource-poor countries to test the feasibility of AZT for PMTCT, and the "acceptability" of routine testing for HIV in antenatal care. Would women be willing to have the test, given that they themselves would not have access to treatment (UNICEF 2003)?

While diagnostic surveillance for PMTCT was proven to be medically effective, it entailed controversy: was it ethical to introduce diagnostic surveillance in resource-poor health systems to prevent mother-to-child transmission when the women themselves did not have access to this life-saving treatment? How would diagnostic surveillance without accompanying antiretroviral treatment for mothers affect the quality of life of their HIV-free children, who may well lose their mothers in the foreseeable future?

During pregnancy, the risks of transmission are relatively low. In most cases, HIV does *not* cross the placenta from mother to fetus. Protection from the placenta may fail, however, if the mother has a viral, bacterial, or parasitic placental infection during pregnancy or if the mother has advanced the immune deficiency associated with AIDS. Children of HIV-positive mothers are at greater risk of being infected *during* childbirth; between 10 and 20 percent will be infected if no steps are taken to prevent transmission. Many infants who acquire HIV during labor and delivery do so by sucking, imbibing, or aspirating maternal blood or cervical secretions that contain HIV. Others can acquire HIV through the mixing of fetal and maternal blood as the placenta separates. Invasive delivery techniques that increase the baby's contact with the mother's blood have been associated with higher risks of mother-to-child transmission during labor and delivery (Msellati 2009; WHO 2002).

ARV prophylaxis aims to prevent transmission during pregnancy, labor, and delivery, but not during subsequent breastfeeding. The prevention of HIV transmission to children was of course an appealing public health objective that fit the global strategy of child-oriented programs, such as immunization (Hardon and Blume 2005). The apparent simplicity of the technology made the intervention appear feasible in resource-poor settings, while the existing infrastructure for antenatal services in the developing world made pregnant women an attractive target for this strategy (Dabis et al. 2000). But the question of whether long-term treatment would be available for HIV-positive women remained unanswered.

Social studies of technology have shown that choices made in the development of new technologies are far from neutral: "Innovators inscribe a specific vision about the world into the technical content of a new object" (Akrich 1992: 208). In the design of new technologies, researchers anticipate the interests, skills, motives, and behaviors of future users; representations of future users thus inform the design of new products (Akrich 1992; Hardon 2006). The PMTCT technology that emerged in the late 1990s assumed the following about pregnant women: (1) they will attend antenatal care services, rather than going to traditional birth attendants and delivering at home; (2) they will submit to being tested, and will return for their test results; and (3) if they are HIV positive, they will adhere to the prophylaxis regime and be willing to bottle-feed their children after delivery. To make PMTCT work, antenatal care workers in resource-poor settings had to enact a broad new diagnostic ideology. They were expected to provide appropriate counseling on PMTCT, conduct HIV testing, and, if their clients were found to be HIV positive, give advice on the use of, and provide them with, ARVs.

Pilot studies conducted by UNICEF in 11 countries (UNICEF 2003) revealed several problems in the implementation of this novel approach to HIV prevention. On average in the 11 countries, 30 percent of women receiving antenatal care were *not* counseled on PMTCT. Of those women who did receive counseling, 30 percent did *not* receive an HIV test. Findings from Kenya and Zambia revealed that one-quarter of the women tested did not return for their test results, while less than half of the women who tested positive for HIV received the recommended prophylactic regime (UNICEF 2003: 5). Women did not receive the full course of AZT for a variety of reasons: they had not yet reached the 34th or 36th week of gestation at the time of their visit; women did not adhere to the twice-a-day for 28 days regime for taking AZT; women's partners opposed the treatment; women delivered at home or reached the facility only when they were in labor; and women were worried about taking drugs during pregnancy.

To improve results, the authors of the report recommended two changes: HIV testing should become routine for *all* pregnant women in antenatal care, and AZT should be replaced by Nevirapine, a less demanding antiretroviral medication. A PMTCT trial had found that providing a single dose of Nevirapine—once *during delivery* to the mother, and once to the infant *postpartum*—could reduce mother-to-child transmission more effectively than AZT (Jackson et al. 2003).[1] This simple regime was considered more feasible, as it did not require "catching" women at their 34th or 36th week of gestation, and it did not require such a demanding treatment regime.[2]

The 2001 Special Session of the UN General Assembly committed its 189 member states to give 80 percent of pregnant women worldwide access to PMTCT care by 2010. The aim was to reduce the proportion of infected children born to HIV-positive mothers by 20 percent by 2005, and by a further 50 percent by 2010. Initially, the WHO and UNAIDS recommended a three-pillar strategy: to prevent (1) new infections among parents; (2) unwanted pregnancies among HIV-positive women; and (3) transmission from HIV-positive pregnant women and mothers to children. PMTCT here was set up as a preventive program. HIV-positive pregnant women would not have access to follow-up diagnostics and care, as was the case in UNICEF's pilot studies.

Only one year later, in 2002, a WHO meeting proposed the inclusion of a fourth pillar: to provide care and support to mothers, infants, and their families (WHO 2002). These aims were endorsed at the PMTCT High Level Global Partners Forum in Abuja, Nigeria in 2005 (UNFPA 2005), by which time global pressure had made antiretroviral treatment available in resource-poor settings. Whereas testing for HIV in the early years of PMTCT was primarily a tool to prevent transmission to children, it now became a gateway to treatment, at least on paper. To implement the fourth pillar of the PMTCT program, antenatal care services needed to ensure the transition of HIV-positive pregnant women into CD4 testing and appropriate long-term medication. As we will see below, referral to further diagnostic services and treatment was institutionalized more rapidly in Africa, where HIV prevalence was high, than in Southeast Asia, where only a small minority of women tested in antenatal care were HIV positive.

In the meantime, HIV testing technologies had evolved. When the UNI-CEF pilot studies were conducted, PMTCT testing facilities would take blood from patients and send it to laboratories for diagnosis; patients had to return for their results, which partly explained the high dropout rates. When PMTCT was scaled up in East Africa, rapid diagnostic tests were available, allowing for results within 30 minutes. At our Southeast Asian study sites, blood was still sent to labs for testing.

OPTING IN VERSUS OPTING OUT OF DIAGNOSIS

The most vocal controversy around PMTCT has to do with how best to prepare pregnant women for the diagnostic event and its impact. With rapid testing available in health facilities—and health services under pressure to meet their targets of testing all pregnant women—global health advocates grew concerned that HIV testing had become routinized as a universal procedure, ignoring the devastating implications of diagnosis and neglecting the counseling component of the program.

Global health advocates argued that pre-test counseling has to be comprehensive enough to help pregnant women consciously choose to be tested, to prepare for a potential positive outcome, and to disclose and commit to prevention should they be HIV positive (Bayer and Edington 2009). They called for continuing the "opt-in" approach that characterized voluntary counseling and testing—the gold standard in the 1990s, when pregnant women who tested positive in resource-poor settings did not have access to life-saving treatment. Voluntary counseling and testing guidelines (CDC 2006; UNAIDS 2000) stipulated that trained counselors should assess the client's sexual risk behavior, discuss coping strategies related to the test results, review prevention options, and reaffirm the decision to test. During post-test counseling, counselors were to give clients their test results, and, in the case of a HIV-positive result, discuss how to reduce sexual risk and how to disclose to their sexual partner(s). Human rights advocates in the U.S. and Europe pushed for extensive counseling and informed consent procedures because of the risks of discrimination and social stigma, and the lack of access to treatment at the time (Bayer 1989; Bayer and Eddington 2009). The proponents of opt-in counseling further argued that people who receive comprehensive counseling are more likely to be committed to preventing HIV transmission and to disclose if they are HIV positive (Weinhardt et al. 1999).

Despite this activism, the WHO guidelines published in 2007 (WHO/UNAIDS 2007) de-emphasized comprehensive pre-test counseling and endorsed an "opt-out" approach to testing in PMTCT. Pregnant women who do not wish to have an HIV test must assertively decline the offer. The main justification for the change to an "opt-out" approach was that—on paper—referral to further diagnostics and lifelong antiretroviral treatment were now part of PMTCT programs. HIV testing, in the view of policy makers, had become a normal diagnostic procedure.

The remainder of this chapter presents ethnographic vignettes from four field sites in Southeast Asia and Sub-Saharan Africa. They describe divergent diagnostic and counseling practices, women's responses to the opt-out approach, and the views of the nurses and counselors conducting the HIV tests within PMTCT programs. Our findings suggest that two issues are crucial for women: whether they have access to and can afford further diagnostic procedures and lifelong treatment with ARVs, and how to tell their husbands that they are HIV positive. The issues at stake thus have less to do with the quality of pre-test counseling than with the consequences of taking the test.

MULTI-SITE FIELDWORK: AN OVERVIEW

The vignettes derive from two multi-site studies on PMTCT. One was conducted in Southeast Asia (Hardon et al. 2009) and the other in East Africa (Hardon et al. 2011). Methods included observations of health facilities, group discussions, semi-structured interviews, and exit interviews.

The studies in Southeast Asia were conducted in 2005 and 2006, in Jakarta and Karawang in Western Java, Indonesia, and in Hanoi and Thai Nguyen in Northern Vietnam. We chose these cities because their PMTCT programs began relatively early, and because the prevalence of sex work and intravenous drug use in these cities means women are at higher risk of contracting HIV. In Indonesia, we worked closely with Yayasan Pelita Ilmu (YPI); in Vietnam, with the Medical Committee Netherlands-Vietnam. Both are non-governmental organizations (NGOs) that aim to improve the delivery of PMTCT services; both also facilitate self-help groups for HIV-positive women. We interviewed 20 pregnant clients of the PMTCT program in an urban-poor community in the Tebet district of Jakarta (where Yayasan Pelita Ilmu was active during our study period); 37 women living with HIV (16 members of a support group in Karawang and Jakarta, and 21 clients of a referral hospital); and 13 health workers involved in the pilot PMTCT program. In Hanoi, we interviewed 38 clients of PMTCT programs, 53 health care workers, and 52 HIV-positive members of a support group. In Thai Nguyen, we interviewed 18 clients and 41 health care workers. In both countries, we attended the regular discussion sessions of the support groups. The sampling of the respondents was purposive.

The ethnographic insights on PMTCT in East Africa are derived from the MATCH (Multi-Country African Testing and Counselling for HIV) study, which conducted in 2008–2009 to compare client experiences with testing and counseling across countries as well as across methods of testing. My role in the MATCH study was to analyze women's experiences of testing for HIV within PMTCT programs (Hardon et al. 2012). The MATCH study included structured interviews with open-ended questions with 74 pregnant women attending antenatal care services in Kenya and 92 in Uganda, and conversations with 10 members of HIV-positive support groups and 10 PMTCT health care providers in each country. In both Kenya and Uganda, the study was conducted in the capital region and one rural province.

PMTCT IN SOUTHEAST ASIA

In Vietnam and Indonesia, HIV prevalence among adults in the general population was below 1 percent at the time of our study. Prevention efforts and awareness campaigns thus focused on "high risk" groups: sex workers and intravenous drugs users. Sentinel surveys show that around 50 percent of intravenous drug users and 10 percent of female sex workers were infected with HIV in both countries (WHO 2008; Nguyen et al. 2008). HIV prevention campaigns therefore associated the virus with immoral behavior and "social evils," thus reinforcing the high levels of stigma attached to HIV/AIDS (Oosterhoff et al. 2008a b; Ogden et al. 2004; Paxton et al. 2005).

Both Vietnam and Indonesia adopted PMTCT policies in response to the 2001 UN Declaration of Commitment. This represented a radical change in AIDS policy, as it meant that prevention programs now reached out to all pregnant women, who, unlike sex workers and drug users, had not been identified as at-risk populations. PMTCT programs further meant that antenatal care providers who previously had nothing to do with AIDS were drawn into AIDS prevention.

Vietnam had already adopted the PMTCT agenda in 2000, when the National Committee for AIDS, Drugs and Prostitution published guidelines on the diagnosis and treatment of HIV/AIDS, which included instructions on antiretroviral prophylaxis. The guidelines indicated that women should be tested for HIV in district-level antenatal care centers and hospitals, and that HIV-positive pregnant women who wanted to continue their pregnancies be referred to obstetric departments at provincial or national-level hospitals. In a 2004 directive, PMTCT—described as a comprehensive program that included care for HIV infected and HIV/AIDS-affected adults and children—was listed as one of the nine core programs in the national strategy to prevent HIV/AIDS. The policy, however, did not mention how, or even whether, informed consent was to be sought, or whether women should be offered an opportunity to opt out.

While Indonesia adopted its PMTCT policy only in 2005, the local NGO, YPI with Global Fund support had been implementing pilot programs in poor urban communities with large numbers of intravenous drug users and sex workers since 1999. Specialist AIDS doctors were members of YPI and helped to set up the PMTCT pilot programs. The YPI model for PMTCT later became the basis of the national PMTCT guidelines published in 2006, which reflect the comprehensive PMTCT framework endorsed in

Abuja. According to the Indonesian guidelines, every woman who visits an antenatal facility should have access to HIV testing and pre-test counseling, following an opt-in approach. The guidelines include providing psychological support and care to HIV-positive mothers and their babies. The policy stipulated that testing should be voluntary, accompanied by quality counseling and informed consent.

To summarize, Vietnam's PMTCT policy entailed routine testing for HIV in antenatal care, while Indonesia chose for an opt-in approach with elaborate pre-test counseling. In both countries, formal PMTCT policies provide HIV-positive women with access to follow-up clinical diagnosis and care. But what happens on the ground in these countries' antenatal care facilities? How do women experience the counseling that they receive? Do health facilities effectively transfer HIV-positive women for follow-up CD4 testing and long-term treatment, especially in low HIV prevalence settings where AIDS care is only offered in specialized centers? What follow are some answers based on ethnographic research.

DIAGNOSIS AS SURVEILLANCE: PMTCT IN VIETNAM

Our fieldwork in Hanoi and Thai Nguyen found that HIV tests are delivered as part of a package set of blood tests that includes tests for blood counts, blood type, blood sugar, hepatitis B, and syphilis, administered by district-level antenatal care services in the eighth month of pregnancy. We observed that when a woman was found to be HIV positive, the test result was confirmed at a national reference laboratory. Upon confirmation, district-level health workers informed the woman of her HIV status, usually at her home, and about how to prevent further transmission. We found that very few women were referred for further diagnosis and treatment. We further noted that women who attended commune-level antenatal care facilities were not tested for HIV, providing women who want to avoid HIV testing an avenue for receiving antenatal care.

At the time of our research, HIV prevalence among pregnant women in Vietnam was around 1 percent. Health workers in PMTCT programs thus rarely had to deal with positive results. The district antenatal care workers whom we interviewed were unanimously positive about the inclusion of HIV tests in the standard package, and stressed the importance of testing for the prevention of transmission from mother to child: "It is easier for us to prevent transmission if we know who among the patients is infected with HIV" (district health worker, Hanoi). In line with Vietnam's comprehensive PMTCT guidelines, district-level health facilities in Hanoi and Thai Nguyen referred HIV-positive pregnant women to the provincial or national hospitals for delivery and to Hanoi for treatment. Health workers at the district level were pleased with routine testing at seven or eight months because the HIV tests would ensure that they did not have to deliver HIV-positive women in their clinics.

While the overall assessment of routine testing was positive, health care workers at both sites said they found it difficult to inform and counsel patients about their positive HIV test results. Some failed to inform the women and instead mentioned their "weak health." These informants emphasized that both their families and the health staff "wanted to protect" the women by *not* informing them. Being "too busy" to inform all patients because the "staff has to focus on the delivery" was also mentioned several times as a reason for not informing the patient. In other words, routine HIV testing did not necessarily deliver the diagnosis to the patient herself.

Like their health care providers, the pregnant women whom we interviewed in the district health facilities valued the integration of routine HIV tests in antenatal care. We frequently heard, from women and their families that the "HIV tests are just like other tests." They saw no difference in principle between being offered an HIV test and any other medical test, like those for hepatitis B or tuberculosis. Many women also mentioned that routine testing was acceptable, because asking for an HIV test would suggest that one was engaged in socially stigmatized behavior. However, all women who tested HIV positive thought that the timing of the tests was too late in the pregnancy.

All the HIV-positive women whom we interviewed in Vietnam complained about the content of the post-test counseling and follow-up care in the hospital. None received information on how to protect their health; there was no information about antiretroviral therapy or about the treatment of opportunistic infections. All but two women complained about the unkind and sometimes discriminatory behavior of the health staff. Some HIV-positive women were informed about their results in front of other people, including in-laws and strangers. One HIV-positive mother in Hanoi told us, "They just shouted the results at me and then they disappeared. I did not know what to do or how I should feel." Another woman in Hanoi complained about their white coats. "When they visited my home, they still wore their white coats; that is unusual so it attracts attention from neighbors which is not good. I prefer to visit the clinics myself and only when somebody is really sick." Our informants further complained about the advice given by health counselors who came to their houses as part of the notification procedure. One woman was told not to eat at local food stalls, and not to have her hair washed at a salon, thus reinforcing the felt stigma.

At our study sites, women were supposed to have a home visit following delivery. According to the 2005 guidelines, they should also have regular CD4 tests to assess whether they need to start antiretroviral therapy. While antiretroviral drugs were available in hospitals at the time of our study, our respondents reported that there was no follow up for either woman or child after delivery.

VOLUNTARY TESTING IN INDONESIA

At the time of our study, the Indonesian government had not yet implemented a nationwide PMTCT program. With support from the Global Fund, the local NGO, YPI had set up a pilot program to provide voluntary counseling and testing in antenatal care facilities in selected Jakarta neighborhoods. These mobile clinics were the entry point for YPI's continuum of care program, during which, between October 2003 and December 2006, 2,771 pregnant women received pre-test counseling. Of these women, 88 percent had an HIV test and 86 percent of the latter returned for post-test counseling and were given their test results. Only eight women (0.4 percent) were confirmed as HIV positive. It is unclear to what extent women who considered themselves at risk avoided the YPI services.

Because attendance is voluntary at YPI clinics, women had to be encouraged to visit community health clinics when the mobile counseling and testing units were present. For this, YPI relied on the cadres of the Family Welfare Movement, which in previous decades had been active in the implementation of the family planning program. Participant observation, however, revealed that the neighborhood housewives of the Family Welfare Movement felt uncomfortable even mentioning HIV. One of our informants admitted, "I told them that you will be called one by one, your baby will be checked whether he is healthy or not. So, I told them it's a test for mother and baby's health, I didn't tell them their blood samples would be taken. I'm afraid they would refuse." Although Indonesia operates an opt-in program for HIV testing, the public health staff who recruit women often avoid informing them about the test that will be offered them, leaving the discussion to the clinic staff themselves. The cadres of the Family Welfare Movement promised pregnant women free medication, formula milk, and transportation fees to entice them: "If we invite her just like that, she has to consider it first. But, if we ask her softly, you know a little bit of luring. . . especially if there's milk. The blood test is free. . . . They should get a transportation fee so that they don't have to think twice."

The pregnant women whom we interviewed at the voluntary counseling and testing sites stated that they were there for the health of their unborn children. They considered attending the clinic to be a part of ordinary antenatal care, and were glad that the services are free. All interviewed women said they were pleased to attend the clinics.

YPI simultaneously trained nurses and midwives in government district health centers to conduct individual pre-counseling sessions with pregnant women. The pre-test sessions focused on the women's health and the risks of HIV infection. We observed that women were only tested if they gave their consent. Their test results were handed back to them two weeks later, confidentially. During post-test counseling, women could choose to discuss their results with the counselors, which they always did. Unsurprisingly, given the low prevalence rates of HIV in the general population, most test results were negative.

When test results were positive, the counselors provided the women with follow-up care and support, facilitated by YPI. But the counselors admitted that they did not always have answers to the women's questions, including information on how to prevent further transmission. YPI staff took responsibility for bringing the (few) women who tested positive to hospitals in Jakarta, where specialized HIV/AIDS doctors who participated in the YPI program were willing to treat them. While these women did not have to pay for antiretroviral treatment, they generally had to pay for their own CD4 tests.

YPI also set up support groups for HIV-positive women, where they received counseling on how to live healthily and received free ARVs (both prophylaxis and long-term treatment), access to free C-sections, formula milk for babies until they were one year of age, and testing for babies' HIV status. "I thank God for this. I am pregnant, and someone has guided me, thank God. This is my condition. I live in the slum area, and I have to accept my status as it is. I get the medicine for free from the hospital, until I deliver my baby" (Mira, HIV-positive pregnant woman in Jatibunder, Jakarta).

But access to treatment was not always easy. The Indonesian government, with support from the Global Fund, has subsidized antiretroviral drugs since 2004, but provision at the time of our study remained erratic. Although there were nine referral hospitals for HIV/AIDS in Jakarta, capacity was limited, as only a few physicians were willing and able to handle the HIV/AIDS cases. Most HIV-positive women whom we interviewed therefore obtained their medication from a variety of sources. For those living in Karawang, there was only one hospital that provided ARVs, where they suffered long waits and high administration costs. The distance to the hospital was also problematic. "At this hospital, the procedures are annoying, we have to wait long . . . we have to pay 20,000 rupiah for the medicine and the administration, 15,000 for the doctor, 15,000 for the ticket, in total 50,000 [approximately USD 5.50] each time we take the medicine. Not to mention the transportation costs" (Tati, HIV-positive mother).

The HIV-positive support group members whom we interviewed stressed that the greatest benefit of the PMTCT program was that it gave women the chance to have healthy children. There is a strong desire to have children among Indonesian women, in part because their social status depends on it. Indeed, most of the HIV-positive women whom we interviewed remained sexually active and wanted to have children in the future. The chance to have a healthy child made them feel like normal women again.

DIAGNOSIS AS SURVEILLANCE: PMTCT IN THE EPIDEMICS OF EAST AFRICA

PMTCT was introduced in East Africa in 2001 when UNICEF conducted trials to test this approach to combat the AIDS epidemic, which was then raging out of control. The Kenyan and Ugandan governments rapidly made PMTCT services available nationwide. After countries in East Africa adopted the World Health Organization's "3 by 5" (three million people on antiretrovirals by 2005) initiative in 2003, most PMTCT programs began offering referrals to AIDS care.

It was in East Africa that the controversy over how to implement counseling and testing arose, spurred by Kevin de Cock who had previously been an advisor to the US Centers for Disease Control in Kenya, and now headed the World Health Organization's AIDS program. De Cock was the most vocal proponent of changing diagnostic testing from "opt-in" to "opt-out" to make it easier for under-resourced health facilities to process large numbers of patients. The raging HIV epidemic was considered a justification for aggressive diagnostic surveillance. We conducted our studies in 2007 and 2008, when the WHO's new counseling guidelines endorsed the opt-out approach but were not yet fully adopted in the region.

In Uganda, a policy that had been formulated in 2005 was still in place, which stated that counseling should be "comprehensive" unless the extra time required "causes a barrier to testing itself" (Uganda Ministry of Health 2005). In contrast, the 2008 Kenyan policy, in line with the new WHO guidelines, placed less emphasis on pre-test counseling, implying a form of triage that was practiced post-test, with those found to be HIV positive entitled to comprehensive post-test counseling.

Kenyan legislation—based on a template drafted by parliamentarians from 12 African countries to protect the rights of individuals infected or exposed to HIV (Sanon et al. 2009)—required HIV-positive persons to disclose to sexual partners. It stated that health care workers should support the choice of their clients to disclose to sexual partners and that "if efforts to encourage the client or patient to disclose their HIV status fail, and the client or patient is placing a sexual partner or other person at risk, a medical practitioner may disclose someone's HIV status to their sexual partner or other person at risk" (Kenya Ministry of Public Health and Sanitation 2008). Refusal to notify one's partner was thus considered an infringement of the partner's right to health and well being.

The new policies on counseling, confidentiality, and disclosure reflect local realities in which HIV testing at health facilities has become routine. While nearly everyone in these countries has a family member with HIV, our fieldwork suggests that being diagnosed with HIV still has major social consequences. While our informants were satisfied with routine HIV testing in antenatal care, their main concern was being blamed for bringing HIV into the family.

Our informants in Kenya and Uganda valued the PMTCT program for helping to protect the unborn child and for providing a gateway to treatment. A young HIV-negative woman tested in a government hospital in rural Kenya told us, "It is good . . . because I was pregnant and wanted to know my status and it is also a must for pregnant mothers." A young woman tested in a government hospital in rural Uganda added, "It is good because if a mother is found positive she is always given treatment."

We asked pregnant women whether it was hard to be tested. Most stated that it was not. When asked why, their responses reflected prior experience with testing (nearly half of our informants had previously been tested) and confidence in a likely negative result due to their awareness of HIV transmission routes. A 26-year-old HIV-negative woman from urban Kenya told us, "I had been faithful to my husband since testing negative in 2002." It was the same story for a married woman from rural Uganda: "Because I had done it before and am also faithful to my husband." Some respondents said it was important for the woman to have "made up her mind" about being tested beforehand. A young educated woman in urban Uganda who refused to be tested told us, "I felt I was not ready for the test that day." Two out of three pregnant women who tested positive for HIV in antenatal care said they were glad to know their status and that good things had happened to them since. One woman reported that she had learnt to live positively and was able to prevent transmission to her child; another said that her health had improved and that she was still together with her husband. Another woman told us, "I started taking ARVs and I am healthy and nobody can suspect I am positive."

In both Kenya and Uganda, nearly all women (regardless of their HIV status) reported that they were treated well and that the PMTCT meeting was helpful overall. We expected that HIV-positive women would evaluate the services more negatively, as they need comprehensive counseling and may have had many questions, and health workers are generally pressed for time. But this was not the case. HIV-positive women reported being given ample time to ask questions; they were advised to discuss their HIV status and to refer their partners. Most HIV-positive women were prescribed medication, and around two-thirds were referred to a support group. The PMTCT programs in these high-prevalence settings in East Africa seem to be doing a good job, and are experienced positively by both HIV-positive and HIV-negative women (Hardon et al. 2012). Our research suggests that HIV-positive women are being effectively referred to AIDS care programs where they can have free CD4 tests and access to antiretroviral treatment when needed.

Given the controversies in the global arena surrounding the need to continue comprehensive pre-test counseling, we examined whether the scaling up of testing came at the expense of women knowing that they can opt out. We found that nearly all pregnant women had been asked if they agreed to be tested; most were told that they had the right to refuse. But in reality, many women did not really feel that they could refuse. Participants in a group discussion who had visited the comprehensive care center at a national hospital in Kenya stated, "You have a choice because you are not being forced." "If you do not want to be tested you can refuse." "There is no pressure to agree to be tested." But one respondent added, "The doctor is very powerful. If he tells you. . . you have to agree. If a doctor or any other medical person tells you to get tested, you do not have any other alternative but to get tested."

Other women said that testing was mandatory. A 23-year-old HIV-negative woman from rural Kenya who had been tested in a government health center told us, "The nurse said it was mandatory when pregnant for PMTCT." A young, uneducated, HIV-negative woman from urban Uganda, also tested in a government hospital, told us, "It was mandatory and a prerequisite for me to get treatment."

Many of our respondents did not oppose mandatory testing. When asked who should be tested, pregnant women were the most commonly mentioned group; other answers included unfaithful husbands and sex workers. But other respondents stressed that forcing women to get the test was not good, reasoning that some would not be able to handle the results, that women should be able to choose for themselves, and that mandatory testing would scare women away from antenatal care.

Opting out by pregnant women burdens health workers, as they then have to keep track of the women and keep offering them tests. As a matron in charge of a maternity ward in Kenya explained:

> There are situations when antenatal mothers come and we are supposed to capture them for testing on their first visit, and when you give the information and counsel them especially on matters related to HIV, some will say, "Look, sister, because I did not come with my husband, I would prefer to take the test when we are together." You just release her but on a subsequent visit she will repeat the same story about the husband not consenting, and she won't tell you she is declining. On another visit she lands on someone else's hands and not you who had counseled her, and the same story is repeated, not knowing that one had been counseled earlier and she is refusing indirectly. Finally, you realize that the mother is approaching delivery and has not been tested, like yesterday we had one, she kept on refusing to take the test, one of the counselors called me and narrated the story, we went to the mother and told her to sign that she has refused to take the test. . . . When we meet such clients we do continue counseling, we never get tired until the client agrees or disagrees.

Recall that in both Kenya and Uganda, diagnostic surveillance is an opt-out procedure. Health workers are not supposed to suggest that it is mandatory. But they do so for pragmatic reasons, to "capture" the target population: "They accept once you explain to them that the test is mandatory," explained an antenatal counselor in a Kenyan health center. An antenatal nurse in Uganda likewise stated, "We talk to them about HIV testing, we tell them about the benefits, we then tell them that it is a government policy for all pregnant mothers to test."

While, overall, the opt-out (mandatory) strategy in East Africa has prevented thousands of mother-to-child transmissions, one worrying finding was that four out of five HIV-positive women reported that they generally kept their HIV status secret. When probed about social stigma, one out of five respondents reported that they felt worthless due to being HIV positive; an equal proportion felt guilty. One out of four had been personally made to feel bad, and around half had heard about other HIV-positive people being treated badly.

In our study, five out of six HIV-positive pregnant women had disclosed to someone. Mostly, they disclosed to family members, usually their sister and/or parents, but only one in three had disclosed to their partners. Given post-test counseling's emphasis on disclosing to partners, it is surprising that only one-third had done so. Some of the women who did not disclose were divorced and therefore saw no reason to do so, but others reported that they found it very difficult to tell their husbands, out of fear of being blamed, abused, and/or abandoned. A 22-year-old woman, who was tested in an urban Kenyan health center and encouraged by health workers to disclose to her husband and convince him to test, told us, "My spouse denied that I was positive and did not take the test. He thought then and still thinks it's a joke." A 29-year-old pregnant woman, who was tested in a government hospital in rural Kenya and had been aware of her HIV-positive status for 16 months, said she was afraid to disclose because she expected her husband to beat her up and leave her. It was a similar story for a 19-year-old pregnant woman in Uganda; she had learned of her status three months prior to our interview and had not disclosed to anybody, including her partner: "My husband would divorce me even if he knows that he is infected."

CONCLUSION

Preventing the mother-to-child transmission of HIV is one of the most ambitious global health programs in history, with a reach equivalent to the global efforts for universal immunization. But whereas the aim of 80 percent coverage for immunization was achieved, the same cannot be said for PMTCT. When the UN reviewed its progress in 2010, it was estimated that only 53 percent of pregnant women living with HIV in Sub-Saharan Africa had received antiretroviral drugs to prevent the mother-to-child transmission of HIV (United Nations 2011). As a preventive health program, the success of PMTCT has been suboptimal.

This chapter explored the dynamics of HIV testing in two regions of the world: in East Africa, where HIV prevalence is high, and in Southeast Asia, where it is low. It examined the way HIV testing is pursued, its underlying logic, and how testing is (not) embedded in further diagnosis and care.

Vietnam, a strong state, adopted guidelines for PMTCT early on. While district health workers conduct HIV testing as a routine part of antenatal care, the tests take place late in pregnancy. HIV-positive women are referred to provincial and national hospitals, which introduces further delays, transportation costs, and absences from home. Our fieldwork revealed a community notification system that does not consider the rights of women to confidentiality and privacy; nor were women provided with appropriate post-test counseling, introducing the psychological burden of diagnosis without adequate health care. The advice given was erratic, reflecting the fact that health workers had not been properly trained in counseling. In Indonesia, the government was slow to introduce a nationwide PMTCT program, leaving it to a local NGO to develop a pilot program with support from the Global Fund. Counselors in the antenatal care services followed a voluntary counseling and testing model, as called for by global health advocates, including safeguards for privacy and confidentiality. But PMTCT coverage within Indonesian antenatal health care leaves much to be desired; women often find out they are HIV positive only when their husbands fall ill. In both Vietnam and Indonesia, women often have difficulties accessing follow-up services and medication.

In Kenya and Uganda, antenatal care services test for HIV on an opt-out basis. Our studies suggest that women generally have no problems with this. In contrast to what we found in Indonesia and Vietnam, HIV-positive women in Kenya and Uganda were referred to AIDS care programs where they can have free CD4 tests and access to antiretroviral treatments when needed.

Comparative analysis of the way PMTCT programs are implemented suggests that their success remains hampered by the social stigma surrounding HIV/AIDS. While AIDS care services exist, some HIV-positive women find it difficult to turn to them (in part, this is because they tend to be diagnosed when they are not yet ill). Our study found that the majority of HIV-positive pregnant women in Kenya, Uganda, and Vietnam did not disclose to their partners; some who did disclose faced rejection by their partners and/or divorce. These findings suggest that the PMTCT strategy of testing pregnant women in antenatal care—and subsequently asking them to refer their partners—comes at a risk that cannot be addressed through good pre-test counseling.

In light of the continuing high levels of social stigma surrounding HIV/AIDS at the sites where we conducted research, how much counseling do women need? Do programs need to emphasize voluntary opt-in procedures or can routine (opt-out) strategies suffice? Our study suggests that pregnant women are generally satisfied with routine testing in antenatal care that does not single out individuals based on their risk profile.

Our findings here echo Mol (2008) in that patient choice is not (always) as liberating as it is advertised to be. Within voluntary counseling and testing, patients are expected to become the masters of their own lives, using medical technologies that promise accurate diagnosis and a return to health and happiness. But the logic of choice, Mol argues, can erode good care by emphasizing the health benefits of choice without sufficient attention to the practices of care. Can routinized PMTCT services with minimal pre-test counseling—as is the case in Uganda and Kenya—be seen as good care, rather than as medical domination that threatens to violate women's rights? In both the routine provider-initiated testing that prevails in Kenya, Uganda, and Vietnam, and the client-oriented system in Indonesia, pregnant women value the provision of HIV tests in antenatal care. As Lock and Kaufert (1998) argue, they are pragmatic users of reproductive medicine. The concerns are raised by the unhappy few who test HIV positive.

Overall, our fieldwork suggests that the diagnostic controversy surrounding HIV testing—whether it should be routine (mandatory, opt out) or a matter of informed individual choice (opt in) misses the point. Pre-test counseling is not the main issue for PMTCT programs. The real issue is whether the services can provide the necessary follow-up social support, treatment, and care when women are identified as HIV positive. While the social needs of vulnerable women are acknowledged in the fourth pillar of the Abuja PMTCT model, the implementation of follow-up care and support for mothers and children is often lacking in practice. When this is the case, pregnant women carry the burden of diagnosis without the necessary resources to act on that knowledge.

In all four countries, pregnant women were easy targets for public intervention, as they were already enrolled in programs for antenatal care. Pregnant women have a long history of being disciplined in reproduction-related screening programs. But in making pregnant women the primary target group for diagnostic surveillance, PMTCT programs run the risk of reinforcing a culture that makes women responsible for ill health and blames them for HIV. Why is the role men play in transmission pathways so often ignored? This question is especially pertinent in countries like Vietnam and Indonesia, where HIV prevalence rates are extremely high among intravenous drug users, who are mainly men. Would it not make sense to raise their awareness of the risk of infecting their girlfriends, wives, and children? PMTCT programs could work with organizations representing intravenous drug users and sex workers to include an arm that focuses on preventing father-to-child transmission. Promoting testing options that reach men might also reduce (self) blame among women for introducing HIV into their families and promote disclosure. If accompanied by good follow-up medical care, home-based testing enables early treatment for both men and women, allowing them to plan for PMTCT before pregnancy.

Achieving the aim of reducing HIV infections among children by 50 percent requires tailoring globally designed public health strategies to local realities. Policy makers need to rethink the way they compartmentalize target groups for prevention, minimize the negative consequences of prevailing stigma and discrimination for those who test HIV positive, and identify local opportunities for follow-up AIDS care and socio-economic support for HIV-positive mothers, fathers, and their children.

NOTES

1 The trial found that the absolute rate of transmission of HIV from mother to child when using this simple Nevirapine regime was reduced to 15.7 percent—meaning that one out of seven infants born to HIV-positive mothers would still be infected. More comprehensive prophylaxis regimes in Europe and the U.S. at the time had reduced mother-to-child transmission to as low as 2 percent.

2 Nevirapine was associated with a 41 percent reduction in the relative risk of transmission through to age 18 months. Economics also played a role: the manufacturer of Nevirapine, Boehringer Ingelheim, had set up a donations program for PMTCT, claiming that the drug was safer and more effective than AZT.

REFERENCES

Akrich, Madeline. "The De-Scription of Technical Objects." In *Shaping Technology/ Building Society: Studies in Socio-Technical Change*, edited by W. Bijker and J. Laws, 205–44. Cambridge: Cambridge University Press, 1992.

Bayer, Ronald. "Ethical and Social Policy Issues Raised by HIV Screening: The Epidemic Evolves and So Do the Challenges. *AIDS* 3, no. 3 (1989): 119–24.

Bayer, Ronald and Claire Edington. "HIV Testing, Human Rights, and Global AIDS Policy: Exceptionalism and its Discontents." *Journal of Health Politics, Policy and Law* 34, no.3 (2009): 301–23.

CDC (Centers for Disease Control and Prevention). Revised Recommendations for HIV Testing of Adolescents, Adults, and Pregnant Women in Health-Care Settings. *MMWR* 55, no. RR14 (2006): 1–17.

Dabis, F., V. Leroy, K. Castetbon, R. Spira, M. L. Newell, and R. Salamonet. "Preventing Mother-to-Child Transmission of HIV-1 in Africa in the Year 2000." *AIDS* 14 no. 8 (2000): 1017–26.

Hardon, Anita. "Biomedical Hype and Hopes: AIDS Medicines for Africa." In *Rethinking Biomedicine and Governance in Africa: Contributions from Anthropology*, edited by P. W. Geissler, R. Rottenburg and J. Zenker, 77–96. Bielefeld: Transcript Verlag, 2012.

———. "Contraceptive Innovation: Reinventing the Script." *Social Science and Medicine* 62, no. 3 (2006): 614–27.

Hardon, Anita and Stuart Blume. "Shifts in Global Immunization Goals (1984–2004): Unfinished Agendas and Mixed Results." *Social Science and Medicine* 60, no. 2 (2005): 345–56.

Hardon, Anita, Emmy Kageha, John Kinsman, David Kyaddondo, Rhoda Wantenze, and Carla Makhlouf Obemeyer. "Dynamics of Care, Situations of Choice: HIV Tests in Times of ART." *Medical Anthropology* 30, no. 2 (2011): 183–201.

Hardon, Anita, Eva Vernooij, Grace Bongololo-Mbera, Peter Cherutich, Alice Desclaux, David Kyaddondo, Odette Ky-Zerbo, Melissa Neuman, Rhonda Wanyenze, and Carla Obermeyer. "Women's Views on Consent, Counseling and Confidentiality in PMTCT: A Mixed-Methods Study in Four African Countries." *BMC Public Health* 12 (2012): 26.

Hardon, Anita, Pauline Oosterhoff, Johanna D. Imelda, Nguyen Thu Anh, and Irwan Hidayana. "Preventing Mother-to-Child Transmission of HIV in Vietnam and Indonesia: Diverging Care Dynamics." *Social Science and Medicine* 69, no. 6 (2009): 838–45.

Jackson, J. Brooks, Phillpa Musoke, Thomas Fleming, Laura A. Guay, Danstan Bagenda, Melissa Allen, Clemensia Nakaiito, Joseph Sherman, Paul Bakaki, Maxensia Owor, Constance Ducar, Martina Deseyve, Anthony Mwatha, Lynda Emel, Coery Duefield, Mark Mirochnick, Mary Glenn Fowler, Lynne Mofenson, Paolo Miotti, Maria Gigliotti, Dorothy Bray, and Francis Mmiro. "Intrapartum and Neonatal Single-Dose Nevirapine Compared with Zidovudine for Prevention of Mother-to-Child Transmission of HIV-1 in Kampala, Uganda: 18-Month Follow-up of the HIVNET 012 Randomised Trial." *Lancet* 362, no. 9387 (2003): 859–68.

Kenya Ministry of Public Health and Sanitation. *Guidelines for HIV Testing and Counselling and Kenya*. Nairobi: National AIDS and STI Control Programme, 2008.

Lock, Margaret and Patricia Kaufert. *Pragmatic Women and Body Politics*. Cambridge: Cambridge University Press, 1998.

Mol, Annemarie. *The Logic of Care: Health and the Problem of Patient Choice*. New York: Routledge, 2008.

Msellati, Phillippe. "Improving Mothers' Access to PMTCT Programs in West Africa: A Public Health Perspective." *Social Science and Medicine* 69, no. 6 (2009): 807–12.

Nguyen, Thu Anh, Pauline Oosterhoff, Anita Hardon, Hien Nguyen Tran, Roel A. Coutinho, and Pamela Wright. "A Hidden HIV Epidemic among Women in Vietnam." *BMC Public Health* 8 (2008): 37.

Ogden, Jessica, Thu Hong Khuat, and Thi Van Nguyen. *Understanding HIV and AIDS-Related Stigma and Discrimination in Vietnam*. Washington: International Center for Research on Women, 2004.

Oosterhoff, P., Anita Hardon, Thu Anh Nguyen, Ngoc Yen Pham, and P. Wright. "Dealing with a Positive Result: Routine HIV Testing of Pregnant Women in Vietnam." *AIDS Care* 20, no. 6 (2008a): 654–9.

Oosterhoff, P., Thu Anh Nguyen, Thuy Hanh Ngo, Ngoc Yen Pham, and P. Wright. "Holding the Line: Family Responses to Pregnancy and the Desire for a Child in the Context of HIV in Vietnam." *Culture, Health & Sexuality* 10, no. 4 (2008b): 403–16.

Paxton, S., G. Gonzales, K. Uppakaew, K. K. Abraham, S. Okta, C. Green, K. S. Nair, T. Merati Parwati, B. Thephthien, M. Marin, and A. Quesada. "AIDS-Related Discrimination in Asia." *AIDS Care* 17, no. 4 9(2005): 413–24.

Sanon, Patrice, Simon Kabore, Jennifer Wilen, Susanna J. Smith, and Jane Galvao. "Advocating Prevention over Punishment: The Risks of HIV Criminalization in Burkina Faso." Reproductive Health Matters 17, no. 34 (2009): 146–53.

Shaffer, Nathan, Rutt Chuachoowong, Phillip A. Mock, Chaiporn Bhadrakom, Wimol Siriwasin, Nancy L. Young, Tawee Chotpitayasunondh, Sanay Chearskul, Anuvat Roongpisuthipong, Pratharn Chinayon, John Karon, Timothy D. Mastro, R. J. Simonds, and Bangkok Collaborative Perinatal HIV Transmission Study Group. "Short-Course Zidovudine for Perinatal HIV-1 Transmission in Bangkok, Thailand: A Randomised Controlled Trial." Lancet 353, no. 9155 (1999): 773–80.

Uganda Ministry of Health. *Uganda National Policy Guidelines for HIV Counselling and Testing*. Kampala: Ministry of Health, 2005.

UNAIDS. *Voluntary Counseling and Testing (VCT): UNAIDS Technical Update*. Geneva: UNAIDS, 2000.

UNFPA. *Call to Action: Towards an HIV-Free and AIDS-Free Generation. Prevention of Mother to Child Transmission (PMTCT) High Level Global Partners Forum*. Abuja, 3 December, 2005.

UNICEF. *Evaluation of United Nations-Supported Pilot Projects for the Prevention of Mother-to-Child Transmission of HIV*. New York: UNICEF, 2003.

United Nations. *Political Declaration on HIV/AIDS: Intensifying Our Efforts to Eliminate HIV/AIDS*. Resolution adopted by the General Assembly on 10 June 2011. New York: United Nations, 2011.

Weinhardt, Lance S., Michael P. Carey, Blair T. Johnson, and Nicole L. Bick. "Effects of HIV Counselling and Testing on Sexual Risk Behavior: A Meta-Analytic Review of Published Research, 1985–1997." *American Journal of Public Health* 89, no. 9 (1999): 1397–405.

WHO. *Epidemiological Fact Sheets on HIV/AIDS: Indonesia and Vietnam 2008 Updates*. Geneva: WHO, 2008.

———. *Strategic Approaches to the Prevention of HIV Infection in Infants: Report of a WHO Meeting*. Morges, Switzerland: World Health Organization, March 20–22, 2002.

WHO/UNAIDS. *Guidance on Provider-Initiated HIV Testing and Counselling in Health Facilities*. Geneva: WHO/UNAIDS, 2007.

———. "Recommendations on the Safe and Effective Use of Short-Course ZDV for Prevention of Mother-to-Child Transmission of HIV." *Weekly Epidemiological Record* 73 (1998): 313–20.

3 Resisting Tuberculosis or TB Resistance
Enacting Diagnosis in Georgian Labs and Prisons

Erin Koch

INTRODUCTION: DIAGNOSING CONTEMPORARY GLOBAL TUBERCULOSIS

This chapter focuses on knowledge production about tuberculosis in post-Soviet Georgia amid the shifting standards of TB management, diagnosis, and treatment. The analysis centers on how TB professionals working in a laboratory produce diagnoses of tuberculosis, and how incarcerated men take up the project of achieving a TB diagnosis as a survival strategy. The ethnographic analysis foregrounds diagnosis as a process of enactment and as a strategic event that is mobilized and transformed, rather than a static nosology or definition. As diagnostic practices travel from laboratories into sites of detention, new meanings of tuberculosis are produced as incarcerated men transform the meanings and effects of a diagnosis into a survival strategy that could potentially improve the conditions in which they are detained. Subsequently, back in the laboratory, their efforts to achieve a TB diagnosis are enacted in ways that call into question the morality of those in detention.

Tuberculosis is one of the most pressing global health issues today, and jails and prisons around the world where conditions are crowded and dilapidated provide incubators for its spread within and beyond sites of incarceration. It is the second leading cause of death from a condition involving a single infectious agent. According to the most recent Global Tuberculosis Report published by the World Health Organization (WHO), in 2013, there were 9 million new cases of the disease, and 1.5 million people died from tuberculosis (2014). These staggering rates are somewhat puzzling, given the scaling up of resources devoted to diagnosing, curing, and managing the spread of the disease since the early 1990s.

In this chapter, I draw on ethnographic research about changes in the production of knowledge about tuberculosis in the country of Georgia following the dissolution of the Soviet Union. I analyze how Georgian service providers working to establish the new National Tuberculosis Program (NTP) navigate changes in what counts as "expert knowledge" to analyze the actual versus the expected results of a so-called technical solution to TB control that is at once cultural, political, and biological. I foreground how TB professionals and prisoners work to achieve TB diagnoses for dramatically different reasons. The diagnosis of tuberculosis is thus something that is achieved not only in laboratories, but also in sites of detention, where incarcerated men actively seek a positive TB diagnosis as a threshold not for naming or obtaining treatment, but to improve their conditions of imprisonment.

Technical and financial support from international organizations was integral for establishing the NTP. On the basis of pilot projects in Georgia, Armenia, and Azerbaijan sponsored by the WHO in 1994 (Zalesky et al. 1999), the Georgian NTP was officially launched in 1995. The pilot projects introduced a highly standardized approach to tuberculosis control known as DOTS, which was established by the WHO in response to the ongoing global TB emergency. The acronym "DOTS" stands for directly observed treatment, short course.[1] The approach is highly dependent upon laboratory-based diagnosis and fixed regimens of first-line anti-TB drugs: rifampicin, isoniazid, ethambutol, and pyrazinamide, with direct observation of medicine ingestion three to seven days a week for six to nine months.[2] The goals of the protocol are to quickly identify people who are actively sick with tuberculosis (and thus spreading bacteria), to treat and rapidly cure those individuals, and to cut the chain of infection. Intensive monitoring at local, national, and international levels also promotes surveillance of the traffic in microbes and contagious individuals within and between countries and continents, and information (largely statistical) about them. Based on fieldwork in labs and prisons, I show that with the implementation of the DOTS approach, tuberculosis is reproduced and takes on new meanings within different sites of the Georgian anti-tuberculosis network, as a paradoxical consequence of standardization.

RESEARCH CONTEXT AND METHODS

The study is based on seventeen months of research conducted during 2001–2007 that was anchored at the NTP in Tbilisi, Georgia's capital city.[3] I conducted semi-structured interviews with more than seventy scientists, health care workers, administrators, and representatives of international donor and aid organizations involved with TB control and health care reforms. Through interviews and informal conversations, I gained firsthand insights into diverse perspectives about tuberculosis and DOTS in Georgia. By taking the concerns people related to me seriously, I learned the nuanced ways in which TB diagnostics are manipulated by professionals, patients, and prisoners, often for different and contradictory reasons.

My research also consisted of long-term participant observation at the National TB Reference Laboratory (NRL) housed at the NTP, at TB training sessions for health professionals, in clinical settings, and in the prison sector,

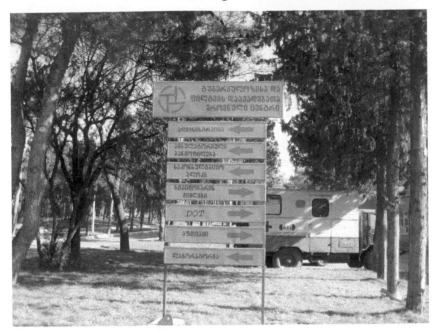

Figure 3.1 Entrance of the NTP. From top to bottom, the different sections of the sign read as follows: National Center for Tuberculosis and Lung Disease; Administration; Ambulatory Department; Consultation Section; Stationary (Inpatient) Recipient; DOT; Pharmacy; Laboratory. Photo by Erin Koch.

where tuberculosis cases are concentrated. As a research methodology, participant observation is both rigorous and flexible; it involves immersion in daily life, be that in communities, homes, workplaces, or other domains of human interactions and experiences. Participant observation also opens up encounters, questions, and perspectives that might not have been anticipated, but that are of fundamental importance to a project's participants, and thus the anthropological enterprise (Wendland 2010: 226). While the NRL's work schedule allowed me to conduct regular participant observation, my access to prisons, clinical settings, and trainings was less amenable to structuring and required flexibility. I often found my conversations and the social interactions I participated in frustrated and confusing. Nonetheless, by embracing these challenges I was able to establish a respected subjective and relational position in a social world. As a researcher, I was thus uniquely positioned to understand the complex yet mundane dynamics of cultural values and political-economic and institutional transformations that affect medical knowledge production for the purposes of diagnosis and treatment of a highly infectious disease in practice. Being able to establish this mode of positionality and subjectivity is one of the greatest strengths of anthropological research because it provides insights into why people do what they do, from the ground up.

In the case analyzed here, grounded ethnographic research enabled me to understand that diagnosis is not a static event that happens at a particular moment, from which the work of treatment can then follow. Instead, diagnosis is an active and strategic process of engagement that is heavily monitored not only by TB administrators and lab workers, but also by prisoners, who work to achieve a diagnosis in an effort to improve their daily lives. Thus, the leviathan of diagnosis is clearly a zone of contention and competition where winning the outcome of a positive TB diagnosis is at once evidence of the correct implementation of new global standards for TB control in the laboratory, and a strategy for freeing oneself from the violent aspects of daily life in prison.

CONTEMPORARY TUBERCULOSIS MANAGEMENT AND ANTIBIOTIC RESISTANCE

The bacterium involved with tuberculosis is *Mycobacterium tuberculosis* (Mtb). From the perspectives of public health and molecular biology, Mtb is widely referred to as a "successful pathogen" and as a "persister" (Hette and Rubin 2008; Vergne et al. 2004). This kind of bacterial success and persistence are attributed to the capacity of slow-growing members of the Mycobacterium complex of bacteria (of which there are more than fifty) to stay alive in the air for hours (especially in the absence of sunlight or ultraviolet rays) and to establish latency in the lungs or other organs and tissues for long periods before reactivating.[4] This type of bacterium is protected from detection by the immune system by a complex wall of lipids (Saunders and Britton 2007: 103). The waxy cell wall also forms a biochemical matrix that renders the majority of available antibiotics ineffective. In this and other ways, Mtb has the capacity to actually exploit the defense of its host to establish latency (Cosma et al. 2003: 666).

The forms of significance of the strains of Mtb and their global circulation dramatically changed in the late 1980s and early 1990s, when social and political events such as the HIV/AIDS epidemic and the demise of the Soviet Union (which increased international traffic in humans and microbes) influenced the rise and spread of antibiotic-resistant strains of tuberculosis.[5] In 1993, the WHO declared tuberculosis a global emergency, bringing about a new era in biomedical standardization for TB diagnosis, treatment, and management. The event was a response to increased rates of tuberculosis—including multi-drug-resistant strains—that began to soar in late 1980s and early 1990s. The framing of an emergency worked to regenerate and redirect public health attention and resources to a disease that had been subject to public health neglect since the 1960s, when international health officials declared that tuberculosis was nearly eradicated (Raviglione and Pio 2002), rendering it "invisible to international donors" (Dye and Williams 2010: 856).

The demise of the Soviet Union demolished centralized health infrastructures, exacerbated poverty, and gave way to higher incarceration rates that created incubators for the disease (Stern 1999). Already facing declining support for health services in the late 1980s (Field 2000), following Soviet collapse, life expectancies in Eurasia and Eastern Europe plummeted (Bazylevych 2011: 1). Georgia, a small country in the South Caucasus that shares borders with the Russian Federation, Armenia, Azerbaijan, Turkey, and the Black Sea, faced particularly high rates of tuberculosis, in part as a consequence of civil wars that led to high populations of internally displaced persons living in crowded and dilapidated housing and a serious energy crisis. Georgia's geopolitical position was a significant factor as well. The region is a historic and strategic crossroads between East and West where people and microbes traffic back and forth on paths previously (and still) crossed by warring empires and important trade routes.

Georgia's separation from the Soviet Union in 1991 was met not only with civil war, but also with a dramatic dismantling of the centralized Soviet medical infrastructure. Abruptly, medical facilities lacked basic supplies, health professionals were "downsized" from their positions or continued working without salaries, and patients lost a highly specialized system that they knew how to navigate. Those factors were particularly favorable to the spread of tuberculosis in Georgia and throughout the former Soviet Union, where the number of cases more than doubled between the mid- and late-1990s (Bonnet et al. 2005; Mdivani et al. 2008). With the exception of Russia, Georgia may have witnessed the most dramatic increase of reported TB rates of all former Soviet Republics (Lomtadze et al. 2009). "With a reported occurrence of about 200 cases per 100,000 inhabitants in the mid-1990s, the Southern Caucasus state of Georgia was said to be the main source of infectious disease among CIS countries" (Peuch 2005).[6] Amid civil wars and the collapse of social safety nets, tuberculosis was running rampant not only in Georgia, but throughout the Caucasus (Abdullaev 2000; Estemirova 2003).

Georgia was one of the first countries in the former Soviet Union to accept technical and financial assistance from Western donors for tuberculosis control, health sector reforms, and other infrastructure and civil-society development programs. But these interventions also challenged the legitimacy of local—and specifically Soviet—approaches to TB control, inciting heated debates about what counts as medical expertise, and fueling rhetoric about the "resistance" of Soviet-trained TB physicians to implementing DOTS (Rechel et al. 2011). In Georgia, these debates emerged within a broader historical context of medical professionalism and TB control that pre-dates 70 years of Soviet socialism. Thus, an anthropological analysis of DOTS implementation reveals the deeply cultural and political nature of diagnosis.

Where diagnostic strategies are made central to disease control, medical and scientific knowledge are bartered, abridged, and contested.

The DOTS strategy is one of the most widely distributed global health interventions in history. The protocol was branded in 1994 and since 1995 has been adopted in over 200 countries. Under DOTS, more than 40 million individuals have been successfully treated for TB, and nearly 6 million lives have been saved (WHO 2014). In 2006, the approach was incorporated as an integral element of the WHO's Stop TB Strategy. The Stop TB Strategy is a consortium of governmental, public, and private organizations and communities that cohere around the problem of global tuberculosis and, increasingly, intersecting cultural, biological, and political dynamics of antibiotic resistance. DOTS has also been adopted as part of the Millennium Development Goals for alleviating major diseases. With such institutional backing, the DOTS protocol has become the global "gold standard" of tuberculosis control (Porter et al. 2002). These standardized procedures for reporting and recording diagnosis, antibiotic treatments, and direct surveillance of medicine ingestion affected a moral economy of medical practice. Here, following the scholarship of physician and medical anthropologist Claire Wendland, moral economy refers to "both process and product: it is the shifting set of values deployed and used to legitimate, evaluate, and potentially alter relations between those seeking medical care, those providing it, and those paying for it or profiting from it" (2010: 197). Despite the common goal of TB control demonstrated in the Stop TB Strategy, limited financial resources and the challenges of implementing globalized standards for disease management on the ground give rise to a range of practices through which TB professionals and patients strategically manipulate the system amid standardization in order to improve their work and living conditions. Each of these is treated in the subsequent sections.

STANDARDIZATION AND ENACTING A DIAGNOSIS

Standardization is a critical element of global health diagnostics. The term refers to processes by which uniformity is established to promote regulation and an allegedly seamless translation (of goods, statistics, policies, protocols, and so on) across geographical and social boundaries. Anthropologists who study standards and their circulations illuminate how abstract models and technologies travel and become meaningful in specific contexts (Bowker and Star 1999; Lampland and Star 2009; Timmermans and Berg 2003). These processes are far from value neutral (Hardon, this volume). They are essential for reorganizing medical services in terms of good management, but establishing "good management" in global health is anything but a value-free enterprise, and in this terrain, market values are particularly powerful (Benatar et al. 2010). In this global standardizing process, achieving a diagnosis through the correct means is a fundamental step that must be enacted by all players, including administrators, lab technicians, physicians, and patients.

In its standardization, the DOTS protocol operates as a biomedical "technology of subjectivity," that "relies on an array of knowledge and expert systems to induce self-animation and self-government" through health management (Ong 2006: 6). However, standardization is a highly variable process. Those standards specific to regimens for the diagnosis, treatment, record keeping, and management of an infectious disease are situated within and informed by a moral economy that is inseparable from political economy (Busch 2000). Standards are also rife with contradictions that shape everyday aspects of disease control for the health workers who produce and distribute TB services. Because standardization can be a fragmented process, "global standards are difficult to enforce. . . . [T]hey are much more than cross-cultural quality assurance mechanisms. . . . [A]s standards travel, their social and economic embeddedness is revealed" (Petryna and Kleinman 2006: 12). Standardization can ultimately prove detrimental to service delivery, systems of classification, diagnosis, and treatment within global health dynamics. This is true in part because tuberculosis is multiplied via DOTS implementation, taking on different forms and meanings within different sites of the Georgian TB network.

Ethnographic research about DOTS implementation provided unique insights about the ways in which standardization paradoxically enacts thresholds of disease management, rather than introducing fixed parameters for diagnosis. I draw attention to Mol's theorization of processes of enactment because it focuses attention on the creative, validating, and affirming effects of diagnosis, and not simply on an unquestioned final diagnostic code and corresponding treatment plan. In diagnostic praxis, standardization encourages rather than discourages debates about modes of knowledge production and what counts as expertise. As professionals and patients grapple over different approaches to TB control, the emphasis on individual responsibility to treatment adherence becomes a zone of enactment (Mol 2002), rather than a fixed object of intervention (Rohden, this volume). With the rise of evidence-based medicine and evidence-based global health (Adams 2010: 51), normative assumptions about management underpin health interventions. The DOTS approach is exemplary of biomedical interventions that focus on management in two senses: first, of patients who will presumably act in their own "self-interest" by pursuing a healthy lifestyle and actively seeking out health services; and second, of information, sputum, microbes, medicines, doctors, laboratory workers, and health administrators. The politics of knowledge and what counts as expert knowledge are ever more intense among stakeholders and participants—including social scientists and anthropologists, whose contributions are often dismissed as anecdotal, or as "too abstract" to count as "science" (Adams 2010). DOTS diagnostics reveal these politics as they emerge from state bureaucracies of care, in laboratory management, and in strategic patient behaviors.

But a clear understanding of the enactment of DOTS must take into consideration local knowledge and experiences "about what it actually means to practice medicine with an unpredictable assortment of donated technologies. . .[and] about the meaning on the ground, in real people's loves, of rules and research ethics formulated at a distance of many thousands of miles . . . and generally about the moral experience of illness, disease and medical practice in places that have little power to make their knowledge heard in decision-making centres" (Feierman et al. 2010: 122). In the sections that follow, I turn to ethnographic views of knowledge production in action, first from the viewpoint of the laboratory, and second from the viewpoint of sites of incarceration. I demonstrate that TB diagnoses are enacted in situated and intersecting contexts, where its achievement is a strategic goal for specific, albeit competing and sometimes contradictory, goals.

ENACTING MICROBES IN THE LABORATORY

In the DOTS protocol, the laboratory is positioned as the central site for definitive diagnosis. I found that the biosocial aspects of diagnosis that emerge in the laboratory through relations between humans, sputum, microbes, and technical devices for knowledge production call into question the forms of laboratory or management introduced with DOTS. The information produced in the laboratory is intended to seamlessly translate across contexts and sites. Ideally, the results of the initial diagnostic tests (smear microscopy) pave the way for next steps within the laboratory, such as growing cultures for a more concrete bacterial identification and for preparing drug susceptibility tests (DSTs). With the authority of a scientific basis, these practices should shape treatment procedures and even what happens in prisons.

However, standardized procedures in the laboratory are not solely in the hands of the workers or machines, and often fall short of these ideals. Meaning comes out of the human-microbe relationships that may call into question assumptions built into changing laboratory work regimens and undermine DOTS.

Analyzing stained and smeared samples from patients or prospective patients produces an initial TB diagnosis. Sputum samples provide a first-order source of information that confirms the presence of bacteria with a level of authority that X-ray images of lungs, examined for visible lesions, no longer hold. As sputum samples are used to culture bacteria, and those cultures are then used for drug susceptibility tests, microbes are rendered visible and knowable for the purpose of diagnosis. However, sputum, cultures, and microbes are not pure forms or substances. Instead, they are infused with meanings that are produced through their manipulation. Such meanings are never determined in advanced, but are generated through human interactivity.

Following sputum as it goes through its diagnostic transformations demonstrates that laboratories are border zones where the "specific needs or demands placed on it" (Clarke and Star 2008: 121) are negotiated. The work of the NRL figures prominently in this sociality of tuberculosis in Georgia, not only because of the knowledge that their work produces, but also because of the ways in which the laboratory is embedded within larger political and economic transformations, and how technicians situate the microbiological within the social.

Although biomedical interventions reify bacterium as static targets of eradication, they are constantly changing in ways that may undermine treatment. The Georgian context further highlights how, within standardized forms of knowledge production, the significance of microbes is made meaningful in practice (Helmreich 2009). Moreover, an ethnographic analysis shows that the significance of the biological attributes is only produced through social relationships, for example, in the local microbiologies (Koch 2011) of diagnostic laboratories and of criteria for getting tested. The microbe is not simply "active" or "latent," as proponents of a standardized technical intervention would have it.

Daily diagnostic work is relatively straightforward, but it is also demanding on the senses. There are limits to the number of samples one technician can process on any given day. For example, ideally, one would prepare a maximum of thirty cultures per week in solid media or twenty to twenty-five per week in liquid media (a procedure that requires less preparation in advance), a maximum of twenty-four DSTs for first-line antibiotics in solid media and ten in liquid media per week, and a maximum of ten DSTs for second-line antibiotics per week in solid media. When I visited Tamuna in the laboratory in 2007, the laboratory technician with whom I worked most closely in the lab updated me on changes to the daily work routines. She showed me a new work schedule more concretely structured around a typical eight-hour workday than previous managers had implemented. On the new sign-up sheet, they are now required to log how many hours they spend on each task to demonstrate how they allocate time over the course of an eight-hour workday. She emphasized that this approach introduced new forms of labor management that do not necessarily correlate with the necessities of their daily work.

Over lunch one afternoon, I asked Dodona and Sopo—two lab technicians who had been working in the TB sector in Georgia since before the Soviet collapse—why, in their opinion, these changes in time management had been introduced, and whether it was to promote higher-quality (more accurate?) test results. Dodona said, "It is because of capitalism." We all laughed, but she was also highlighting the issue that market-oriented worldviews, which push for greater efficiency and rationality in labor production and management, do not necessarily result in higher-quality test results. In fact, these changes might even undermine efforts to produce faster results of diagnostic tests because the managerial worldview does not account for the role of microbial life cycles or human-microbe relations in daily laboratory work. "This is because there is concern from 'above' [indicating both hierarchy and the administrative offices upstairs from the laboratory] that there is what they are calling 'idle time' in the laboratory," Tamuna chimed in. In this way, the schedule also functions as a time card. She emphasized that this managerial task does not make sense in the laboratory. Daily work can vary because of the quality and quantity of sputum samples, and the quality of work will drop if technicians push themselves too hard. "Today is a good example. We prepared cultures all morning. How long were we in the box working?" Tamuna asked me. I replied, "Almost three and a half hours." She countered, "In theory, we could do another set before the eight-hour workday ends. The managers think that we should, but that is not a good idea. The quality will not be good. And something might go wrong, and we might not have enough time to repeat the steps. Sometimes I feel like they are becoming more concerned with the number of samples we process and not the quality of [the] work. And the administrators do not know what it is like to actually perform these tasks. The head of the laboratory does not understand why, after three to four hours of work, a technician might not be able to perform the entire procedure again merely to fill the workday." Tamuna clearly understands the managerial rationale for tracking labor time and output under the new system: the resources used in the lab are costly, and efficiency must be maintained. However, these rationales also seem irrational, given the potential for making mistakes because a tech's eyes are tired, or because they have to rush through the steps or cannot complete a full cycle of sample preparation because the official work day has concluded and they are forced to "clock out." Thus, the managerial concerns are often outmoded by the local microbiology in which they work.

This gap between administrative perceptions and everyday work habits recalls E. P. Thompson's argument that capitalist labor regimes rely upon "time thrift" for productive efficiency that becomes a marker of the temporal characteristic of modern labor practices. In his analysis of the effects of Industrial Era timekeeping devices and practices, Thompson argued that more "natural" and "task-oriented" ways of organizing labor and social life were displaced by time thrift, which to a certain extent responded to a need "for the synchronization of labor" (1993: 71). But even if post-Soviet time management is important to synchronize work in the laboratory, the imposition of "time-discipline" (90) and clock time will not necessarily overlap with microbial time. While changes in labor management bring about new forms of surveillance and self-discipline, the bacteria that workers are attempting to render and typify also have a disciplinary role in daily laboratory work (Landecker 2007).

From the vantage point of the laboratory, we see that nuances of host-pathogen interactions emerge on a threshold that is not simply biological or cultural, but a shifting political and economic terrain in which diagnostic regimes create obstacles to effective care. Molecular aspects of Mtb actively shape laboratory-based diagnostic procedures and outcomes that are at the heart of TB management strategies for identifying individuals who are actively sick with tuberculosis, and for ascertaining whether or not their strains of Mtb are susceptible to antibiotics. But the processes of diagnostic standardization, shifts to a market economy, and control by the institutions that mediate these diagnostic practices all but erase the cultural meanings, uses, and currency of sputum, the key diagnostic material. The relationship of sputum to disease categories and control is contingent and emergent. Sputum mediates and traverses concerns over national bodies politic, and the boundaries between local populations (sick and healthy, civilian and incarcerated) through standardization, although not necessarily in the ways that the administrators who attempt to order everyday practices by mapping clock time onto microbial time desire.

New techniques for preparing DSTs bring these contingencies into sharp relief. Like cultures, DSTs are monitored on a weekly basis for growth. DSTs are read against the controls. If there is growth in any of the tubes treated with S (streptomycin), H (isoniazid), R (rifampicin) or E (ethambutol), it means that the patient has a strain of tuberculosis resistant to that drug, which they indicate by writing "R" in the column for that antibiotic. If there is no growth, the bacterium is most likely sensitive to the antibiotic, which they indicate by writing an "S" in the appropriate column. Growing cultures and DSTs in solid media can take as long as eleven weeks to produce results.

However, faster methods are available.[7] One method commonplace in resource-rich research laboratories is to grow specimens in liquid media, using small test tubes that contain the liquid media at the time of purchase. Growth can be measured by a computerized device called a BACTEC that automatically reads tubes for growth and contamination hourly. It can also be measured by hand using a black light that illuminates the bacteria growing in the fluorescent broth. With support from the Global Fund, in 2006, the NRL adopted liquid growth methods using BACTEC. The adoption of this automated system for incubating and analyzing bacterial growth marks the influence of industry in global science. Automation is a significant aspect of both standardization and efficiency in science and industry, and could significantly improve TB diagnostics (Palomino 2012). However, such techniques are not necessarily well suited for under-resourced countries or for all clinical or research laboratories. The reagents in the liquid media speed up the bacterial growth cycle of Mtb.

But, is faster necessarily better? For example, one worker expressed concern about the assumption of faster being better precisely because Mtb is a naturally slow-growing microbe. "They [the administrators] do not want us to spend money on fluorography. They are waiting for someone to invent a little tablet that will treat TB patients in two weeks. But that is impossible because of the biology of the TB microbe."

In the fall of 2007, a total switch from previous methods was made. Unfortunately, due to a power outage one night, the lab lost 160 tubes—drug susceptibility tests for seventy patients. Although the power outage would have similarly compromised cultures growing in solid media, the financial loss in this case was much greater because the materials for liquid growth are more costly. As a result, the lab workers were not able to either fully abandon prior methods or fully adopt the new methods for growing cultures to diagnose tuberculosis and its potential resistance to antibiotics. Instead, they ran DSTs in both solid and liquid media as a backup and only grew cultures on solid media.

I talked with the laboratory technicians about the benefits and burdens of this "upgrade." Tamuna explained the new processes in detail. A pre-mixed reagent that, once opened, has to be used within twenty-four hours catalyzes decontamination. Cultures are prepared from sediments that are similar to solid media. Technicians add two additional components to the liquid broth that comes already prepared in the tubes: a growth-promoter and an anti-contaminant. Sediment is re-suspended in saline and added to the tubes. If workers are preparing drug-susceptibility tests, additional steps are taken to treat the broth with antibiotics. The main advantage is temporal: not only are the media prepared in the tubes in advance, but also, the test results are available much more quickly. In liquid media, growth can be established in eight to fourteen days. In running drug-susceptibility tests, liquid media afford results in four to thirteen days, rather than three weeks.[8] Indeed, this is the main reason why the administration of the NTP decided to adopt liquid media and BACTEC. It is especially important to be able to rapidly identify patients who have drug-resistant forms of tuberculosis, despite the fact that treatment might not be available for everyone. A definitive "negative" can only be diagnosed if there is no growth in the liquid after forty-two days. Moreover, liquid media are 15 to 20 percent more sensitive than solid media, meaning that because some species may in fact *only* grow in liquid media, not solid egg-based media, the tests will be more reliable.

In the Georgian context, these advantages are challenged by local infrastructural and economic constraints that are not necessarily taken into consideration with the push for diagnostic standardization. Not only are the materials in which growth is fostered more expensive, the computers that automatically monitor growth are expensive as well. Repairing or acquiring a new BACTEC machine in Tbilisi would be difficult, especially because much of their laboratory equipment that is shipped from overseas can, for example, get held up in Georgian customs for months due to insufficient paperwork, or accusations thereof. When I was there, only one of the two BACTEC machines was functional. No one was sure when it would be repaired. Because the focus is on inserting "upgrades" to the DOTS approach as it has been implemented in Georgia, rather than recognizing and valuing the local dynamics of diagnosis in action, the DOTS program is undermined at its diagnostic threshold.

Another critique of the homogenized diagnostic regimen is the risk it poses for local workers, many of whom may be under-equipped for safe laboratory practice. Liquid media pose a higher risk for contamination than solid media for both laboratory technicians and for samples. The bacteria growing inside liquid media are more mobile than those growing in colonies and affixed to solid media. These conditions are more dangerous for laboratory technicians because of the nature of interaction with pathogens. There is also a higher risk of sample contamination, 7 to 8 percent in liquid versus 3 to 5 percent in solid media.

In liquid media, it can be difficult to distinguish other bacteria from Mycobacterium. Fluorescence (in liquid media) shows all bacteria, including both Mycobacterium and bacteria that may contaminate samples. "We can sort of tell by looking at the liquid media. If Mtb is growing there are probably grains on the silicone base in the tube. If there are flakes floating in the broth it is probably some type of Mycobacteria. But not Mtb." Again, as Lela explained, here, the growth cycle of Mtb is a factor: "In the laboratory it takes two to three weeks to grow visible colonies. It takes at least two weeks to get an adult organism that has the ability to divide and form colonies, so you can confirm that you are witnessing Mtb. This is because [Mtb] is a slow-growing bacterium. You need this time in the laboratory. With BACTEC you can see them earlier, but you cannot see them mature into colonies. In the liquid medium they are very young. All you can see is that something is growing." For Lela, the key question is not how quickly do they get results, but what is the nature of those results?

There are also concerns about the accuracy of the results. Sometimes BACTEC gives false negative results from a sputum smear. As a result, each tube of liquid media that the BACTEC machine registers for positive growth must then be smeared and stained to confirm the presence of Mycobacteria. The BACTEC machine is computerized; each tube is pre-labeled with a barcode that is scanned before it is entered into the machine. The computer monitors for growth automatically on an hourly basis. Any tubes that register positive growth are registered on the display and compiled in a report that the computer also generates. Technicians check the temperature of the machine daily. "We have to check the growth in liquid media on a daily basis, and we have to smear every culture to double-check. In our conditions, with limited space, it is also difficult for us to routinize the tasks related to BACTEC, compared to solid media."

When Tamuna explained this to me, I told her that it sounded like a lot more work that resulted in even more work and ambiguity. She agreed that the "faster" methods also nearly double labor time. At the time of this research, the laboratory staff included enough technicians to perform the work, but not enough space. The additional labor required by the new approach also keeps the safety cabinets (hoods) occupied, so that other work cannot be performed in a timely fashion. I sat watching her scan the barcodes that come pre-affixed to the small liquid-filled tubes. The culture room had become a much more crowded environment, especially because they are still running DSTs in both solid and liquid media. Because the test is faster, they are now culturing all diagnostic specimens and testing them for drug susceptibility, whereas previously, they only ran culture tests for smear-positive cases and susceptibility tests on clinicians' requests. Because the procedure bears a higher risk of contamination, all TB-sensitive cultures must also be smeared and read under a microscope for confirmation. For these reasons, Tamuna explained, this process is "difficult to routinize in our conditions. Our technical expertise is fine, but we do not have the space or the time [because they are the only laboratory in Georgia with access to this technology] . . . For *this laboratory in this country*, BACTEC could be good for research experiments, but it is not good for routine diagnostic testing and laboratory work."

The technologies and techniques for manipulating samples in the laboratory, along with infrastructural, political, and economic forces, impact the meanings and relevance of the newer technologies. Clearly, microbes do not simply shape social aspects of infection and treatment; local cultural politics of scientific (and biomedical) expertise also shape the status and meanings of microbes, and how they relate to laboratory cultures, bodies, and protocols. These processes are particularly contentious as the status of laboratory-based knowledge moves from spaces of knowledge production to clinical, prison, and other administrative realms.

ENACTING TUBERCULOSIS IN PRISONS

In the late 1990s, the International Committee for the Red Cross (ICRC) identified tuberculosis as a serious health threat in Georgia's prisons, which are also a reservoir for the spread of the disease into the larger population. With a total prison population of 24,187 (536 per 100,000, at 101.8 percent of official capacity), Georgia currently has the fourth-highest number of prisoners per capita worldwide (International Centre for Prison Studies 2011). Prison conditions have been under the spotlight of local and international organizations that are critical of human rights violations. Prison reform has also been a highly politicized terrain in post-Soviet Georgia, particularly since former president Saak'ashvili's 2004 presidential campaign, in which ending corruption in the criminal justice system took center stage in his platform. But in Georgia, incarceration has become what one member of the ICRC TB team described to me as "Americanized." By this, he was referring to the fact that Saak'ashvili had adopted a "zero tolerance" approach to crime and, like the United States, increasingly relied on incarceration as punishment. Tuberculosis is part of the punishment (Farmer 2003). The conditions of overcrowding make a prison sentence into a probable death sentence as well (Stern 1999).

Poverty (and a growing gap between economic classes, with no middle class), unemployment, and the withdrawal of social safety nets led to increases in crime. At the same time, amid market reforms, incarceration increasingly became the state's response to crime. "First, widespread and sudden poverty led to an increase in crime. Second, economic insecurity led to a fear of crime and a public demand for greater protection. So, the number of arrests rose" (Stern 2003: 182). This led to a serious overcrowding problem in prisons, which in turn fueled the spread of tuberculosis.[9] At the time of writing, debates about introducing alternatives to incarceration into the criminal justice system are still underway in Georgia.

The shifting roles of both the ICRC and the government of Georgia in managing tuberculosis in the prison system reveal how tuberculosis is decisively institutionalized in the prisons. Paradoxically, as DOTS implementation unfolds—with great success under ICRC supervision—the strategies of TB control that define that approach create multiple meanings of tuberculosis under conditions of incarceration. Tuberculosis remains and becomes a form of punishment, an opportunity for improving one's conditions of detention, and a site for the management and surveillance of both the prison population and the government. All prisoners, not just those with TB, are thereby enrolled in this regime of standardization, as moral diagnostics are produced and circulated through disease-oriented interventions. The multiplicities of tuberculosis in the prison system are all produced through the disciplinary techniques exercised in the very bodies of those detained.

Administering DOTS appears to be more straightforward in prisons, at least from the perspective of getting the bugs to the drugs, because the population is physically immobile. Case finding, when pursued, might be active or passive, and because detainees are highly visible, it might be more difficult for them to avoid the regime of medicine ingestion under direct observation than someone who is not detained. While the direct observation tactic of DOTS aligns well with the bodily control one expects in prisons, there are unexpected consequences to diagnostic practice.

Despite the tremendous benefits of ICRC involvement in the prisons, and DOTS implementation in that context, the protocol's narrow emphasis on treating—and continuing to treat—individuals who test positive by smear microscopy means that a lot of individuals with latent TB fall under the radar. In prisons, overcrowding exacerbates the limited diagnostic gaze of smear microscopy. In highly overcrowded conditions, it is necessary to conduct yearly X-rays to increase detection of cases beyond those found by smear microscopy alone (Legrand et al. 2008). But in Georgia's prisons, X-ray screening is largely unavailable, and diagnosis based on single sputum samples is insufficient for determining whether an individual is actively sick. According to Nana, who works with a prison rights group in Tbilisi, this is because serum-positive prisoners only get a couple of months of treatment. "After smear conversion [from positive to negative in looking for microbes in the sputum], they are returned to the same social conditions, and it is very likely that these cases will be reactivated. This is the main reason why there are a lot of antibiotic-resistant cases in the prisons." But the limitations of smear microscopy as a diagnostic tool also call the legitimacy of some prisoners' illness claims into question.

During our interview in 2008, Nana explained, "There are a lot of inmates who have a latent form of tuberculosis, but in these cases the smear test will be negative. These prisoners are automatically excluded from the program." As a population, prisoners are seen as non-citizens, not subject to the rights of "civilian" populations or the right to medical care under conditions of incarceration. This exacerbates latency and the invisibility of disease in relation to such a morally compromised population. Beatings are justified in the minds of prison guards because it is easy to lie about something one cannot see (under the microscope). For example, the bacteria might not be concentrated in the sputum because the disease is so far advanced that it is in the bloodstream. The hidden costs of globalizing interventions, and their slippages, are perhaps most explicit in the prisons; despite the efforts and positive effects of ICRC involvement, the very conditions that perpetuate the rise and spread of tuberculosis and drug-resistant tuberculosis are either neglected or beyond the reach of the ICRC and the Georgian prison administration. In Georgia, these processes unfold in the larger context of rapidly rising rates of incarceration, managerial incapacities, and the lack of accountability for the prisoners' health.

CHEATING DIAGNOSIS

One afternoon in the summer of 2001 when I was working in the National Reference Laboratory, I watched and listened as laboratory workers participated in producing a unique meaning of tuberculosis at the intersection of the laboratory and prison domains. Tamuna, the technician who was also my primary teacher at the laboratory, was on the microscopy team rotation that month, responsible for registering sputum samples, preparing slides, and analyzing them under a microscope. It was a hot August morning and already almost 30 degrees Celsius outside, making us uncomfortable in our laboratory coats, masks, and gloves. During the time of research, there were air conditioning units in the kitchen/eating area of the lab and in some of the offices, but there was no air conditioning in the slide preparation rooms or in "the box," where cultures and DSTs were prepared. I was perched in my usual seat next to Tamuna at the small table where technicians prepared slides, and I was trying to help her by writing patient registration numbers onto each slide before she smeared and stained the samples.

That day, the microscopy team would be analyzing thirty-two samples, twenty-six of which were collected from prisoners. Tamuna placed all of the samples on the worktable to record the patients' registration numbers. The samples from the prisoners were distinguishable from those of "civilian" patients because all of them were collected and transported in containers with red lids. Interrupting the seamless flow of her work routine, Tamuna paused with one of the samples and held the container up to the light. She frowned a little and wrote "cheated" in English on the container next to the patient's registration number. A few minutes later, she paused over another sample and again wrote "cheated" on the cup. Curious about both her use of English during a process that usually took place entirely in Georgian and the meaning of the term, I asked her to explain why she distinguished those samples, and what she meant by "cheated."

As she carried the cups from the table to the hood, where she would be protected from bacteria that might become airborne when she opened the containers, Tamuna said that sometimes the laboratory technicians notice something "abnormal" about the appearance or consistency of a sample. I took my regular seat on the stool next to the hood, still unaccustomed to the notion that a sample of infected sputum could ever be considered normal. She went on to explain, "Sometimes the sample does not look right. Maybe part of it seems really clear and thin but the rest is thick and yellow or green [a sign of infection]. Or maybe there is something that does not belong, like a black particle." She pointed out a black spot in one of the samples she had labeled as "cheated." For Tamuna and her colleagues at the NRL and the ICRC, these abnormalities in a bodily substance might point to illicit behavior; they might indicate that someone tried to mix fresh or dry sputum from someone else into their sample. "Some prisoners want to be diagnosed with tuberculosis so they can be sent to the hospital." At that time, I had not yet visited any sites of detention, but I assumed things must be pretty abysmal to drive people to barter in sputum. "That makes sense to me," I thought and jotted in my notes, "I would probably do the same."

About four hours later, after Tamuna and the other technicians on the microscopy team had finished analyzing the slides, the two of us retreated to the laboratory's small kitchen area for a coffee break, and to wait out the rest of the workday. Lela, one of the biologists, burst through the hallway doors, clearly frustrated. *"Ra mokhda?"* (What happened?) I asked. Waving one of the patient registration forms, she said she was very upset about one of the three sputum samples that had been collected from a prisoner and delivered to the laboratory that morning. As part of the diagnostic process, "TB suspects" give sputum samples over two to three consecutive days, according to WHO guidelines. Lela had just been comparing this individual's results to those from the preceding day. The registration form showed that his sample from the day before had tested negative for Mtb, but that the sample from that day was *ochti plusi* (four plus), indicating a very high number of bacteria in the sputum and a highly infectious individual. She said it was impossible to have such a discrepancy in the number of bacteria from one day to the next. "He must have cheated," she grumbled, as she took the small electric coffee maker and a bag of Turkish coffee out of the cabinet.

As Lela joined us with her coffee and a novel that she would devour during a brief break, I asked her and Tamuna if they could elaborate on what they meant by "cheating." Lela put down her book and explained that many prisoners falsify their sputum samples by putting the sputum from someone else in their collection cup. "Maybe they put it in a shirt sleeve or something, or circulate things through networks. No one really knows because they hide this behavior, and the ICRC does not try to find out because they do not want to get any prisoners in trouble." They told me that people who are positive (for tuberculosis) exchange their sputum for vodka, cigarettes, and so on. People who are TB negative barter for the sputum because they want to achieve a TB diagnosis. At that time, TB treatment was only available in a TB prison colony located in Ksani, approximately thirty kilometers outside of Tbilisi. A TB diagnosis would result in a transfer to that hospital.[10]

Although they seemed annoyed about the wrench such practices threw in the diagnostic process, both Lela and Tamuna emphasized that they understand why people "cheat," as did many ICRC staff with whom I spoke about the intersections of tuberculosis and incarceration in Georgia. The conditions in the prison colonies and pre-detention centers are deplorable. But at the Ksani prison TB hospital, which had then recently been renovated by the ICRC and was at that time referred to as the "five star hotel" of Georgia's prison system, everyday life was relatively better than at the other sites. The rooms were less crowded, detainees had more freedom of movement, they were allowed to spend time outside, there was less violence between detainees and guards and among detainees, and the food was better. "But what makes it cheating?" I asked, still not sure how a term that sounded to me like a moral judgment applied to a set of practices that seemed to me more like a survival strategy than illicit behavior.

Lela put down her novel again, and took a sip of her coffee. She folded her hands on the table, unfolded them, and covered my hands with hers. Leaning forward and squeezing my hands gently, she said, *"chemo Erini"* (my Erin), before switching from Georgian to English, as if this would help me understand the logic. "It is *cheating* because they are trying to cheat the system. They are trying to get access to something that they do not have a right to." To be clear, that something—whether Tamuna and Lela meant to convey this or not, and I do not believe they did—included not only medicines for an illness they did not have, but also fresh air, sunlight, relatively decent food, and a reprieve from interpersonal violence.

Lela, Tamuna, and I continued our discussion for a few more minutes before we walked down the hill from the TB center to the Metro station and parted ways for the afternoon. As we talked, they highlighted some of the health concerns that such "illicit" sputum exchange could pose. If, for example, a prisoner successfully "cheated," he might find himself in better living conditions. But he might also risk increased exposure to TB infection at Ksani, and be required to take the difficult treatment regimen for six to nine months. Not only would he probably feel sick from the antibiotics, but also, if that person were to become actually actively sick with tuberculosis at a later date, the prior months of exposure to the standard antibiotics would put him at a higher risk for developing a drug-resistant strain. I conceded that it seemed like a lot to gamble. At the same time, I felt uncomfortable with the moral judgment they seemed to be passing with the label "cheating."

The term "cheating," it seemed to me, was being deployed by the ICRC and laboratory staff as a moral diagnostic—that is, as a barometer for norms and presuppositions about the rights, responsibilities, and conduct of individuals and institutions that are in part produced and circulated through health interventions in prisons, and that are anything but value neutral (Koch 2006). "Anyway," Lela said as we descended the escalator to catch our trains, "now we have been alerted to this behavior by the ICRC. They are on the lookout for suspicious behavior at the point of sputum collection. And they have trained us to be on the lookout for suspicious samples in the laboratory. So there is not much chance for getting away with it. Eventually TB treatment will be available at all the prisons in Georgia, and there will be no point in trying to cheat."

In 2001, DOTS was still centralized at Ksani, and attempts to cheat were prevalent within the prisons because a TB diagnosis would basically ensure being sent to that facility. "Some prisoners 'cheat' on their sputum test to GET IN to a TB programme, giving 'positive' sputum from someone else whereas they do not have TB because the TB programme is seen as advantageous . . . Others, who have been cured, 'cheat' on their sputum test by giving someone else's 'positive' sputum, so as to STAY ON in the programme, for the same perceived (and real) advantages" (Reyes 2007: 58). To control the "cheating," the ICRC team implemented a heavy system to monitor the samples and the prisoners that extends throughout the prison system, the ICRC's efforts, and the work done in the laboratory.

I asked the expatriate doctor, who was then head of the ICRC's TB program, how prisoners "cheat" exactly, and how the ICRC monitors these practices. He replied, "Aahh, there are many ways to cheat, some of them are very sophisticated, and they traffic dry and fresh sputum between the colonies, . . . so the sputum collected in Ksani and the colonies is seriously observed by ICRC staff. . . . They [the detainees] have to wash their mouth in case they are keeping dry or fresh sputum inside. They have to wash their hands, they do not touch the cup, and they spit. If we suspect that there is a particle of dry sputum that does not belong, we ask them to produce another [sample]." He also emphasized that he "understands why" they try to cheat their way to Ksani, but that getting there under false pretenses risks taking resources away from people who are "really" TB positive, and exposes them to toxic antibiotics.

Over the course of my long-term research in Georgia, I have participated in numerous informal conversations with ICRC staff about cheating, as well as issues of language specifically concerning the use of the word to describe these practices. As in English, this suggests that a cheater—*mat'q'uara*—is someone who knows the rules of the game and breaks them to gain access to resources to which they are not entitled, and would not have access to if they played by the rules. My inquiries about exactly who is being cheated, and out of what they are being cheated, often brought about heated responses concerning detainees who are milking resources to which they do not have a right. However, this position is always held in tension with the experiences of working in the penitentiary system. As Shota, a Georgian physician who held a high position on the ICRC TB team until the organization turned over the prison TB program to the government in 2010, so poignantly said about cheating, "It is unbelievable for any non-sentenced or any civilian or any person who is outside. It is unbelievable for me. But to tell you honestly, I am not sure if I were [one of] them, if I would not do the same. It is very difficult to judge them. But cheating remains a serious problem." Medical staff also clearly advocate through their individual actions and interactions for improved living and health conditions among prisoners. Nevertheless, cheating is seen as immoral behavior that threatens resource management and rational TB control.

In the prisons, DOTS implementation made "cheating" possible, rendering a positive TB diagnosis into a possible survival strategy, from my perspective, and as a moral diagnostic of the prisoners' behavior. As described here, "cheating" is a slippage born of DOTS implementation. This is not to suggest that within the Soviet centralized prison system and its social hierarchies, detainees did not similarly feign or marshal disease status or other biological conditions to improve their situation under detention. The point here is that cheating—as a form of unofficial expertise concerning the meanings and uses of sputum—disturbs a standardized flow of knowledge and resources, and reveals the limited TB diagnostic and managerial capacities. What, after all, is the meaning of "cheating" under circumstances of such intense duress that prisoners will permanently risk their health to avoid the greater violence and hazards of prison existence?

Over the course of my long-term research, the ICRC estimated that instances of cheating have been decreasing, largely because DOTS was being implemented throughout the prison system, not just at one facility. Nonetheless, sputum collection remained highly routinized and conducted under heavy surveillance. Looking for TB "suspects"—a clinical term that points to the potential risk they pose to others—among individuals who are already positioned as morally suspect in their criminality adds the job of policing sputum samples and the quality of samples to doctors and laboratory technicians. These forms of surveillance in the TB network reconfigure the work of sputum collectors and laboratory technicians whose work duties come to include looking for suspicious sputum samples and "cheaters."

During my visit to Ksani in 2001, I interviewed Dr. Gamsaxurdia, the head doctor, and observed and participated in routine sputum collection. The government of Georgia had recently followed through with ICRC recommendations to renovate the facility, and to create separate buildings for drug-sensitive and drug-resistant patients. At that time, treatment for MDR-TB had not yet been started in the prisons or in the so-called civilian (non-incarcerated) population.

As we toured the facility, the doctor who was at that time head of the ICRC's prison TB program pointed out the handful of small buildings that housed offices, clinical examination rooms, and the colony-style cells where groups of prisoners were contained together. As our general tour ended, he pointed to a wall that separated the two remaining buildings for TB-positive patients (those who were in the first phase of treatment and still considered infectious) and prisoners with MDR-TB. There was also a building with a small chapel and the kitchen where food was prepared, and an open court-yard where prisoners were allowed to be outside for fresh air and sunshine. This access to fresh air and sunshine is among the most prominent character-istics that distinguished Ksani from other prison facilities and made a posi-tive TB diagnosis desirable as a possible route to better prison conditions.

In accordance with WHO guidelines, sputum collection takes place in a special room built by the ICRC for sputum collection, as part of their larger project of the rehabilitation of the facilities there. The room was approxi-mately twelve by twenty feet, with a sink and acrylic plastic dividers creat-ing stalls where prisoners stand while they produce samples.

I arrived at the room with the team of nurses and doctors who run the collection procedure. There were about twenty men milling around outside, waiting. When we entered the room, the five nurses took their places: the first at the door that stands at the beginning of one long wall, the second against the center of that same wall, the third at the sink, and one each behind the outer walls of the stalls. On both sides, there is a space between the wall of the room and the outer sheets of acrylic plastic.

Following sputum and prisoners, the process unfolds as follows: first, the prisoner gives his name to the nurse at the door, who makes sure he is on the list for that day, and checks his face against a photograph. Is he who he says he is?

She tells the second nurse his prison ID number, and the second nurse writes it on the collection cup. Meanwhile, the prisoner goes to the sink, where he shows his hands to the third nurse, washes them, and rinses his mouth out. Next, the second nurse hands his cup to one of the nurses sta-tioned behind the divider. He stands in the stall while she hands his cup around a space between the wall and the acrylic plastic and holds it for him as he coughs up sputum. Finally, the nurse brings the cup to the doctor standing in the middle of the room. He checks it for "suspicious particles" and puts it in a cooler for transport to the laboratory in Tbilisi.

Members of the ICRC team with whom I spoke about these matters over the course of my research question the extent to which sputum is actually "sold" or "bought." When I asked Shota about whether sputum circulates in commodified form, he replied, "On the one hand you probably have to think that there is a reasonable amount of that. . . . It might be informal. I cannot really say that it costs something or if there is trade going on . . . because usually if it is the case, if people are exchanging [sputum for goods] it is so confidential that we cannot know about it. Otherwise, it would not be cheating. It would be business."

Here, the distinction between cheating and business speaks to the links between the conditions in Georgia's prisons and the broader social, political, and economic transformations. The term "business" suggests a legitimate exchange between a seller and consumer. "Cheating," on the other hand, reeks of illegitimacy and an individual who is attempting to access something to which he does not have a right, and in the process manipulating a system to ends for which it is not intended.

ICRC staff members also assert that individuals who try to cheat are not punished on these grounds. Although the term "cheating" suggests that the recalcitrance of detainees is taken for granted, there is no point in reporting cheaters to prison administrators given the deplorable conditions that drive inmates to barter in sputum samples in the first place. Second of all, they are aware of the risks. "Certainly there are still people who try to cheat. We try to identify them, explain to them [why this is a problem], and work with them. Sometimes people are fully aware of that they are doing or what kind of risk they are taking, but they still decide to cheat . . . to try to improve the living conditions at the risk of exposing [themselves] to TB." Through their interactions with ICRC TB program staff, prisoners are educated about the risky nature of tuberculosis: how the bacteria spread, why uninterrupted treatment is crucial for curing the disease, and the potential side effects of anti-TB medicines.

Detainees use their knowledge of incarceration and tuberculosis as a diagnostic survival strategy. As a result, their moral integrity is called further into question, and they are subjected to additional modes of suspicion and surveillance. The focus on medicine ingestion at the heart of the DOTS protocol perpetuates the institutionalization of TB—the very disease it is intended to control—within the penitentiary system.

In an effort to control the "cheating," the ICRC slowly started decentralizing DOTS: that is, implementing the protocol in other sites of incarceration, so that a positive TB diagnosis would not guarantee transfer to Ksani. In 2002, DOTS was implemented at Kriti, Georgia's high-security prison, and SIZO No. 5, the largest detention site in the country, both located in Tbilisi. By the time the government of Georgia took over control of the TB control program in the prisons in 2010, the ICRC had almost entirely decentralized the DOTS program within the prison system, and a TB diagnosis will not necessarily provide a route to better conditions at a separate facility. According to Shota, this means that each of the sixteen non-medical facilities has the staff and material resources to implement DOTS. "There is no longer a prison where you cannot be treated because of staffing issues. It is not necessary to transfer every detainee who has tuberculosis to Ksani for eight or nine months of treatment."

When I asked Shota if these ongoing efforts of decentralization were to eliminate the traffic in sputum, he replied, "This is exactly why we are doing this. Now, no one will be motivated to try to get transferred from one place to another. Decentralization is also good because if they are being housed and treated in one facility, but they do not behave well or need to be transferred for another reason, their treatment will go uninterrupted. In every prison facility there is a possibility to be treated [under DOTS] and to continue treatment. We are no longer interfering with administrative aspects of detention. The conflict of interest between incarceration and medical treatment is gone."

Cheating is thus cast as more of a threat to resource management and rational TB control than a public health issue. If, for example, cheating was officially recognized as a highly problematic survival strategy—rather than deviant behavior—efforts to stop cheating could also be marshaled to push for radically changing conditions within the prisons that fuel the spread of tuberculosis to begin with. At the same time, it is important to note that such transformations demand resources that the government cannot provide (Carter 2006). Implementing the DOTS protocol on the ground intersects a terrain where violence, filth, bureaucratic (ir)rationality, and the expanding public/private health system clash. This social suffering illuminates the tangled impediments and necessities behind globalized health care. At the same time, in this context, the prison operates as a laboratory for testing DOTS on a population whose movements are restricted, and the ways in which achieving a diagnosis can create new opportunities for resource competition.[11] However, the power regimes of DOTS and the surveillance of sputum collection are not perfectible. The unintended side effects of DOTS implementation, such as managerial insufficiencies and inconsistencies that undermine the approach, and the ways in which the implementation makes a positive TB diagnosis desirable, similarly highlight how the institutionalization of diagnosis and biomedical standardization propel new forms of moral personhood.

The limits of DOTS diagnostics are revealed wherever the control and regulation of disease intersects with judicial governance. These forms and practices of sovereignty are brought to bear on prisoners whose bodies are already vehicles for different forms of harm. Georgian prison practices challenge the flawless status of Western biomedical rationalities and standards that slip at particular levels of surveillance and regulation. DOTS implementation in that region has produced more effects than merely providing detainees with medical services they desperately needed. Standardizing new regimes of sputum collection and diagnosis also gave way to meanings of tuberculosis and strategies for its management that are both unique to the prison context and firmly embedded within Georgia's expanding National Tuberculosis Program.

"Having" tuberculosis entails not only a medical diagnosis of a very serious, potentially fatal disease, but also an unofficial form of expert knowledge put into motion by detainees who mobilize the exchange of sputum samples. The ambiguities of the sputum smear as the main diagnostic in Georgia's DOTS apparatus support the idea that such bold attempts to improve one's situation are morally reprehensible. Within the prison system, TB control with the DOTS approach is a contradictory process that, in Georgia, jeopardizes the potential of the protocol to provide a long-term sustainable response to tuberculosis. Diagnosis is enacted in a multiplicity of ways in different sites of the TB network, not fixed as a singular event within the TB life cycle.

CONCLUSION

While the DOTS approach marks a watershed in globally distributed disease-specific interventions, I found that in its implementation, the standardized nature of the protocol might, paradoxically, also be perpetuating conditions that sustain the very disease that it has been designed to eliminate. At the very least, as the specific Georgian example shows, DOTS implementation has introduced new management ideologies that create a hierarchy of knowledge in which TB professionals and prisoners both debate meanings of tuberculosis and navigate a shifting and often competing terrain upon which both work to achieve a positive TB diagnosis.

This chapter has highlighted how both laboratory technicians and prisoners work to achieve a positive TB diagnosis. The point is not that they are seeking a fixed or static object, but that they are engaged in dynamic processes of negotiation enabled by the implementation of the standardized DOTS approach. In both the laboratory and sites of detention, diagnosis is a threshold and an achievement. For lab workers, enacting a diagnosis—in the sense of enactment that Mol (2002) provides—of active and possible antibiotic-resistant tuberculosis is something that they achieve against the odds of market-oriented worldviews, which push for greater efficiency and rationality in labor production and management. As the laboratory technicians and scientists with whom I worked all made painfully clear, such effects of standardization do not necessarily result in higher-quality test results. Instead, such transformations in the standards for producing reliable diagnoses can undermine efforts to produce faster results of diagnostic tests because the managerial worldview does not account for the role of microbial life cycles or human-microbe relations in daily laboratory work. From the vantage point of prisoners, and the ways in which detainees work to achieve a diagnosis as a strategic survival strategy, it is also clear that DOTS programming, tied as it is to prisons, is about prisoner resistance to the inhumane conditions of incarceration. Here, resistance refers not to how social contexts breed antibiotic resistant strains of Mtb, but instead to the resistance of prisoners to the inhumane conditions in which they live, and to the fact that tuberculosis is part of the punishment. A strategically achieved diagnosis—even a falsified one, morally diagnosed as such as "cheating"—could provide an opportunity to free them from conditions of interpersonal violence, poor nutrition, overcrowding, and a lack of fresh air and sunlight.

On the basis of these ethnographic findings, it is perhaps ironic to demonstrate that the DOTS approach—which remains the foundation of the WHO-housed Stop TB Partnership—is marketed and implemented as the most rational and efficient strategy for managing tuberculosis, microbes, sputum, diagnostic and treatment practices, and relationships, recording and reporting techniques, and patients.[12] Instead, it is clear from the analysis presented here of how diagnosis is strategically enacted that a "standardized bureaucratic product" (Bowker and Star 1999: 1) such as DOTS will not function in uniform fashion in any context, as a focus on human-microbe interactions, for example, can show. Over the course of my research, numerous representatives of international organizations and Georgian TB professionals contended that the DOTS approach has become an unofficial requirement for national TB programs that seek financial and technical support from governments and aid organizations. Its implementation carries symbolic capital, without which it would be even more difficult for under-resourced health systems to compete for funds on the global market. The anthropological analysis presented here highlights the challenges of DOTS implementation in a range of contexts that collectively ask whether "one size fits all" in global health management (Bonnet et al. 2005). Public health and social science scholars have found that DOTS simultaneously creates the conditions for alleviating and perpetuating TB burdens around the world. However, these accounts often focus on the compliance (or lack thereof) of either doctors and administrators, patient populations, or both, as they imagine and fix geographies in terms of health and disease management (Tekle et al. 2002).

As a counterpoint to such approaches, this chapter's focus on the strategies laboratory technicians and prisoners strategically employ to achieve and enact a TB diagnosis calls into question the focus in DOTS and DOTS-Plus on antibiotic distribution and treatment outcomes for active cases. Insights from these nodes on the TB network illuminate diagnostic ideologies and values of prevention and testing in contemporary global health (Hardon, this volume). There are no universal pre-packaged solutions to the conundrums that fuel tuberculosis and make the disease, in all of its multiplicities, so challenging to control.

NOTES

1 "Short course" refers to the relatively short duration of the fixed antibiotic regimen at the heart of DOTS, which is usually six to nine months for patients being treated for antibiotic-susceptible strains.
2 The average cost of one full course of treatment under DOTS can be as low as $10. But this does not include direct or indirect (i.e. transportation) costs that patients might incur in seeking a diagnosis and prior to the onset of

treatment, regardless of whether diagnosis should officially be free of cost according to the National TB Program. Costs incurred by NTPs will vary widely based on local political and economic factors, including governmental and international financial and technical support. Treatment for drug-resistant tuberculosis is managed by the approach known as DOTS-Plus, which provides guidelines for administering second-line antibiotics. In the late 1990s, one full course of treatment to cure one person infected with MDR-TB with the necessary second-line antibiotics could cost as much as US $20,000, for a regimen that lasts, on average, two years. To make the second-line antibiotics used in treating MDR-TB (and eventually XDR-TB) more affordable and readily available, they helped to establish the Green Light Committee (GLC) in 2000. The GLC is a public-private partnership now integrated into the Stop TB Partnership that brings together donor organizations, governments that apply for GLC support, academic and research institutions, and civil society in the fight against antibiotic resistance. Currently, the cost can be as low as UD $2,000.

3 The research for this project would not have been possible without the generosity and assistance of the employees of the NTP and the NRL, as well as the members of the ICRC team in charge of TB control in prisons. I am responsible for any and all errors. Research for this project was supported by a Dissertation Improvement Grant from the Science and Technology Studies Program of the National Science Foundation; the Eurasia Program of the Social Science Research Council, with funds provided by the US Department of State through the Title VIII Program; the Graduate Faculty of Political and Social Science at the New School for Social Research; and the University of Kentucky. Following standard anthropological practice, all names are pseudonyms, except in the case of public officials, such as national political figures. Versions of some of the analyses and ethnographic material in this chapter have appeared in the journals *American Ethnologist* and *Medical Anthropology* and in my book *Free Market Tuberculosis: Managing Epidemics in Post-Soviet Georgia*. I thank Carolyn Smith-Morris for her generous and insightful feedback on this chapter.

4 Reactivation means that an individual transitions from being infected but not actively sick or contagious to an active case of the disease. Reactivation can be triggered by immunosuppression, which is why there are such high rates of TB among those living with HIV/AIDS.

5 Resistant forms of Mtb include multidrug-resistant tuberculosis (MDR-TB) and extensively resistant tuberculosis (XDR-TB). Strains of MDR-TB are resistant to both rifampicin and isoniazid—two of the most powerful and widely prescribed first-line antibiotics. The WHO defines XDR-TB as bacteria that are resistant to at least four antibiotics: rifampicin, isoniazid, any fluoroquinolone (a class of antibiotics that inhibit DNA replication and transcription in the microbe), and at least one of three injectable second-line drugs: capreomycin, kanamycin, and amikacin.

6 The Commonwealth of Independent States (CIS) is a regional group of states committed to promoting democracy and cooperation in anti-crime activities, trade, and so on. Georgia is no longer a member.

7 In July 2008, the WHO endorsed a diagnostic that tests for MDR-TB in two days. It costs eight dollars and consists of a line-probe assay that investigates DNA from bacterial strains for mutations linked to drug resistance. The test is not technically demanding, and can be easily implemented in resource-poor settings.

8 In liquid media, reagents treated with pyrazinamide may take a week longer to grow than those treated with other first-line drugs.

9 As numerous ICRC representatives informed me in formal and informal conversations, Shevardnadze's administration granted several amnesties to prisoners. In most cases, they were political prisoners who had been incarcerated during the civil war. They were pardoned if they had been fighting for Georgia's territorial integrity. Amnesties can create difficulties for the control of TB, because there are no resources in place to track detainees once they are released into "civil society."

10 An individual is unlikely to actually contract pulmonary tuberculosis by placing someone else's sputum in his/her mouth—the means through which many individuals attempt to forge sputum samples—as this does not provide the bacteria access to the lungs. However, if one's efforts to secure a false TB diagnosis to either be sent to or to prolong a stay in a prison hospital are successful, that individual will be exposed to active tuberculosis, and will be placed under treatment with antibiotics that they might develop resistance to and that might produce iatrogenic effects.

11 This is not a unique situation. For example, in the United States, there is a history of using prison populations for medical experiments. The same can be said of Holocaust victims, who were subject to medical and scientific experimentation in the concentration camps. Finally, there is a long history of using incarceration *as* a public health tool, most recently in the MDR-TB outbreak in New York in the late 1980s (Coker 2000). It has recently been suggested that, under the DOTS protocol, prisoners in Siberia were given anti-TB drugs that had far exceeded their expiration date (Farmer 2003).

12 News about the financial and managerial crisis within the Global Fund underscores the business-oriented worldview in the contemporary global health industry. After Round 11 of funding was canceled, the organization put in its place a temporary "Transitional Funding Mechanism" to maintain support for existing programs. Gabriel Jaramillo, its new general manager, is a former chair and chief executive of Sovereign Bank whose goal is to reconfigure the managerial goals and structures of the organization, and downsize to a "leaner and meaner" Global Fund to prioritize grants management (Boseley 2012).

REFERENCES CITED

Abdullaev, Nabi. "Tuberculosis Rages in the Caucasus." *Prism* 6 (October 31, 2000). Accessed June 19, 2003. www.jamestown.org/pubs/view/pri_006_010_007.htm.

Adams, Vincanne. "Against Global Health? Arbitrating Science, Non-Science, and Nonsense through Health." In *Against Health: How Health Became the New Morality*, edited by Jonathan M. Metzl and Anna Kirkland, 40–58. New York: New York University Press, 2010.

Bazylevych, Maryna. "Health and Care Work in Postsocialist Eastern Europe and the Former Soviet Union." *Anthropology of East Europe Review* 29 (2011): 1–7.

Benatar, Solomon R., Graham Lister, and Strom C. Thacker. "Values in Global Health Governance." *Global Public Health* 5 (2010): 143–53.

Bonnet, Maryline, V. Sizaire, Y. Kebede, A. Janin, D. Doshetov, B. Mirozoian, A. Arzumanian, T. Muminov, E. Iona, L. Rigouts, S. Rüsch-Gerdes, F. Varaine. "Does One Size Fit All? Drug Resistance and Standard Treatments: Results of Six Tuberculosis Programs in Former Soviet Countries." *International Journal of Tuberculosis and Lung Disease* 9 (2005): 1147–54.

Boseley, Sarah. "Can the Global Fund's New Management Change its Fortunes?" *The Guardian*. Accessed April 19, 2012. http://www.guardian.co.

uk/society/sarah-boseley-global-health/2012/apr/18/can-jaramillo-change-global-fund-fortunes.

Bowker, Geoffry C., and Susan Lee Star. *Sorting Things Out: Classification and Its Consequences*. Cambridge, MA.: MIT Press, 1999.

Busch, Lawrence. "The Moral Economy of Grades and Standards." *Journal of Rural Studies* 16 (2000): 273–83.

Carter, Stephen A. "Rainy Night in Georgia: Managing Change in the Conditions of Confinement." *Corrections Today Magazine* 68 (2006): 56–60.

Clarke, Adele, and Susan Leigh Star. "The Social Worlds Framework: A Theory/ Methods Package." In *The Handbook of Science and Technology Studies*. 3rd ed., edited by Edward J. Hackett, Olga Amsterdamska, Michael E. Lynch, and Judy Wajcman, 113–37. Cambridge, MA: MIT Press, 2008.

Coker, Richard. J. *From Chaos to Coercion: Detention and the Control of Tuberculosis*. New York: St. Martin's Press, 2000.

Cosma, Christine, David R. Sherman, and Lalita Ramakrishnan. "The Secret Lives of the Pathogenic Mycobacteria." *Annual Review of Microbiology* 57 (2003): 641–76.

Dye, Christopher, and B.G. Williams. "The Population Dynamics and Control of Tuberculosis." *Science* 328 (2010): 856–61.

Estemirova, Natalya. "Chechnya Stricken by TB." Institute for War and Peace Reporting, Caucasus Reporting Service No. 180, May 22, 2003. Accessed May 22, 2003. www.iwpr.net/index.pl?archive/cau/cau_200305_180_3_eng.txt.

Farmer, Paul E. *Pathologies of Power: Health, Human Rights, and the New War on the Poor*. Berkeley: University of California Press, 2003.

Feierman, Steven, Kearsley Alison Stewart, Paul E. Farmer and Veena Das. "Anthropology, Knowledge-Flows and Global Health." *Global Public Health* 5(2010): 122–28.

Helmreich, Stephan. *Alien Ocean: Anthropological Voyages in Microbial Seas*. Berkeley: University of California Press, 2009.

Hett, E.C. and E.J. Rubin. "Bacterial Growth and Cell Division: A Mycobacterial Perspective." *Microbiology and Molecular Biology Reviews* 72 (2008): 126–56.

International Centre for Prison Studies. *World Prison Brief*. London: International Centre for Prison Studies, 2011.

Koch, Erin. "Local Microbiologies of Tuberculosis: Insights from the Republic of Georgia." *Medical Anthropology: Cross-Cultural Studies in Health and Illness* 30 (2011): 81–101.

———. "Beyond Suspicion: Evidence, Uncertainty, and Tuberculosis in Georgian Prisons." *American Ethnologist* 33 (2006): 50–62.

Lampland, Martha, and Susan Leigh Star, editors. *Standards and Their Stories: How Quantifying, Classifying, and Formalizing Practices Shape Everyday Life*. Ithaca, NY: Cornell University Press, 2009.

Landecker, Hannah. *Culturing Life: How Cells Became Technologies*. Cambridge, MA: Harvard University Press, 2007.

Legrand, Judith, Alexandra Sanchez, Francoise Le Pont, Luiz Camacho, and Bernard Larouze. "Modeling the Impact of Tuberculosis Control Strategies in Highly Endemic Overcrowded Prisons" *PLoS One* 3 (2008): e2100. doi:10.1371/journal.pone.0002100 Accessed March 15, 2010.

Lomtadze, N., R. Aspindzelashvili, M. Janjgava. V. Mirtskhulava, A. Wright, H. M. Blumberg, and A. Salakaia. "Prevalence and Risk Factors for Multidrug-Resistant Tuberculosis in the Republic of Georgia: A Population-based Study." *International Journal of Tuberculosis and Lung Disease* 131 (2009): 68–73.

Mdivani, Nino, Ekaterina Zangaladze, Natalia Volkova, Ekaterina Kourbatova, Thea Jibuti, Natalia Shubladze, Tamar Kutateladze, George Khechinashvili, Carlos del Rio, Archil Salakaia, and Henry M. Blumberg. "High Prevalence of

Multidrug-Resistant Tuberculosis in Georgia." *International Journal of Infectious Disease* 12 (2008): 635–44.

Mol, Annemarie. *The Body Multiple: Ontology in Medical Practice*. Durham: Duke University Press, 2002.

Ong, Aihwa. *Neoliberalism as Exception: Mutations in Citizenship and Sovereignty*. Durham, NC: Duke University Press, 2006.

Palomino, J. C. "Current Developments and Future Perspectives for TB Diagnostics." *Future Microbiology* 7 (2012): 59–71.

Petryna, Adriana, and Arthur Kleinman. "The Pharmaceutical Nexus." In *Global Pharmaceuticals: Ethics, Markets, Practices*, edited by A. Petryna, A. Lakoff, and A. Kleinman, 1–32. Durham, NC: Duke University Press, 2006.

Peuch, Jean-Christophe. "Georgia: Official Says TB Epidemics Contained, but Warns Against Too Much Optimism." *Radio Free Europe/Radio Liberty (RFE/RL)* (October 29, 2002). Accessed March 13, 2005. www.rferl.org/features/2002/10/20102002171916.asp.

Porter, John D., Kelley Lee, and Jessica Ogden. "The Globalisation of DOTS: Tuberculosis as a Global Emergency." In *Health Policy in a Globalising World*, edited by Kelley Lee, Kent Buse, and Suzanne Fustukian, 181–94. Cambridge, UK: Cambridge University Press, 2002.

Raviglione, Mercedes C., and A. Pio. "Evolution of WHO Policies for Tuberculosis Control, 1948–2001." *The Lancet* 359 (2002): 755–80.

Rechel, Boika, Colin Kennedy, Martin McKee, and Bernd Rechel. "The Soviet Legacy in Diagnosis and Treatment: Implications for Population Health." *Journal of Public Health Policy* 32 (2011): 293–304.

Reyes, Hernan. "Pitfalls of TB Management in Prisons, Revisited." *International Journal of Prisoner Health* 3 (2007): 43–67.

Saunders, Bernadette M., and Warwick J. Britton. "Life and Death in the Granuloma: Immunopathology of Tuberculosis." *Immunology and Cell Biology* 85 (2007): 103–11.

Stern, Vivien. "The House of the Dead Revisited: Prisons, Tuberculosis and Public Health in the Former Soviet Bloc." In *The Return of the White Plague: Global Poverty and the 'New' Tuberculosis*, edited by Matthew Gandy and Alimuddin Zumla, 178–91. London: Verso Books, 2003.

———, editor. *Sentenced to Die? The Problem of TB in Prisons in Eastern Europe and Central Asia*. London: International Centre for Prison Studies, 1999.

Tekle, B.D., H. Mariam, and A. Ali. "Defaulting from DOTS and its Determinants in Three Districts of Arsi Zone in Ethiopia." *International Journal of Tuberculosis and Lung Disease* 6 (2002.): 573–79.

Thompson, E. P. "Time, Work-Discipline and Industrial Capitalism." *Past and Present* 38 (1967): 56–97.

Timmermans, Stefan, and Mac Berg. *The Gold Standard: The Challenge of Evidence-Based Medicine and Standardization in Health Care*. Philadelphia: Temple University Press, 2003.

Vergne, Isabelle, Jennifer Chua, Sudha B. Singh, and Vojo Deretic. "Cell Biology of Mycobacterium Tuberculosis Phagosome." *Annual Review of Cell and Developmental Biology* 20 (2004): 367–94.

Wendland, Claire L. *A Heart for the Work: Journeys through an African Medical School*. Chicago: The University of Chicago Press, 2010.

World Health Organization. *Global Tuberculosis Control: WHO Report*. Geneva: WHO, 2014. Accessed November 15, 2014.

Zalesky, R., F. Abdullajev, G. Khechinashvili, M. Safarian, T. Madaras, M. Grzemska, E. Englund, S. Dittmann, and M. Raviglione. "Tuberculosis Control in the Caucasus: Successes and Constraints in DOTS Implementation." *International Journal of Tuberculosis and Lung Disease* 3 (1999): 394–401.

Part II
Medicalization and Resistance to Diagnosis

Part II

4 Promotion of Andropause in Brazil

A Case of Male Medicalization

Fabiola Rohden

INTRODUCTION

In recent decades in Brazil, there has been a marked medicalization and pharmacologization of sexuality centered around the development of new technologies, diagnostic categories, and intervention methods, including the creation of public policies. This phenomenon is related to the emergence of a scenario characterized by certain key elements, namely medications, medical societies, the pharmaceutical industry, the media, consumers, and events that range from the prescription of medications in the doctor's office to the running of campaigns and formulation of policies in the Brazilian public health system.

This study approaches the problem of the recent construction of new medical diagnoses and their corresponding potential consumer markets by considering the emergence of androgen deficiency in the aging male (ADAM), or andropause. This is a "disease" that supposedly affects men from the ages of 35 and 40, and would be characterized by the loss of libido or sexual desire, reduced muscle mass, weakness, depression, erectile dysfunction, and other symptoms caused by a decrease in testosterone levels.[1]

This account of the creation of andropause as a new entity in the male health care scene, a process observed more recently in Brazil, prompts a deeper debate on the construction of new diseases. In this regard, an analytical scheme can be proposed for recognizing the context, the process, the most important means, the main characters, and the final outcomes. Of course, I am not affirming the inexistence of andropause nor of the elements perceived by subjects as related to the physical dimension, such as hormonal levels measured in the lab, or the very sensations described by men. Similarly, I do not intend to question the rights of men to better health care. What I have tried to show was the play of various interests associated with the production of andropause as a new category of diagnosis and treatment.

Thus, the context includes a broader process of the medicalization of life based on a tenacious association between health, youth, beauty, and sexual activity. This has translated into a series of bodily attributions and forms of care that have been especially salient during the last few decades. The increasing reach of diagnoses on various life stages and conditions, along with technological developments permitting deeper scrutiny of the body as well as new therapeutic possibilities, have been important factors (Smith-Morris, this volume). For andropause in particular, there are other aspects pertaining more narrowly to a connection between sexuality and aging. Firstly, it is about the successful transformation of erection problems into a specific medical category—erectile dysfunction—, which emerged concomitantly to the "discovery" of new drugs for treating it. A path had already been opened, then, for men to pay more attention to sexuality (understood reductively as erectile function), as well as for various forms of advertising encouraging them to seek the resources available (Rohden 2013). Thus, a new cultural atmosphere and a powerful medico-pharmaceutical infrastructure were already in place for supporting the creation of the andropause diagnosis (Marshal 2007).

Secondly, one also finds the configuration of a new way of representing the body centered on the importance of hormones for defining individual characteristics, especially those related to sexual differentiation and sexuality (Hoberman 2005; Oudshoorn 1994; Rohden 2008). Related to that, there was the successful medicalization of menopause, which, in spite of the associated risks, has been largely described by biomedical and lay discourses as a period of loss that should be stopped or retarded by means of hormone replacement therapies. Finally, there was also the development of a public agenda of greater attention to male health promoted by an articulation of various actors, most prominently the urologists. This agenda has even been translated into new governmental policies. As Carrara et al. (2009) have remarked, this movement was founded on a new view of men's vulnerability, according to which men, far from appearing as rights-claiming subjects, figure as victims of their own nature and carelessness.

Beyond this broader approach, the study of new pathologies demands the consideration of processes of medicalization based on a definition of diseases as ontologically real and specific entities. Inasmuch as diseases become social entities with which we come to interact in increasingly quotidian forms, it is not surprising that the dimension of diagnosis and its capacity to spark heated political tensions have become important. This becomes evident, for instance, when different social groups—from doctors to governmental agencies to activists—entertain lengthy disputes on the appropriateness of a certain diagnosis. Moreover, the operationalization of the diagnosis becomes a fundamental piece of the entire process of therapeutic care, from the organization of health care systems and drug use to the bureaucracy that is formed in its the wake (Rosenberg 2002; Myers, this volume).

The term "medicalization" has been used by authors such as P. Conrad (1992, 2007) to define the process whereby problems previously defined as non-medical come to be conceived and treated as medical problems and characterized as diseases or disorders. This phenomenon increasingly encompasses behaviors regarded as deviant, as well as vital processes or life conditions such as birth, aging, death, sexuality, and so forth. An important claim I make, however, is that doctors are not always the central or most powerful agents in this play of interests. Many times, patients themselves take active part in the search for the institutionalized medicalization of a certain condition, thus adding even more complexity to this sociocultural process.

Pharmaceutical labs have played a major role in this process by influencing research agendas, medical training, and doctors' prescription practices. In many cases, for instance, the investment in advertising is greater than that in research, and new drugs are a recombination of previously known substances (Angell 2007; Fishman 2004; Moynihan 2010; Tiefer 2006b). Some authors have even regarded the promotion and commercialization of new diseases as cases of disease mongering: that is, the execution of a set of sequential strategies to be deployed in order to convince people who are not necessarily "sick" that they have health problems that are treatable by the medical-pharmaceutical apparatus. Among such strategies there is the definition of a large share of the population as diseased, its association with problems linked to a generic idea of hormone imbalance, the selective use of statistics and symptoms with little evidential power, the valorization of technology, and the promotion of skilled expert doctors especially trained for communicating with the press (Payer 1991).[2]

With respect to the particular association between aging and sexuality, it should be noted that the promotion of new drugs and resources goes side-by-side with an encouragement of behavioral models that value the young, healthy, and sexually active body. In the case of men, students on the medicalization of so-called male menopause, such as B. Marshall (2007, 2010), have suggested that we are witnessing the creation of new narratives that associate aging men with a feminine model. This model suggests a body that is more vulnerable and subject to medical intervention as well as to a continuous process of "virility watch." Marshall, a major reference on the issue, proposes that the main task for the critical studies of science, health, and aging would be to investigate the stories on sexuality and aging told by what she calls the "pharmaceutical imagination." It is about acknowledging how, in the promotion of new diagnoses and treatments, narratives that activate values and representations sensitive to particular cultural contexts are also produced. In this case, the "pharmaceutical imagination" has been successful in redefining the course of sexual life in terms of the effects of drugs used in the treatment of sexual function (Marshall 2010).

The foundation for such a transformation would be a change in the standard used for thinking about the body and its functions. The normal-abnormal binary was replaced by a new one, the functional-dysfunctional. As an example, Marshall remarks that the decline in erectile function or testosterone levels during a man's lifetime was considered "normal" for a long time. But these have come to be regarded as "dysfunctional," as something to be "demonstrated" by the existence of treatments capable of improving function. Thus, the "functional" comes to be defined by what is treatable.[3] The most evident instance of this is the role Viagra has played in the creation of the very category of erectile dysfunction, and, more recently, how testosterone replacement became the marker for redefining andropause (Marshall 2010).

Based on this framing, and on the acknowledgement of the new movement of medicalization of male aging and its increasing association with the valorization of sexuality, in what follows, this study will map out the emergence of andropause or ADAM[4] in biomedical publications and its subsequent public popularization in the media, including its absorption by government initiatives, calling attention to the evident growth in investment in this sector by pharmaceutical labs.

Because the goal of this study is to analyze the creation of the phenomenon called andropause—which involves a spectrum that ranges from cutting-edge research to urologic exams in public to the interest of pharmaceutical labs, attention from the media, and the crafting of public policies—the methodological strategy is multiple. This socio-anthropological study articulates different qualitative research techniques, such as participant observation, interviews, and documental research. Articles in scientific journals have also been analyzed, as have the websites of medical societies, news reports, television programs, and publicity material, as well as the ethnography of medical conferences and campaigns, and interviews with professionals in the related areas. A broad range of sources is essential to capture the full extent of the processes studied and the intricacy of the sociotechnical networks set into play. It is necessary for showing the contrast between the discourses produced in science and in the popularization strategies aimed at increasing the consumption of new representations and products.

ANDROPAUSE IN BIOMEDICAL RESEARCH AND LITERATURE

According to B. Marshall (2007), the so-called male climacteric began to emerge as an organic and treatable disease in the 1930s. But it was not until the 40s that scientific treatment was proposed, with the definition of climacteric hypogonadism as a clinical disorder caused by the decline in testosterone that affected a relatively small share of older males. Sexual dysfunction already appeared as the main symptom, but not as a focus of treatment; after all, at that time, to promote sexuality in older men was considered problematic or even immoral. Testosterone therapy was thus used along with repeated and firm admonitions that sexual benefits were not a priority. It is only from the 60s onwards that the passive acceptance of changes in sexual capacity caused by aging began to be questioned, and sexuality itself became central in the reconsideration of andropause. That, however, would have to wait until the 90s to take off in biomedical research, in association with the discoveries associated with the treatment of erectile dysfunction.

In general, this scenario is manifested in the scientific literature on this topic. References were searched using keywords such as andropause, male climacteric, ADAM, late male hypogonadism, and others in the database of the Virtual Health Library,[5] which aggregates data from MEDLINE (International Literature in the Health Sciences) and LILACS (Latin American and Caribbean Health Sciences). It was found that, even though there have been some references to male climacteric or andropause from the beginning of the MEDLINE catalogue (1966), it is only at the turn of the century that this occurs in a more significant number of papers. If, during the 70s, 80s, and 90s, there was a more or less stable amount of papers—respectively, 56, 39, and 50 pieces—, between January 2001 and September 2009, there were 321 publications. Most of these were published in urology and endocrinology medical journals, and bring information broad discussions on concepts or even on the very existence of andropause, or ADAM, to considerations about its possible symptoms, treatments, hormone replacement therapies, associations with other conditions, comparisons with menopause, and an emphasis on the problems related to sexuality, such as erectile dysfunction and loss of desire.

Such an excessive increase in the number of papers relates to the international release of a tool for identifying and measuring ADAM is not simply due to chance. The Aging Males' Symptoms (AMS) scale was originally developed in Germany in 1999, and was based on the assumption that, just as women do during menopause, men would also develop similar symptoms (Heinemann et al. 2003). According to the authors, Heinemann et al. (2003), the scale could be used to identify symptoms of aging among groups of men with different conditions, assess the severity of symptoms in time, and measure changes pre- and post-androgen replacement therapy. It was developed based on the analysis of over 200 variables measured in more than one hundred men who were "medically well characterized." After statistical analyses, three dimensions of symptoms were identified: psychological, somatic-vegetative, and sexual, which would account for 51.6 percent of the total variance.

This allowed for a decrease in the number of items on the scale to 17. This new version was immediately applied to a sample of 992 German men in order to establish reference scores for the severity of symptoms in men older than 40. The scale was then translated into English, and the article published by the authors in 2003 contained versions of the AMS in twelve languages (Heinemann et al. 2003). It encouraged those interested in making use of the instrument to go ahead and do it without the need for formal permission. In their conclusion, the authors reasserted that the scale was an important instrument, as it was already being used across the world (Heinemann et al. 2003). Moreover, they declared that the study involved no conflict of interest.[6]

The AMS Questionnaire asked respondents to inform the presence of the following symptoms: (1) Decline in your feeling of general well-being (general state of health, subjective feeling); (2) Joint pain and muscular ache (lower back pain, joint pain, pain in a limb, general back ache); (3) Excessive sweating (unexpected/sudden episodes of sweating, hot flushes independent of strain); (4) Sleep problems (difficulty in falling asleep, difficulty in sleeping through, waking up early and feeling tired, poor sleep, sleeplessness); (5) Increased need for sleep, often feeling tired; (6) Irritability (feeling aggressive, easily upset about little things, moody); (7) Nervousness (inner tension, restlessness, feeling fidgety); (8) Anxiety (feeling panicky); (9) Physical exhaustion/lacking vitality (general decrease in performance, reduced activity, lacking interest in leisure activities, feeling of getting less done, of achieving less, of having to force oneself to undertake activities); (10) Decrease in muscular strength (feeling of weakness); (11) Depressive mood (feeling down, sad, on the verge of tears, lack of drive, mood swings, feeling nothing is of any use); (12) Feeling that you have passed your peak; (13) Feeling burnt out, having hit rock-bottom; (14) Decrease in beard growth; (15) Decrease in ability/frequency to perform sexually; (16) Decrease in the number of morning erections; (17) Decrease in sexual desire/libido (lacking pleasure in sex, lacking desire for sexual intercourse) (Heinemann et al. 2003).

The AMS scale allowed for the production of the first data for the new diagnosis, as well as for the diffusion of the condition. This became a fundamental instrument in research protocols and academic debates, in the production of figures to be insistently repeated as reference standards, in its own diffusion as an explanatory tool for the new "disease" or "dysfunction," and, at the level of self-diagnosis, in mediating between the potential patient and the search for medical care and treatment. For the physicians, the scale facilitated and made viable a diagnosis that was new and little known, allowing for and encouraging the prescription of a particular kind of treatment.

Another important aspect of this process is the association between andropause and hypogonadism or androgenic deficiency, a biochemical state. The redefinition of a complex of ill-defined symptoms with accurate diagnoses has also occurred with other health problems (Warren and Manderson, this volume; Smith-Morris, this volume). It is possible to suggest that the promotion of a new name—androgen deficiency in the aging male—would be related to such purposeful association with hypogonadism. But if, early on, androgen deficiency was only part of the focus on a broader symptomatic picture, the urologists' effort today is towards narrowing the scope on testosterone. This trend—the association between andropause and hypogonadism—has manifested in international journals; for instance, a 2006 editorial of *European Urology* supports the term "testosterone deficiency syndrome" by arguing that "[t]estosterone is clearly understood by the medical community and by the public at large as the chief male hormone" (Morales et al. 2006: 408–409). Moreover, this term would not carry the negative and erroneous perception that the problem would be limited to older men, which is currently suggested by the terms andropause, male climacteric or menopause, or even androgen deficiency in the aging male.

As highlighted by Marshall (2007), the use of testosterone was approved in the United States only for the treatment of hypogonadism, and not for andropause itself. It thus became necessary to construct a specific relationship between hypogonadism and andropause in order to justify the use of these drugs by a new group of people. Between 1997 and 2002, prescriptions of testosterone, especially by means of new transdermic products, increased by 400 percent, and were provided mostly to men between the ages of 45 and 55. Marshall (2007) affirms the success of this strategy and how, more than the medicalization of andropause, it achieved the medicalization of middle-aged men themselves.

ANDROPAUSE AS A MEDIA PHENOMENON

With respect to the reverberation of such themes in the media or even the creation of andropause as a culturally significant category, *Veja* issues published between 1990 and 2009 carried out a survey of andropause and similar topics. This magazine was chosen due to its position as the best-selling weekly periodical in Brazil; the total number of readers is estimated at 10 million. One could start with the news report by Glenda Mezarobba published in the *Veja* magazine on May 28, 1997. Poignantly entitled "The male autumn: a growing number of men seek the vigor of youth in hormone replacement therapy," it showed how andropause has led more and more men to seek urologists, endocrinologists, or specialists in orthomolecular medicine, especially in the United States, where 200,000 men were already users of hormone replacement. The male version of menopause, characterized by a decline in hormone production, would affect 30 percent of US males between the ages of 50 and 60 (Mezarobba 1997: 90). It would be thus necessary—this was the message to the reader—to recognize the symptoms and to perform a testosterone dosage exam. In Mezarobba's story, this hormone is presented as fountain of youth of sorts, which, besides encouraging the development of male sexual traits, would command libido. The piece's tone manifests some doubts in the different stances taken by the experts interviewed, but only with respect to the need for hormone replacement. There is even a box highlighting replacement therapy's benefits (reduction of irritability, anti-aging, increased resistance against infections, increased muscle mass, and improved sexual performance) and risks (anxiety, sleeping problems, increased body hair, liver and prostate cancer, testicular atrophy).

With regards to the creation of this diagnosis, the prevailing idea is that it is a problematic condition to be investigated and treated. In the words of urologist Cristiano Santana, a researcher at the State University of Campinas, "even though the arrest in hormonal production is never complete, the male climacteric does exist, and many are its symptoms" (Mezarobba

1997: 90). The final part is dedicated to testimonials from men who felt they benefited from replacement therapy, and to a description of the available treatments—pills, injections, and transdermal patches. The latter were presented as the most effective, albeit more costly. There is also reference to the fact that Dr. Santana had been prescribing patches imported from the United States and England for the previous eight months. The story ends by noting that men would be "experiencing a bit of the dilemmas facing women with regards to how to control menopause," and that replacement therapy would have to be maintained for the rest of one's life (Mezarobba 1997: 92).

If this "pioneer" 1997 news report left some room for doubt, the cover story by Gabriela Carelli published on February 13, 2002 had a different focus. This time, the title was "The ages of sex: the post-Viagra era promises new treatments in order to retard the biological clock of both men and women and improve sexual performance." For men, it highlighted that, with the solution to penis irrigation provided by Viagra and similar drugs, expert attention had turned to issues that indirectly affected male sexual performance. The new revolution in sexual health was presented as having two pillars: re-establishing hormone normality, and stimulating sexual disposition. The "hormonal domain" would thus be a promising one for maintaining libido for longer—an indispensable follow up because the decline in bodily hormones could begin as early as 35 years of age. The box entitled "Men's weapons" affirmed that hormone replacement had been the established method for fighting testosterone reduction since 1999, and that some doctors were prescribing treatment to men showing testosterone reduction from the age of 45. The piece is filled with assurances such as this: "The most positive action in medicine during the 90s was to replace hormones in the hope of restoring health and avoiding diseases associated with the loss of such substances—including almost all sexual dysfunctions such as impotence or lack of sexual desire" (Careli 2002: 75). There is also the reproduction of a 30-question test to evaluate the readers' so-called sexual age, authored by Boston University urologist Irwin Goldstein, one of the champions of the diagnosis and treatment of sexual dysfunctions.

The following year, the magazine brought a subtle half-column, uncredited note published on July 23 entitled "Pure invention: andropause would be just an excuse for laziness." It asserted that the "theory" that the male sex would also have its menopause was losing ground, and that an increasing number of experts would be affirming that "andropause simply does not exist." It referred to declarations by the researcher at the New England Research Institute in the U.S., Professor John McKinlay, made at the annual meeting of the British Fertility Society. He claimed that the symptoms observed in men in their fifties would have nothing to do with declines in hormone production; rather, they would stem from a lazy and careless lifestyle. This researcher was also quoted as saying that andropause would be "an invention of the pharmaceutical industry in order to sell more drugs" (Pura Invenção 2003).

In spite of such occasional sparks of doubt, the supplement "*Veja* Special—Man" published in October that same year would resume the previous direction. This was dedicated to charting the condition of contemporary men and providing a sort of guide to them on various fronts, including behavior, health, and sexuality. One of the full-page explanatory boxes discussed the subject "Penis + Prostate," and presented the characteristics and problems of males between the ages of 20 and 70. In reading it, one finds out that the thirties are the "apex of sexual potency;" at the age of 30, the erection angle (shown in a graphic illustration) is at twenty degrees. When one turns 40, this angle is drastically reduced to five degrees, and may reach less than one degree at the age of fifty, and minus twenty-five degrees at seventy. The forties thus appeared as a key moment, as explained in the box "What happens throughout the years." According to the information provided, this would be the phase where andropause beings, and, since then, there would be a 1 percent annual decline testosterone production; "only" 20 percent of males, however, would need hormonal replacement therapy (*Veja Especial Homem* October, 2003: 75). In spite of what is suggested by the text, I point out that 20 percent of males over 40 represents a significant contingent of people who would be obliged to seek exams and treatments for a lifelong condition that is occasionally called into question.

Since 2005, in the analyzed magazine, there has been a consolidation of social representations around andropause and its connection with issues related to sexuality. This is due to the deployment of expert arguments, the diffusion of quantitative studies, and the triumphant tone in the marketing of new drugs. It should be remarked that the search for alternative treatments like psychotherapy has lost ground to the proposition of new drugs or the rediscovery or old ones, like antidepressants for treating sexual problems like difficulty achieving an erection, premature ejaculation, and lack of desire. This may be again illustrated by a *Veja* cover story from January 19, 2005. In the cover picture's background, there is a thermometer in between a woman's breasts, along with the headline, "Sexual health: science shows that physical and psychological well-being depends much more on sexuality than one would have thought" and the announcement of a "Test: find out your 'sexual IQ'." The long story, written by Anna Paula Buchalla, began by recalling the saying, "sex: when it is good it's great, and when it is bad, it's still very good." It then presented the sexual quotient test for evaluating one's "quality of sex life," created by the psychiatrist Carmita Abdo,[7] coordinator of Prosex (sexuality project of the São Paulo State University Hospital). This test resulted from interviews with 630 men and 580 women between the ages of 18 and 70 that indicated ten basic criteria to discern between "satisfactory sex" and "disappointing sex." According to Carmita Abdo, it would help couples to identify problems and solutions for improving their sex life. Further on, this researcher affirmed "[the] objective is to apply it [the test] in all medical appointments, in order to inform the doctor about possible problems with their patients, both physical and emotional" (Buchalla 2005: 75). After the importance of the test was ascertained, the text presented an argument seconded by the World Health Organization that included sex as a parameter for defining quality of life. It claimed that "safe, frequent and pleasant sex, doctors affirm, may protect the heart, avoid insomnia, alleviate stress, strengthen the immune system, fight anxiety, regulate humor, help lose weight, and even retard aging" (Buchalla 2005: 75). Virtually all problems related to the health and quality of life of modern individuals are listed in this sentence, thus indicating the unavoidable need to seek "improvement" in one's sex life.

Next, more data was introduced without referencing sources, neither date nor research methodology: for instance, the statement was made that "eight in ten Brazilians (men and women) [who are] victims of sexual problems declared that their anxieties affect work, relationship with their children, social relations, and leisure," besides, of course, the relationship with the partner, without crediting the source of the information (Buchalla 2005: 75). It also made reference to a study presented simply as "carried out by FIOCRUZ at Bahia" with 77,000 men from 24 Brazilian states with an average age of 52, which found that 66 percent of Brazilians presented, to a greater or lesser degree, with erection difficulties. Moreover, "the higher the age range, the greater the prevalence and severity of the dysfunction" (Buchalla 2005: 76). On the following page, the data that men would suffer a decline in testosterone production (now referred to as the "hormone of libido") since 40, 20 percent of which is beyond normal levels, reappeared. Without presenting or discussing the issue of hormone replacement therapy, the text further cited a new testosterone-based drug called the Nebido that has been recently released by the German lab Schering AG (Buchalla 2005: 77–78).

This quote was followed by large, two-page box entitled "Chemical aid: drugs that promise to fight male and female sexual dysfunctions." For men, besides drugs for erectile dysfunction and premature ejaculation, there were testosterone patches, injections, and pills ("the trigger of sexual desire") already available for consumption. These were in addition to those scheduled to be released during the second semester of 2005, which included the well-presented Nebido. The source was attributed to Sidney Glina, the then-president of the Brazilian Society of Urology (SBU), and Luiz Otávio Torres, president of the Latin American Society for the Study of Impotence and Sexuality (Buchalla 2005: 73–74). Finally, two pieces of information were also insisted upon. One stated that "[t]hanks to the anti-impotence oral drugs, during the last five years the number of Brazilians who seek help for their sexual problems has increased fourfold" (Buchalla 2005: 77). The box bearing the suggestive title "More freedom" affirmed that in the year 2000, only 10 percent of Brazilians with erectile dysfunction sought treatment, and that in 2005, this share had increased to 40 percent. The second piece of relevant information is that these men's companions would have been key to the search for medical help, by encouraging their partners to get treatment in 56 percent of cases (Buchalla 2005: 78).

The following year, when the Brazilian Society of Urology formulated a consensus with respect to testosterone replacement therapy for ADAM, the tone in the media indicated that the category of andropause and the notion of efficacy associated with testosterone replacement had been consolidated. The same journalist, Ana Paula Buchalla, authored another lengthy report entitled "The hormone of youth: doctors lose the fear of prescribing testosterone replacement therapy for middle-aged men with accentuated loss in physical vigor" (Buchalla 2006: 116). The story opened with a two-page graph showing the variation in testosterone levels during the life of a man, indicating as sources the *Male Aging Study* and the New England Research Institutes in the U.S. This time, we were informed that the apex of testosterone production takes place at twenty, and that at thirty the "virility hormone" begins to decrease on average 1 percent each year. At 40, 20 percent of men would present symptoms caused by hormonal decline such as fatigue, irritability, and loss of libido. From sixty onwards, 30 percent of males and from seventy onwards, 50 percent of them, would suffer declines in testosterone (Buchalla 2006: 116–117). It is worth noting that hormone reduction and its supposed effects were attributed to increasingly lower ages. If previously the yearly rate of 1 percent reduction began at 40, it now receded to thirty.

The story informed the reader that andropause would affect 20 percent of males who were suffering from irritability, sleeping problems, pain, physical fatigue, general discouragement, loss of sexual desire, and lower potency. It explained that such symptoms "were found by a study funded by the Schering lab in Brazil [and] coordinated by the psychiatrist Carmita Abdo from the Sexuality Project (Prosex) at the São Paulo State University Hospital," and went on to add that "[a]s one can see, man is indeed his testosterone" (Buchalla 2006: 117). The text affirmed that, if not too long ago there was no consensus on hormonal replacement, in the past five years, more than a hundred scientific studies validated it. Moreover, no research would have been able to "prove with rigor" the association between testosterone replacement and prostate cancer and, little by little, science would have also began to "debunk another myth," that replacement could also be a risk factor for cardiovascular diseases. Among the experts consulted, there is again Carmita Abdo, declaring that "[e]verything indicates that the extra hormone allows for a longer and better life" (Buchalla 2006: 118).

Testosterone is then turned from risk factor into a protection factor against disease, as well as a fundamental addition to those seeking longevity and an active sex life. The story goes on to affirm that "testosterone is so much in evidence that, only last year, around sixty studies were published about replacement treatments" (Buchalla 2006: 119), and that the most striking of them had shown that men with testosterone deficiency presented

a higher death risk, and that 88 percent had a higher risk of developing serious chronic illnesses. A statement from the urologist Sidney Glina, from the
Institute H. Ellis in São Paulo, followed: "On the face of such evidence, we,
the doctors, lost the fear of prescribing testosterone" (Buchalla 2006: 119).

The construction of testosterone replacement as "fact and evidence" is
also achieved by the use of figures regarding consumption, to make evident
the creation of a new, profitable market. The magazine stated that, according to the IMS Health Consultancy, American pharmacies received 2.4 million prescriptions in 2005—that is, twice as much as in the two previous
years. It also cited, without referencing, an article in *The New England
Journal of Medicine*, which found a 500 percent increase in sales of testosterone supplements since 1993. It then concluded, "According to projec-
tions by the pharmaceutical industry, within five years this will be a billion
dollar market" (Buchalla 2006: 119). This is an explicit indication of the
interest of pharmaceutical labs in the medicalization of andropause.

Another piece of "evidence" deployed by the story was that, in developed
countries, the testosterone exam would already be a routine procedure,
something that confirmed the need for promoting it in Brazil. The text ends
by proposing that the "absorption of testosterone" may encourage men to
take better care of their own health, because less than 60 percent of males
over 40 see a doctor regularly, and when they do so, they are taken by their
partners. This reinforces the idea—which was to become more recurrent in
the following years—of men's concern about sexuality and their growing
interest in using testosterone, as well as their more consistent participation
in the universe of care and consumption of exams and health treatments.
Once again, women figure here as strategic allies.

The report included statements illustrated by photos of two businessmen, ages 44 and 68, who attested to the benefits of hormone replacement
therapy. Besides that, there were two boxes. One of them cited indications,
warnings, and contraindications to the use of synthetic testosterone, and
explained how it should be administered. It referred to transdermal patches
(30 percent of patients reported local irritation), pills (which have to be
swallowed twice a day and bring the risk of sharp metabolic alterations),
hypodermic implants (contraindicated for senior patients due to the risk
of infection), and gels (no problems reported). At the top of the list are
the intramuscular injections, presented as the most widely used method for
replacing hormones. If the old injections had the inconvenience of requiring
on average twenty-two annual applications, "a new testosterone injection
has been recently released in Brazil, the Nebido, which requires only four
shots a year. Another advantage is that it avoids drastic changes in hormone
rates" (Buchalla 2006: 120). Besides the fact that Nebido was mentioned
only for its advantages, it should be noted that it was the only drug whose
commercial name was made explicit.[8]

Another box entitled "How are your hormones?" included a test. The
source was not cited, but it is a reproduction of the well-known AMS scale.

The questionnaire was presented as an instrument to measure the degree of male aging since the forties, based on an analysis of the symptoms that reflect a decline in testosterone production. The difference here was that, besides the test's traditional seventeen questions, there was an evaluation of the scores. Those who scored between 17 and 26 points learned that they belonged to the "category of men who have not yet felt the effects of low testosterone production." Those who scored between 27 and 36 points found out that "the first symptoms of testosterone reduction are starting to appear," and that they should "pay attention to the signs sent by your body." A score between 37 and 49 indicated that symptoms "are still moderate, but it should not prevent someone from seeking guidance from an expert" to indicate the need for hormone replacement or not. Finally, for those who scored 50 or more, "quality of life is severely compromised by the low production of testosterone." Moreover, "the test's result suggests that you should seek a doctor in order to assess what would be the best hormonal replacement therapy in your case" (Buchalla 2006: 119). First, it should be remarked that almost anyone would check at least "little" or "moderate" for topics as generic as "lower sensation of general well-being," "sleeping problems," "tiredness," or "irritability." One only needed to check the option "none" seven times and the option "little" ten times to fall in the category of those who are feeling the early symptoms. Thus, men could very easily reach the subsequent categories and find out that they were suffering from andropause and should seek guidance and treatment. Also, for those who scored over 50, which can be achieved just by checking "moderate" in all criteria, the indication of replacement was decisive; the doctor would only have to decide the best therapy in each case.

In the following year, this questionnaire was reproduced in widely read magazines such as *Época*, where it appeared on November 26, 2007.[9] This was in fact a publicity ad by Schering, which printed the lab logo on the top left-hand side of the page. To the right, there was the picture of a man no older than 50, and at the center, the acronym ADAM, followed by call: "Men over 40: if the lack of disposition and sexual desire is already part of your life, this will interest you." Below, there was an explanation:

> ADAM means androgen deficiency in the aging male (also known and andropause), and is directly related to a decline in testosterone after 40. Symptoms include the loss of libido (sexual desire), reduction of muscle mass, loss of energy, depression, erectile dysfunction, and there may also be a risk of cardiovascular disease. If you are over 40 and wish to find out if you have symptoms associated with ADAM, fill in the scale below and take it to a doctor (*Época*, Mars 26, 2007: 11)

This time, the source was quoted as being the AMS scale. The scale was presented as an important tool to help doctors evaluate the health and quality of life of mature males, besides being used worldwide and standardized according to psychometric norms. Finally, there was a reference to two websites, and to Schering's customer service phone number.

It is important to highlight here the role of the media. More than conveying information or translating the intricate and complex discoveries of science to the public at large, what it does is it effectively participates in the construction of new social realities. It is on the pages of magazines and newspapers or on TV shows that figures gain colors and images that allow for self-framing by the public. Here, one sees pictures or statements by "common" characters who recount their suffering and moments of redemption and success following the treatments; this may suggest an identification and approximation by the public with such trajectories. It is also in these spaces that the validity of such propositions, be they diagnoses or treatments, is tested via the scientific and medical authority.

In this respect, a commentary should be made on the very idea of the creation of interests. Various news stories, brochures, and interviews raised the idea that andropause had become a topic of great interest without, of course, acknowledging their own function as promoters of this process. This circular discourse helps to cement the idea that there would be a concomitantly constructed demand for knowledge and treatment of the problem.

ANDROPAUSE: POPULARIZATION ON TV

The pieces of the picture described above were woven together even tighter at another occasion for diffusing andropause, or ADAM, that was broadcasted on August 28, 2007, during the TV show *Saúde Brasil* (Brazil Health). This was a thirty-minute episode about ADAM produced by the Brazil Health Project, and was broadcasted on public channels like TVE Brasil and TV Cultura.[10] Presented by journalist Lina Menezes, who shared the shows' direction with Gilney Rodrigues, the story was structured around the definition of the problem, its symptoms and risks, as well as possible solutions—all supported by statements from experts and interviews with "common folks." The presenter began by announcing that it was a topic of growing interest: the relationship of testosterone to the health of men over 40, what happens to the male body, and the care that men should take in order to maintain their health and quality of life. A comparison with menopause was introduced by explanations from the endocrinologist Ruth Clapauch and the urologist Geraldo Eduardo Faria. The latter affirmed that, in men, the hormone decline is slow and gradual, so the symptoms are not identified as clearly as in women. Moreover, he added, "Today we know that it is very important that, in the event of reduction in [the] male hormone, men need to be treated in order to restore their quality of life."

Next, there is the participation of Sidney Glina, who declared that "some men will suffer significant decline from the age of fifty, the estimate is between 10 and 15 percent of them. So, this is a disease which today has a name—some people call it andropause, but I don't like this name—, we call it androgenic aging deficiency." According to Ruth Caplauch, it is estimated that 20 percent of men between the ages of 60 and 69 have andropause, and this percentage would increase significantly with age. Between 70 and 79 years of age, this number would be 30 percent, and above 80 years, 50 percent. According to Glina, ADAM, or andropause, "is a disease, and it has to be treated. Those who have similar symptoms should seek a doctor in order to be appropriately treated, because testosterone is an important hormone." As an "extremely important hormone" produced by men, it is responsible for various bodily functions such as sexual differentiation, sexual desire, erection, conservation of muscle mass, and memory. This thesis was further reinforced by psychiatrist Carmita Abdo, who affirmed, "Testosterone is a sexual hormone par excellence;" it is what "triggers sexual desire," and when it is lacking, "desire will of course suffer." She also added that "the loss or reduction of libido, so much in focus today, is due to declines in blood levels of testosterone both in men and in women." Besides jeopardizing "erectile competence," low levels of testosterone could harm reproductive capacity. The show's narrator informed viewers that men's difficulties in their sex lives that are related to ADAM "damage conjugal relations," and that "the couple has no idea that the reason is an illness which can and should be treated."

Lina Menezes then opened a discussion on how testosterone decline could affect various organs or bodily functions. This was illustrated by a comment made by Geraldo Eduardo Faria: "when you look at the individual man who has hormonal deficiency, it is that figure of the individual with a very thin arm, the muscle is already atrophied." According to this doctor, in this condition, men lose the capacity to transform the protein they ingest into muscle mass. Ruth Caplauch went on to say that testosterone "acts also at the level of the nervous system, promoting a more appropriate mood. Finally, it acts on the prostate, bones, skin, red blood cells. I would say that it acts in the entire body." The presenter then added that testosterone has a direct impact on the brain, something which was further confirmed by Faria when he declared that, as a result of lower testosterone levels, the individual's capacity for concentration and intellectual activity is reduced, it becomes harder to understand and learn, and he feels drowsy more often—typical manifestations of impaired brain activity. She also talked about the "various negative impacts affecting quality of life" as well as depression, tiredness, drowsiness, apathy, irritability, abdominal fat, increase of cardiovascular risk and osteoporosis, as well as its association with diabetes and metabolic syndrome.

The show proceeded to tackle the difficulties involved in recognizing the symptoms. It conveyed the image of a silent threat, which called for the need to seek an expert able to recognize the symptoms and provide appropriate treatment. Both Glina and Faria remarked on the importance of considering individuals on a case-by-case basis. But this was soon replaced by an emphasis on testosterone measurement exams and lab scenes. There was then an account of available treatments, mediated by a quick statement from Caplauch on the balancing of risks and benefits. Geraldo Eduardo Faria explained that in Brazil, the vast majority of treatments involved testosterone injections applied every twelve or fifteen days, but that "more recently, a new product arrived at the Brazilian market with testosterone injections of prolonged action. It is much more practical because the individual will receive a shot every three months." They then discussed the use of gel and oral pills, but both were associated with absorption problems.

Towards the end of the show, the importance of testosterone for the couple as well as the women's role in aiding diagnosis and treatment were reinforced. According to Faria, women are instrumental in helping identify the problem when their partners begin to show clinical evidence that may suggest andropause: "[it is] important that the partner, the wife, encourages her partner to seek a doctor in order to check if it is indeed andropause, so he may benefit from treatment." It also approached the topic of possible prejudice against treatment. There was the testimony of a 73-year-old man, who said, "[N]o doubt, I have no prejudice against it, much to the contrary; I think everything that can increase your performance in life, be it physical, intellectual or sentimental, because these things are all related aren't they? I think it is worth doing it." This opinion was supported by psychiatrist Carmita Abdo, who declared, "[T]here should be no prejudice against the so-called andropause, the androgen deficiency in the aging male, because there is a cure, there is a remedy." She further added that "andropause, or androgen deficiency in the aging male, as it should be called, has a solution, and it is up to men to go and search for it." The duties that should characterize the contemporary man, informing oneself and taking care of one's health, were thus introduced. This point was synthesized by the narrator, who affirmed, "Taking care of one's health is a commitment by each of us; especially today, when the rise in life expectancy is a reality." Finally, after the recommendation of some resources—above all, the Brazilian Society of Urology —the presenter concluded:

> Well, if you are a man over 40, watch out for the symptoms. They may indicate androgen deficiency in the aging male, also known as andropause. And as we have seen, deficiency of testosterone, the chief male hormone, which may occur at this stage can be treated with replacement therapy. That can help men restore their quality of life and live longer and happier (*Saúde Brasil*, August 28, 2007).

It is possible to conclude that the show fulfilled its objective of informing viewers about ADAM or andropause, a problem that had been the object of "growing interest;" moreover, it remarked on the need to see a doctor and be evaluated on an individual basis. What is most salient, however, is the certainty with which ADAM is presented as a "disease" or "illness" that "has a cure," the widely broadcasted hormone replacement therapy via the recently released long-duration testosterone injections. It is also worth noticing with respect to the shots used that, besides the experts and passers-by interviewed, on twelve occasions, there were scenes shown of doctors or doctors writing prescriptions, often zoomed in on their pen-holding hands, or on the prescription itself. Certainly, these images reflect the show's more general framing, which seems to be focused on medicalization.

I would like to point out that the SBU appeared quite saliently in the acknowledgements at the end of the show; this is another indication of the consolidation of this body as the main legitimate source of information on andropause. On the Society's website, this topic already appeared quite frequently. Beginning in 2008, the main image at the top center of the home page was the logo "ADAM"—the exact same logo appearing in the ads and on the scale dispersed by Bayer Schering Pharma AG.

If the long news reports in magazines such as *Veja* and *Isto é* broadcasted andropause to a public with "superior" financial and educational capital, which is reflected in the kind of written and graphic language used, and in the images of businessmen undergoing replacement therapy, there is a progressive inclusion of that topic in new scenarios and with new framings.[11] The TV show described above has this characteristic, in relation to both the participation of people from the lower classes and the repetitive and simple language used. This is in tandem with the strategies pursued by the SBU during the last few years to encourage attention to male health.

MEDICAL CONFERENCES, PUBLIC CAMPAIGNS, AND GOVERNMENT INITIATIVES

From 2007 on, it is possible to find data that indicate a constant presence of the issue of andropause in medical conferences held in Brazil. Urologists especially emphasize the importance of andropause diagnosis and promote the organization of public awareness campaigns. At the same time, they have pressured the Brazilian government to include the topic in its health policy.

At medical conferences, the subject was highlighted, not just in the talks, but also in the publicity materials prepared by the drug companies. A publicity ad by Schering about ADAM with the AMS scale was distributed in conferences on sexuality and urology that year, such as the 11th Brazilian Conference on Human Sexuality, held in October 2007 in Recife. In the stands set up by Schering, there was ample distribution of tablets with reproductions of the scale. There were even conferences specifically dedicated to this topic, such as "Sexuality and ADAM," which was organized by the Brazilian Association for the Study of Sexual Inadequacies on July 6, 2007, in Campinas.

But it was at the 31st Brazilian Conference of Urology, which took place during Sidney Glina's SBU presidency, that the theme was approached with even greater enthusiasm. This event took place between September 27 and October 1, 2007, in Salvador, and assembled over 5,500 participants. There, Bayer Schering Pharma AG (a lab created after the acquisition of Schering by Bayer) announced a specific field of male health centered on the promotion of Nebido for the treatment of ADAM and of Levitra, for treating erectile dysfunction. In the press conference held during this launch, new data produced by the research effort coordinated by Carmita Abdo and funded by Bayer Schering Pharma AG was presented. This was the Aging Population Study, undertaken with 10,161 participants in 18 Brazilian capitals between February and June 2006.[12]

The article, which presented early research results for men, explained that the investigation used self-administered questionnaires filled by voluntary subjects aged 40 or older, who were passers-by on streets and beaches and in squares, parks, and shopping malls. It included questions regarding general and sexual health, life habits, and AMS scale questions. According to the results, the parameters obtained indicated that 13.3 percent of the subjects presented "symptoms suggesting ADAM" (Abdo and Afif-Abdo 2007: 381). Moreover, the article repeated a few times that men "with moderate to serious AMS presented twice as much erectile dysfunction (in general) and three times as much complete erectile dysfunction than those with lower AMS scores" (Abdo and Afif-Abdo 2007: 382), thus reinforcing the connection between ADAM and sexual dysfunctions. Another piece of information insisted upon was that "the vast majority of these men did not take testosterone measurements during the past twelve months, and, of those who did, a significant share (about 9.0 percent of all males) presented low levels of the hormone, if the proportion of 1.8 percent for each 20.0 percent were maintained for the remaining 80.0 percent of those who did not take the measurement" (Abdo and Afif-Abdo 2007: 382). This estimate is curious to say the least, but it supports the idea that men should do more exams; the study also recommended campaigns targeting these individuals in order to intervene earlier to prevent disease.

In 2009, the SBU carried out campaigns supported by Bayer Schering Pharma AG exclusively targeted to educating the public about ADAM in the cities of Goiânia, Porto Alegre, and Natal, in public squares and supermarket parking lots. According to the then-president of the SBU, José Carlos de Almeida, the purpose was to explain to the population the "diagnosis, symptoms and treatments for this problem, which is present in 20 percent to 30 percent of men aged 40 or older" without them knowing it; he described ADAM as a "silent disease" (Sociedade Braisleiria de Urologica accessed June 21, 2010). That same year, the SBU radio channel, which broadcasted information that was also accessible via the SBU website, made available talks on such topics. One of them, entitled "Evils of aging," described the problems associated with the progressive decline in levels of testosterone, the "male hormone," and state that decline accelerated in 20 percent of men, who should thus seek replacement treatments (Sociedade Brasileira de Urologia accessed September 15, 2009).[13]

In 2010, there was an intensification of the strategy to carry out broader diffusion campaigns, which included the SBU's Movement for Male Health. This campaign was aimed at educating the population on the need to prevent and treat male illnesses such as erectile dysfunction, andropause, and prostate problems. The Movement's Mobile Unit (a truck equipped with a medical clinic and a team made up of three urologists and other health workers), supported by the Lilly lab, would go around the country's largest capital cities providing medical orientation free of charge.

This strategy of carrying out campaigns directly targeting the population of large cities by offering immediate access to urologists needs to be contextualized as part of a broader movement of public activism by the SBU. This also included the Society's participation in the creation of a National Policy for the Integrated Care of Male Health, which officially launched in August 2009. As Carrara et al. (2009) have remarked, since at least 2004, the SBU has been putting pressure on government, parliamentarians, health councils, and other medical societies to elaborate on such a policy. In 2008, these efforts were consolidated in the signature of a technical cooperation agreement between the SBU and the Ministry of Health, with the aim of promoting assistance to men in the public health system through medical guidance and the promotion of educational campaigns, the first of which was carried out between July and September 2008 and was dedicated to erectile dysfunction (Carrara et al. 2009: 663–665).

A last piece of evidence related to the process whereby ADAM was created and legitimized in Brazil is the presence of this category and its definition in the Health Portal (section "male health") on the Ministry of Health's official website. Here, ADAM is presented as a gradual decline in the male sexual hormone (testosterone), accompanied by the following explanation:

> The reason for such [a] decline is that [the] levels of testosterone, the chief male hormone, begin to recede by up to 1 percent each year since the age of thirty. This reduction is gradual but permanent. Therefore, at around the age of fifty, about 10 percent of males present low testosterone levels. At the age of seventy, over half of them suffer hormone deficiency. At eighty, most men present levels of testosterone and behaviors similar to boys before puberty (Ministério da Saúde, accessed July 29, 2010).

The Ministry therefore subscribed to the 1 percent yearly reduction from the age of thirty statistic, as well as to the claim that the decline in testosterone levels is associated with "behaviors" similar to those of boys before puberty. Moreover, this definition described symptoms such as intense fatigue, depression, irritability, anxiety disorders, inexplicable mood fluctuations, sensitivity, insomnia, lower libido, weakness, loss of muscle mass, and erection difficulties. In the item "diagnosis," the proposal is that once the symptoms are recognized, a dosage of free testosterone should be given. If "levels are below 200 nanograms/dl and the individual does not present significant risks, a testosterone replacement therapy (or TRT) may be initiated"—of course, under medical supervision Ministério da Saúde, accessed July 29, 2010). At this point, the absence of any significant debate on the existence of ADAM or on the validity of hormone replacement therapy is evident; there are only admonitions regarding the need for professional follow-up and the tailoring of diagnosis and treatment for each patient, which are common to informative materials about any "disease."

As for the outcomes of this process, it can be suggested that the construction of andropause as a public category and a new entity of diagnosis and treatment has been fully successful. Its inclusion in the Ministry of Health's website and the way it was defined indicate the extent of its current legitimacy. Moreover, the terms used to define it—as a disturbance, disease, infirmity, silent illness—lead to an assumption that there are no more doubts about its nature, nor are there suspicions over its character as a pathology. Certainly, the reference to increasingly lower ages as points of onset of testosterone reduction and andropause lends further support to the picture of prevalence and irreversibility.

ANDROPAUSE: A CASE OF MALE MEDICALIZATION

Barbara Marshall and Stephen Katz (2002) argued that in the 20th century, the process of medicalization was focused on men and circumscribed male sexuality to erectile dysfunction. Through a general problematization that links sexuality and age as fundamental dimensions to the modern subject, it is worth noting the importance of cultures and lifestyles prevalent in the end of last century, such as the emphasis on health, on activity, and on staying young to a process that will produce a vast field of studies and interventions around the penetrative capacity of the masculine organ. To begin with, the diagnosis of erectile dysfunction is defined exactly as the function of the (in) capacity to penetrate a vagina, thus marking the heterosexual inclination of those definitions (Marshall and Katz 2002). The great novelty of the 20th century, according to the authors, was the shift that happened going from the admission of the decline of sexual vitality over the course of time, when there was even a certain pejorative suspicion regarding sex in old age, to a period when one is expected to perform well sexually until the end of life. Moreover, sexual activity is portrayed as a necessary condition for a healthy life and the erectile capacity defines male virility during the whole life span of men (Marshall 2006: Marshall and Katz 2002).

The ascension of diagnoses of erectile dysfunction comes from ancient concerns with impotence, which was mostly approached as a problem of psychological origins, including in the works of Masters and Johnson. Until the 1980s, it was a common belief that the fear of impotence was what caused impotence, and that the treatment should include therapy and counseling, even in conjunction with hormonal treatments, prosthesis, and vitamin supplements. During this period, urological research in the field started to deliver innovative results. New discoveries, such as the intra-cavernous injection of papaverine, contributed to the transformation of the erection into an eminent physiological event in detriment to its psychological aspects. Therefore, impotence became a disorder with organic causes, and that is how it should be treated. An important development was the Consensus Development Conference on Impotence that took place in 1992, organized by the U.S. National Institutes of Health. Among the recommendations contained in its final document was the substitution of the term "impotence" for "erectile dysfunction," in order to characterize the incapacity of obtaining and/or maintaining an erection long enough for a satisfactory sexual performance. In addition, it also promoted the ideas that it is an organic disease that is treatable and that it is also a matter of public health. It was instrumental to have the epidemiological data in order to address it as a public health issue. The most cited study was the Massachusetts Male Aging Study, which interviewed 1,700 men between the ages of 40 and 70 living in the Boston area between 1987 and 1989. The study found that 525 of the men had some degree of erectile dysfunction, defined as the inability to obtain and maintain an erection strong enough to perform sexual intercourse (Feldman et al. 1994). Despite being criticized (Lexchin 2006), the study prevailed: it widened the concept of the disease through the idea of stages, and by conceptualizing these symptoms as a progressive disorder. The study was cited and served to create the notion of the risks and the responsibilities that should be carried by the individuals, thus promoting the idea of constant vigilance and the consumption of products to guarantee erectile health, the symbol of masculinity and of physical and emotional health (Giami 2004; Marshall and Katz 2002; Tiefer 2006a).

It is exactly in this context that we watch the launch of Viagra (sildenafil citrate), produced by Pfizer and aimed at facilitating and maintaining an erection, which illustrates the development of a molecular science of sexuality (Marshall and Katz 2002: 60). Viagra has been a success in commercial terms, a blockbuster, and a drug that rakes in at least one billion dollars annually (Tiefer 2006a: 279). It is important to mention that it is precisely the construction of Viagra as a medication to treat a disease and not to be used as an aphrodisiac, as observed by Alain Giami (Giami 2004), that has made it such a success. Viagra was approved for consumption by the Food and Drug Administration in the United States in 1998. Shortly after that, the first studies financed by Pfizer were published, confirming the efficacy of the medication and how well it was tolerated. The foundation of these studies was the International Index of Erectile Function, which was created in 1997. It contained 15 questions designed to examine the erectile function and do away with the difficulties in establishing a diagnostic of dysfunction, as well as to evaluate the results of the trials with new medicines (Giami 2004).

An important facet of this process is the degree of institutionalization that the field was acquiring with the evident predominance of urologists. In 1982, the International Society for Impotence Research was created, aimed at the scientific study of erection and its functional mechanisms, with its official publication, the International Journal of Impotence Research, starting in 1989. In 2000, the Society changed its name to the International Society for Sexual and Impotence Research, leaving an obvious opening to the inclusion of other aspects of male sexuality and also female sexuality. According to Giami (2004: 14), this was a strategy to broaden the limits of intervention with sexual activity on a global scale and to depart from the confines of erectile dysfunction. In 1999, the International Consultation about Erectile Dysfunction was organized in Paris under the auspice of the World Health Organization and the International Urology Society. The conference was sponsored by the pharmaceutical industry, and it marked the process of the internationalization of the medicalization of impotence and the alliance between urologists and the pharmaceutical industry. Similarly, the World Association for Sexual Health conference that happened in Paris in 2001, translates, according to Giami (2004: 16), into the entrance of the pharmaceutical industry and urologists into the world of sexology, which was traditionally fragmented between doctors and non-doctors and between issues of sexual education and prevention, besides the treatment of sexual disorders. According to Leonore Tiefer, the process of the medicalization of sexuality goes beyond the phase of the creation of systems of classification and enters the stage of institutionalization and professionalization of "sexual medicine" with the support of organizations, conferences, training centers, scientific journals, clinics, and medical departments. This new branch of sexual medicine went side by side with "sexual pharmacology" (Tiefer 2006a: 275).

In an article entitled "Bigger and Better: How Pfizer Redefined Erectile Dysfunction," Joel Lexchin (2006) problematizes the strategies adopted by the pharmaceutical industry to promote Viagra. The main argument is that it was necessary, on the one hand, to transform erectile dysfunction into a problem that may afflict any man, at any time in his life, and that there was a medicine already available to solve or to prevent this difficulty. In this sense, Viagra integrated the broader collection of lifestyle drugs or comfort medications destined to enhance individual performance, a market clearly in the process of expansion. Viagra's success came exactly from that, according to Lexchin (2006: 1). If it had been restricted to the treatment of erectile dysfunction associated with organic causes, it would have been a failure in terms of sales. On the other hand, Pfizer also worked to promote the idea of erectile dysfunction as an acceptable subject in public discourse, which also led to a higher demand for treatment (Lexchin 2006).

Meika Loe (2001, 2004) makes another interesting argument. She argues that Viagra is a cultural and material technology that is related to the construction of a new possibility of intervention with the male body, in contrast with the traditional history of medical intervention with women's bodies. Loe is pointing here to the possible use of diagnosis for tapping an unexplored market among men. This has become possible thanks to the propagation of an idea of masculinity in crisis, illustrated above all by the metaphor of the erection (Loe 2001). The idea that the erection, the symbol of virility and masculine identity, is effectively unstable, subject to many types of misfortune, seems to gain more and more notoriety. It is precisely to combat this lack of control or the unpredictability of the male body that the industry offers a cure like Viagra, capable of fulfilling the expectation of a better performance always (Grace et al. 2006).

Furthermore, there is the history of Viagra advertisement campaigns in several countries, which clearly shows how the medicine has been converted into something destined to improve sexual performance without any restrictions and without being destined to a specific group. It was initially geared to an older public and in the context of a heterosexual union, but it started being offered to younger and younger men and it started to be featured without a presumable partner (Marshall and Katz 2002: 61). What was behind this commercial trajectory was the creation of a feeling of masculine vulnerability that led to the search for the control and enhancement of potency and of sexuality in general (Vares and Braun 2006).

I would underline that physical and mental instability have been frequently associated more with female bodies, governed by variable hormone cycles and by different stages linked to the reproductive life, which also justifies the sexual instability of women (Oudshoorn 1994). The novelty is that now this representation has also reached the male body, and it threatens the notion that men are "naturally" potent. Whereas female sexuality has historically been focused on and been encapsulated by reproduction, male sexuality is viewed obliquely through penetration in sexual intercourse.

Loe (2001) suggests that the development of technologies associated with reproduction and, especially, the contraceptive pill, which was created in the middle of the 20th century, were precursors of a new pharmacology of sex. The same thread connected the pill, which liberated women's sexuality from its reproductive consequences, and Viagra, which supposedly guarantees male sexual satisfaction (Loe 2001: 101). Furthermore, Alain Giami and Brenda Spencer (2004) argue in favor of three models of sexuality that characterize the last decades: liberated sexuality, in the context of the pill; protected sexuality, to the extent of the HIV/AIDS epidemic and condom use; and functional sexuality, in light of the medications for sexual dysfunction (Giami and Spencer 2004).

Based on the above observations, it could be argued that a new wave of the medicalization of male sexuality is particularly apparent in the promotion of the diagnosis of sexual dysfunction and andropause, or ADAM (Rohden 2013; Rosenfeld and Faircloth 2006). The assumption is that sexual activity is a precondition for a healthy life and that erectile function is what defines virility throughout a man's life (Giami 2002). It is precisely in this context that Viagra was brought out by Pfizer (Marshall 2006). In the wake of Viagra, some new testosterone-based medications for the treatment of andropause have been brought out, which are also associated with combatting sexual dysfunctions. Such is the case of Nebido, developed by Bayer Schering Pharma AG, which has also been promoted in large-scale campaigns in Brazil.

The public and political campaigns about erectile dysfunction and andropause illustrate how, in the last two decades, a new focus on masculinity has taken shape via the pharmacologization of sexuality. This has been either through the use of drugs to achieve erection or the prescription of testosterone. Although a degree of critical perception can now be noted, especially with the publication of data that call into question the efficacy and safety of such therapies, it can be supposed that medicalization has won the day, both in medical practice and in the lay representations that are taking root. In the specific case of the conjunction of aging and sexuality, it should be noted that the promotion of the new drugs and resources has gone hand-in-hand with the absolutely unquestioning promotion of modes of behavior centered around the veneration of a young, healthy, sexually active body.

For andropause, it is significant that the entire process whereby the disease has come to be recognized, and its diagnosis and treatment promoted, revolved around testosterone. In tune with the pervasiveness of hormone-focused discourse as a prevalent explanatory source in medicine since the 20th century, testosterone was given a pivotal role inasmuch as it was presented as a sort of essential synthesis of masculinity and virility. It is by means of a model of external improvement of the self and by the consumption of testosterone that men are to be convinced of this new capacity for administering the body biochemically. This would offer them an inexhaustible source for renewing their own masculinity.

NOTES

1 This chapter stems from the research project *Gender differences in the recent medicalization of aging and sexuality: the creation of the categories menopause, andropause, and sexual dysfunction*, coordinated by Fabíola Rohden and funded by the National Council of Scientific and Technological

Development. I would like to thank Carolyn Smith-Morris for her suggestions and comments.

2 The journal *Plosmedicine* released on a special issue about medicalization in April 2006, with articles by researchers such as Tiefer (2006b). See also Cassels and Moynihan (2005) and Kassirer (2005).

3 See Smith-Morris (2010) for a discussion about the chronicity of an illness experience as a technological, political, and economic fact.

4 The two terms as well as others will be used here in tandem with their current usage in the field.

5 According to data available at http://bases.bvs.br, accessed September 2009.

6 In 2006, L. Heinemann published another paper seeking to confirm the clinical capacity of the AMS scale to measure the effects of testosterone treatment based on research with 1,670 men with androgen deficiency who were treated with testosterone gel. This time, the paper's second author, Claudia Moore, declared that she was an employee at the company manufacturing the testosterone. The authors nonetheless claimed that there had been no conflict of interest in the investigation and data production (Heinemann et al. 2006).

7 That same year, Carmita Abdo, a female psychiatrist, was granted the honor of becoming a member of the SBU, then headed by Sidney Glina. These two doctors would become central characters in the movement for the publicizing of so-called sexual dysfunctions and their treatments in Brazil.

8 This kind of story and the explicit mention of Nebido would be repeated in other magazines, for instance, in a report published in *Isto é* (2006) entitled "Men's fragilities: scientific discoveries are changing our understanding of what takes place in the bodies and minds of individuals over 40." It called attention to treatments for andropause, which was presented as having important consequences for men's lives, such as a decline in force and energy, damaged cognitive function, and lower desire and sexual potency. Of the alternatives surveyed, it mentioned that the "classic option" was testosterone replacement, and that the latest novelty in this respect was the release of Nebido in Brazil.

9 Andropause became prominent even in female magazines, such as in the report "Andropause: men on the verge of a nervous breakdown" published in *Claudia* (Nabuco 2007).

10 According to TV Cultura, "*Saúde Brasil* is a series of educational documentaries on health, with a focus on prevention. Besides basic orientations, the show de-mystifies prejudices and myths involving various diseases. Produced by Aguilla Productions and Communication, the show presents the disease, its causes, risk factors, treatments, cares and orientations". It is supported by the STD/AIDS National Program and the São Paulo state and city governments. Available at http://www.tvcultura.com.br/saudebrasil, July 29, 2010.

11 See, for example, the report "To replace testosterone is an option after sixty" from the *O Globo* October 2, 2008 issue. It highlighted the necessity of replacement for the 10–13.3 percent of males over 40 who presented ADAM symptoms (Marinho2008).

12 The complete results were released in 2009 in the *Population Study of Aging in Brazil* (Abdo 2009).

13 The discussion and promotion of ADAM as a salient topic in medical conferences persisted in 2009. In the 32nd Conference in Goiânia, described as the largest event of its kind in Latin America, new orientations for the diagnosis and treatment of ADAM were presented with the aim of unifying procedures in Brazil. In the 10th Conference of the Latin American Society for Sexual

Medicine in Florianópolis, Brazil, this topic was also at the foreground. In this event, a booklet entitled "Sexual health as a portal for male health" was distributed. The booklet, published by Bayer Schering Pharma AG, stressed Nebido's benefits through the slogan "In ADAM, look for the first and only quarterly testosterone injection."

REFERENCES

Abdo, Carmita. *Estudo Populacional do Envelhecimento no Brasil.* São Paulo: Editora Segmento Farma, 2009.

Abdo, Carmita and João Afif-Abdo. "Estudo Populacional do 2007. (EPE): Primeiros Resultados Masculinos." *Revista Brasileira de Medicina* 64, no. 8 (2007): 379–83.

Angell, Marcia. *A Verdade sobre os Laboratórios Farmacêuticos.* Rio de Janeiro: Record, 2007.

Buchalla, Ana Paula. "O Hormônio da Juventude." *Veja* (December 13, 2006): 116–22.

———. "O Termômetro da Vida Sexual." *Veja* (January 19, 2005): 70–78.

Carelli, Gabriela. "As Idades do Sexo." *Veja* (February 13, 2002): 74–79.

Carrara, Sérgio, Jane Russo, and Livi Faro. "A Política de Atenção à Saúde do Homem no Brasil: os Paradoxos da Medicalização do Corpo Masculino." *Physis. Revista de Saúde Coletiva* 19, no. 3 (2009): 659–78.

Cassels, Alan and Ray Moynihan. *Selling Sickness: How the World's Biggest Pharmaceutical Companies Are Turning Us All into Patients.* New York: Nation Books, 2005.

Conrad, Peter. *Medicalization of Society: On the Transformation of Human Conditions into Treatable Disorders.* Baltimore: The Johns Hopkins University Press, 2007.

———. "Medicalization and Social Control." *Annual Review of Sociology* 18 (1992): 209–32.

Feldman, H. A., I. Goldstein, D. Hatzichristou, R. Krane, and J. Mickinlay. "Impotence and Its Medical and Psychosocial Correlates: Results of the Massachusetts Male Ageing Study." *Journal of Urology* 151 (1994): 54–61.

Fishman, Jennifer. "Manufacturing Desire: The Commodification of Female Sexual Dysfunction." *Social Studies of Science* 34, no. 2 (2004): 187–218.

Giami, Alain. "De l'Impuissance à la Dysfonction Éretile: Destins de la Médicalization de la Sexualité." In *Le Gouvernement des Corps*, edited by Didier Fassin and Dominique Memmi, 77–108. Paris: Éditions EHESS, 2004.

———. "Sexual Health: The Emergence, Development, and Diversity of a Concept." *Annual Review of Sex Research* 13 (2002): 1–35.

Giami, Alain and Brenda Spencer. "Les Objets Techniques de la Sexualité et l'Organisation des Rapports de Genre dans l'Activité Sexuelle: Contraceptifs Oraux, Préservatifs et Traitement des Troubles Sexuels." *Révue Epidemiologique de Santé Publique* 52 (2004): 377–87.

Grace, Victoria, Annie Potts, Nicola Gavey and Tiina Vares. "The Discursive Condition of Viagra." *Sexualities* 9, no. 3 (2006): 295–314.

Heinemann, Lothar, Claudia Moore, Juergen Dinger, and Diana Stoehr. "Sensitivity as Outcome Measure of Androgen Replacement: the AMS Scale." *Health and Quality of Life Outcomes* 4 (2006): 4–23.

Heinemann, Lothar, Farid Saad, Thomas Zimmermann, Annoesjka Novak, Eric Myon, Xavier Badia, Peter Potthoff, et al. "The Aging Male's Symptoms (AMS)

Scale: Update and Compilation of International Versions." *Health and Quality of Life Outcomes* 1 (2003):1–15.

Hoberman, John. *Testosterone Dreams. Rejuvenation, Aphrodisia, Doping.* Berkeley: University of California Press, 2005.

Kassirer, Jerome. *On the Take. How Medicine's Complicity with Big Business can Endanger your Health.* Oxford: Oxford University Press, 2005.

Lexchin, Joel. "Bigger and Better: How Pfizer Redefined Erectile Dysfunction." *Plosmedicine* 3, no. 4 (2006): 1–4.

Loe, Meika. *The Rise of Viagra: How the Little Bleu Pill Changed Sex in America.* New York: New York University Press, 2004.

———. "Fixing Broken Masculinity: Viagra as a Technology for the Production of Gender and Sexuality." *Sexuality and Culture* 5, no.3 (2001): 97–125.

Marinho, Antonio. "Repor Testosterona é Opção após os 60 anos." *O Globo* (February 10, 2008): 39.

Marshall, Barbara. "Science, Medicine and Virility Surveillance: 'Sexy Seniors' in the Pharmaceutical Imagination." *Sociology of Health & Illness* 32, no. 2 (2010): 211–24.

———. "The New Virility: Viagra, Male Aging and Sexual Function." *Sexualities* 9, no. 3 (2006): 345–62.

———. "Climateric Redux? (Re)Medicalizing the Male Menopause." *Men and Masculinity* 9 (2007): 509–29.

Marshall, Barbara and Stephen Katz. "Forever Functional: Sexual Fitness and the Ageing Male Body." *Body and Society* 8, no. 43 (2008): 43–70.

Mezarobba, Glenda. "O Outono do Macho." *Veja* (May 28, 1997): 90–92.

Morales, Alvaro, Claude C. Schulman, Jacques Tostain, and Frederick C. W. Wu. "Testosterone Deficiency Syndrome (TDS) Needs to be Named Appropriately—The Importance of Accurate Terminology." *European Urology* 50 (2006): 407–409.

Moynihan, Ray. "Female Sexual Dysfunction: Merging of Marketing and Medical Science." *British Medical Journal* 341 (2010): 698–701.

Nabuco, Cristina. "Andropausa: Homens à Beira de um Ataque de Nervos." *Claudia* (May 2007): 154–57.

Oudshoorn, Nelly. *Beyond the Natural Body, an Archeology of Sex Hormones.* London: Routledge, 1994.

Payer, Lynn. *Disease-Mongers: How Doctors, Drug Companies, and Insures Are Making You Fell Sick.* New York: Wiley and Sons, 1991.

Pura Invenção. "A Andropausa Seria Apenas uma Desculpa para Preguiçoso." *Veja* no. 64 (July 2003): 23.

Rohden, Fabíola. "O Império dos Hormônios e a Constituição da Diferença entre os Sexos." *História, Ciências, Saúde—Manguinhos* 15 (2008): 133–52.

———. "Gender Differences and the Medicalization of Sexuality in the Creation of Sexual Dysfunctions Diagnosis." In *Sexuality, Culture and Politics: A South American Reader*, edited by Sívori, Horacio, Sérgio Carrara, Jane Russo, Maria Luiza Heilborn, Anna Paula Uziel and Bruno Zilli, 620–38. Rio de Janeiro: Latin American Center on Sexuality and Human Rights, 2013. http://www.clam.org.br/en/south-american-reader/default.asp.

Rosenberg, Charles E. "The Tyranny of Diagnosis: Specific Entities and Individual Experience." *The Milbank Quarterly* 80, no. 2 (2002): 237–59.

Rosenfeld, Dana and Christopher A Faircloth. *Medicalized Masculinities.* Philadelphia: Temple University Press, 2006.

Smith-Morris, Carolyn. "The Chronicity of Life, the Acuteness of Diagnosis." In *Chronic Conditions, Fluid States: Chronicity and the Anthropology of Illness*, edited by Lenore Manderson and Carolyn Smith-Morris, 21–37. New Brunswick: Rutgers University Press, 2010.

Tiefer, Leonor. "The Viagra Phenomenon." *Sexualities* 9, no. 3 (2006a): 273–94.
———. "Female Sexual Dysfunction: A Case Study of Disease Mongering and Activist Resistance." *PLOS Medicine* 3, no. 4 (2006b): 1–5.
Vares, Tiina and Victoria Braun. "Spreading the Word, but What Word Is That? Viagra and Male Sexuality in Popular Culture." *Sexualities* 9, no. 3 (2006): 315–32.
"Veja Especial Homem." *Veja*. October Special Issue. 2003.

5 Making Sense of Unmeasurable Suffering

The Recontextualization of Debut Stories to a Diagnosis of Chronic Fatigue Syndrome

Lisbeth Sachs

INTRODUCTION

Today, fewer and fewer people in the Western world feel "healthy and bodily well despite undeniable progress in their objective state of health" (Barsky 1988: 414; Naraindas 2011; also Nichter, this volume). Barsky tries to account for a widening gap between what he calls objective health status and subjective health experience—a phenomenon he dubs "the failure of success." The success lies in advances in medical technology, which make it increasingly possible for people in general as well as for medical professionals to interpret somatic or psychological disturbances in terms of medical diagnosis. The "failure" lies in the tendency for people in general to use medical diagnosis for life experience and thereby translate social signs into bodily dysfunctions. In a discussion on "medical tourism" (ibid.), the authors take up those constraints and shortages that may be directly responsible for unresolved health issues. They are also due to a therapeutic impasse resulting from orthodox medicine's inability to provide a solution for many patients' problems. The patients described in this chapter have been called "the tired nomads" (Evengård and Sachs 1994) due to the complex situation they find themselves in as a result of the failure of success.

One such diagnostic "success story" has been chronic fatigue syndrome (CFS). The disturbances represented by this syndrome have been given a medical diagnosis, but no pathology has yet been found to account for them. The diagnosis is based instead on negative findings in diagnostic testing. In this chapter, I discuss such testing in relation to recontextualization/re-narrativization, modes of interpretation, and the discursive body, together with the criteria for the syndrome.

BACKGROUND OF THE CFS DIAGNOSIS

During the 1980s, fatigue emerged as a recurring symptom in the clinical picture of several modern syndromes: fibromyalgia, multiple chemical sensitivity, myalgic encephalomyelitis, chronic fatigue syndrome, and several others (Ware 1998). In the case of chronic fatigue syndrome, a feeling of fatigue is the central symptom in the syndrome.

The definition of CFS stresses the appearance of somatic symptoms that have not been subject to objective measurements, but have only been reported by the patient.[1] Following the diagnostic criteria set forth by Fukuda et al. (1994), a consensus was reached on which tests would be necessary before making a diagnosis: complete blood count, erythrocyte sedimentation rate, alanine aminotransferase, total protein, albumin, globulin, alkaline phosphatase, calcium, phosphate, glucose, blood urea nitrogen, electrolytes, creatinine, thyroid stimulating hormone, and urinalysis (Evengård et al. 1999). The main purpose of this testing was to rule out viruses and infections of various kinds as well as a pathology caused by deficiencies that may present the same symptoms. CFS is a condition characterized by the impairment of neurocognitive functions and poor quality of sleep as well as by somatic symptoms such as recurrent sore throat, muscle aches, arthralgias, headache, and post-exertional malaise.

Advances in medical technology having to do with the microanalysis of all kinds of somatic samples are a prerequisite for making this negatively determined diagnosis. The first descriptions of the syndrome probably appeared during the middle of the 19th century, when an American neurologist named Charles Beard popularized the diagnosis of neurasthenia. His descriptions of that illness bear a strong resemblance to what is now referred to as CFS (Beard 1869). Since the label "neurasthenia" fell out of favor in the early 20th century, other illness labels have been applied to similar conditions; however, the label "CFS" was recommended by the United States Centers for Disease Control and Prevention (Fukuda et al. 1994), and is now commonly used.

The diagnostic dilemma posed by a chronic disease without any demonstrable evidence of serious physical disorders or pathology, as in the case of CFS, is being discussed among medical and social scholars alike. Some of the issues have to do with whether syndromic diagnoses (such as CFS) are, themselves, disabling because the label prompts people to identify with the diagnosis. At times, both physicians and patients seem to be uneasy about the possibility of a self-fulfilling prophecy that might have deleterious consequences. Yet a diagnosis of CFS may allow people to name, and hence to legitimize, their suffering, and this may well help them to cope with their respective social worlds. A diagnosis can thus contribute to identification with a legitimate sick role.

Consequently, one of the most relevant questions in this situation seems to be in what way the participants make sense of the arbitrary; namely, suffering without a biomedically established pathology. How is the medical interpretation of the patient's suffering and diagnosis introduced and negotiated, and what kind of interpretative framework is it superseding?

In this chapter, I use material (interviews and observations) from 21 men and women who are in the diagnostic process for CFS to examine the varying modes of interpretation offered by biomedicine on the one hand, and personal (or everyday) sense-making of bodily experience on the other. Through descriptive analysis of professional and lay ambivalence about causality, including how this negative diagnosis is interpreted and made sense of, I consider CFS as a diagnostic dilemma (Evengård et al. 1999; Evengård and Sachs 1994, 2000; Hydén and Sachs 1998; Sachs 1998, 2001a, b, 2012).

OBJECTIFICATION OF CHRONIC SUFFERING

CFS poses a dilemma in that biomedically trained practitioners tend to search for a specific disease, whereas patients tend to discuss their sufferings in terms of their total life situation. In the communicative act, the discursive body is constituted through various means (e.g., diagnostic and therapeutic talk) within specific contexts. With regard to persons with CFS, two types of context are of particular interest: the everyday context and the biomedical context. The everyday context is characterized by unquestioned assumptions and shared ways of reasoning; the biomedical context is characterized by assumptions and ways of reasoning that are connected to the specific needs and rules deemed relevant to diagnosis, treatment, and cure.

The clinical encounter talk about bodily sensations often provides an example of recontextualization (Linell 1995). This involves extracting the aspects of discourse from one context (e.g., the everyday) and moving them to another (e.g., the biomedical). Aspects of discourse that can be recontextualized include causal stories, assessments, knowledge, and theoretical constructs (Adelswärd and Sachs 1996, 2001; also Potter on giving uptake to bodily and personal experience, this volume). Within this perspective, it does not seem reasonable to present states of health and states of disease as ontologically different. Rather, it makes more sense to present physiological changes as developing into pathological symptoms along a health-disease continuum. This involves a process that begins with the pre-objective body and eventually leads to various symbolic interpretations of physiological changes. Such interpretation begins when people start to construct illness and, in so doing, objectify the body, a process that is evident in the descriptions of suffering offered by the ill (Good et al. 1992). The words used for these descriptions are dictated by language and culture (Manderson and Smith 2010).

Both the everyday view and the biomedical view are culturally constructed modes of interpretation that, as such, shape perception, labeling, and modes of seeking help. In industrialized Western countries, disorders entailing psychological and emotional distress are psychologized, with somatic manifestations of these disorders being treated as, at best, secondary. With regard to CFS, research and practice attach great importance to somatic dysfunctions. With CFS, causality, as described by the patient, includes both life situation and bodily dysfunction. The biomedical diagnosis, however, is based solely on the latter. Yet it is precisely the absence of a specific bodily dysfunction that underpins the diagnosis of CFS (Hydén and Sachs 1998; Evengård and Sachs 1994; Sachs 1996).

When medical questions are asked concerning the physiological, mechanical, chemical, pathological, or other causes of chronic pain, such suffering can be verbally elaborated upon. In some cases, however, sufferers from chronic pain complain that the pain "resists objectification" (e.g., Jackson 1994: 215), which means that they are unable to relate to the body and its functions in an objective way. Biomedical consultation provides a situation within which people are helped to objectify their pain. Within this situation, people are led to believe that their pain can be defined in medical terms. And, indeed, simply by being defined, CFS becomes an entity that affects how people start relating to their bodily symptoms.

A considerable body of research within a wide range of disciplines has shown that social factors are generally capable of influencing the onset and development of certain diseases (as well as life expectancy and general well-being). Research in medical sociology and anthropology discusses how illness is conditioned by the body's interaction with society (Fassin 2007; Sachs 2012). Studies of the social origins and development of neurasthenia (regarded as a predecessor of CFS) in China reveal that the Cultural Revolution, together with certain basic principles of Chinese culture, informed this disorder's constellation of symptoms (Kleinman 1980, 1982, 1986, 1988) Similarly, American studies of CFS have tried to find common factors among sufferers (Lin 1989; Wessley 1990). Attempts to derive the cause of suffering from people's life histories raise the issue of how such experiences may be expressed symbolically (Sachs 2012). Researchers have found connections between how symptoms are described at the micro-level. Ongoing dialectical discourses between these levels also illustrate the social implications of suffering and show that social processes may affect the occurrence and development of disease (Ware 1992; Ware and Kleinman 1992a, b; Sachs 1998, 2001a). Thus, symptoms can express the embodied experiences and cultural sources of suffering, and this raises the issue of how society, culture, our bodies, and our lives are interwoven so as to generate suffering and disease (Nissen and Manderson 2013).

BACKGROUND AND METHODS

A CFS clinic, which was attached to the Department of Infectious Diseases and employed three physicians, opened as a project in 1992 at one of the major hospitals in Stockholm, Sweden. The work at the clinic was based on research grants. The aim was both to try to find a biomedical cause of the illness and to try to help long-suffering persons by giving then information about their condition, arranging meetings with persons having the same condition, and offering physiotherapy. I was engaged to conduct research on how a diagnosis of CFS was understood over time, as well as on the clinical encounter between patient and physician.

My study involves 21 patients, four men and 17 women. I met with these people for one year, from autumn 1995 to spring 1996. The majority of the patients were young, between the ages of 25 and 35 at the onset of their illness. The mean duration of suffering before they visited the CFS clinic was between three and five years. CFS was diagnosed in almost half of these cases. The other half involved people who either had an undetected pathology or who did not fulfill the criteria used to be able to diagnose the syndrome (Fukuda et al. 1994).

I interviewed each patient before she/he met the doctor. I was also present at the consultation, during which a doctor read the patient's documents and discussed all prior somatic and psychological events. All interviews, as well as consultations, were audiotaped and transcribed. In addition, I tracked the 10 people diagnosed with CFS over a period of almost two years following their first consultation at the clinic. I began with the consultation and the ambivalent diagnostic process, and then moved on to the post-consultation interviews and the follow-up material.

During the consultation, the patient and the doctor have to cooperate in order to understand the nature of the former's suffering. Their means of accomplishing this task are mainly discursive. This is because, given the long history of the patient's suffering, most physical tests have already been conducted. The consultations all lasted one hour or more.

DIAGNOSTIC AMBIVALENCE

From the transcripts of these discussions, it is clear that the cause of suffering is shrouded in ambivalence. Biomedicine's impact and reputation are so powerful that even its many failures to resolve chronic illness do not discourage sufferers from turning to it. CFS sufferers frequently devote between five to ten years, and sometimes even longer, to searching for biomedical answers to their questions (Evengård and Sachs 1994; Sachs and Evengård 2000; Sachs 2012). The doctors are clearly frustrated by not being able to diagnose and treat their patients. In fact, one of the doctors became so disturbed that she left the clinic. The suffering of the patients was enormous, and aside from recommending the activities associated with the clinic, the doctors could only provide advice about sick leave and/or painkillers.

In the clinical encounter, the patient's bodily problems and sufferings are presented within two interpretive frameworks: the everyday (consisting of the patient's narration of the history of his/her pain) and the biomedical (consisting of the doctor's analysis of the patient's narration).

DEBUT NARRATIVES AS DIAGNOSIS

Fairly early on in each of the 21 encounters, the doctor would start by asking the patient to describe how his/her problem or illness began. Sometimes this would provide a clue as to whether a particular infection or incident may have triggered the process. All patients responded with what we may call a debut narrative, relating how they first identified and related to their problem. These debut narratives differed in length, elaborateness, and detail, but they all presented physical suffering as both ongoing and troublesome. In these narratives, patients connect with their everyday life and worlds, which form the background against which they present their physical problems. They relate their symptoms and their attempts to understand them both in terms of everyday explanations and in terms of biomedical explanations.

One female patient was in her early 30s and had been ill for almost one year. Her symptoms were severe, involving constant pain and swelling of the lymph nodes, dizziness, and grave fatigue. She had searched all over to find a doctor who would confirm the reality of her illness. She was regarded as healthy and she reported that doctors met her concerns with disbelief and even rudeness. Sometimes, she tried to work, but other times, she just had to rest. Her life was miserable and her marriage was under enormous strain. Below is a description of her story. Some background information was already known from a questionnaire she had filled in before her encounter with the doctor.

> DOCTOR: You write that you think your complaint. . . began less than a year ago. . . .
>
> PATIENT: Yes, you see we were on holiday; we have a cottage, so we were there two and a half weeks. We had added to it and then last year, well, we extended the garage and added another shed. . . We were there you see and worked and I ran the household plus looked after my elderly parents-in-law. It was rather like the home-help service plus not having any holiday, as it were, lying and relaxing, you know. Instead it was full speed ahead all the time. And the first, I don't know. . . it was when we returned home, it was a Saturday, then . . . let me see. . . the 11th. . . no, the 13th I think, then we went back to my parents' home, and it's 240 kilometers, I sat as a passenger. And when I was to get out of the car it was as though I had no legs to stand on. They were there, of course, but it was as thought they didn't feel, or what can I say.
>
> DOCTOR: Mmm.
>
> PATIENT: And later that evening too I was kind of so odd, it was . . . I don't know how to describe it, it felt like electric shocks both here and there or something of that sort. But then I went to bed and slept and . . . next day it's as though I have no memory of being poorly in the legs because then I tested my niece's moped, for instance, and things like that. And then you see we traveled another 320 kilometers to my hometown and we helped each other with the luggage we had and that

sort of thing and tidied up and . . . Then the morning when I woke up and was to go downstairs—we have a bedroom on the first floor—I was so stiff I could barely go down the stairs. So then I said to Rolf, my old man, "My, oh my, it must be. . . all that exercise." Because we had been at it, painting, among other things, the outside of that new building and I'd painted all round twice over. It had meant standing on ladders and on the Friday I'd cycled five kilometers and things like that, you see. . . . But I still went to work and worked there and . . . and I swelled up then in the left leg. My left leg became twice as large then for 14 days (laughter).

DOCTOR: And whereabouts was the swelling then?

PATIENT: Yes all the way down here, and here. . .

DOCTOR: The lower leg and all of the foot and. . .?

During the first part of the narrative, the woman describes how her body was incapable of carrying out her intentions, such as getting out of the car or going downstairs. She takes this as a clear sign that something is wrong and she presents her narration within an everyday framework. During the second part of the narrative, she describes additional problems and complaints. She talks about certain bodily sensations, saying, "It felt like electric shocks both here and there." Back in her own home, the problem with her leg and foot recurs, something that prompts her, together with her husband, to try to understand and explain her complaints with reference to what she has been doing over the past few days. In other words, she presents her account within an everyday interpretive framework, explaining certain types of bodily pain by associating them with certain types of mundane activity.

She concludes her narrative by bringing events up to date. She goes to work, but one leg swells up to twice the size of the other; the swelling lasts for a fortnight and prompts her to see a doctor, eventually bringing her to her present situation. The doctor terminates the narrative by taking up the matter of the swollen leg and foot. Thereby she is moving from the everyday interpretive framework to the biomedical interpretive framework. At this point, the focus moves from the body's dysfunction within an everyday social context to a particular part of the body in relation to itself.

In this and all the other debut narratives, the patient focuses on certain bodily phenomena and non-functioning body parts. These phenomena force themselves on the patient, commanding her attention and action. In this way, they become objects of her consciousness. The narrative form enables the patient to make connections between bodily phenomena and everyday situations; indeed, the narrative form seems to be a common instrument for introducing everyday experiences into a biomedical context (Mattingly 1989; Mishler 1984; Garro 1990).

The patient defines her complaints within an everyday context and thus identifies them and gives them meaning. She defines her body as dysfunctional in relation to the performance of everyday activities. This dysfunction gives rise to suffering in the form of pain and fatigue, which she also describes in relation to an everyday context. However, when her problems continue for an unacceptable period of time, accounting for them within an everyday interpretive mode ceases to yield an acceptable explanation. It is this temporal dimension that transforms her suffering from being minor or acute to being chronic. It is now that she turns to the medical institution for help in explaining and making sense of her bodily suffering.

When the woman tries to define her complaints, she turns from the temporal dimension and relates to her body as herself; she does not have a body, she is her body, and it is only through her body that the world will appear (Manderson 2010; Sachs 2012).

In the last line of the above excerpt, the doctor focuses on something that can be represented within a biomedical mode: the patient's swollen leg and foot. This initiates a long sequence of medical questions concerning symptoms, medication, and so on. In other words, this part of the consultation follows a traditional question-and-answer format in order to secure the patient's problems more firmly within a strictly biomedical framework. Consequently, the themes of suffering and dysfunction that the patient has formulated and discussed within an everyday interpretive mode are now devalued under the biomedical diagnosis and named pathologies. This is a clear example of how the debut narrative of the patient is recontextualized within the medical encounter.

THE MEDICALIZED BODY

The doctor presents the patient with a lengthy account of how various signs of bodily disorders and fatigue can be categorized as elusive phenomena that medical science is endeavoring to decode and understand. This account presents a notion of medical progress as a struggle to decode the body's as yet indecipherable signs. In other words, biomedicine offers the patient another diagnostic framework within which to interpret his/her symptoms.

The three doctors at the clinic concluded their respective communication in a similar manner. They offered a general introduction to the problem of CFS and then linked it to the patient's problem, thus contextualizing the latter within a biomedical mode.

> PATIENT: I don't know if it's that I've had . . . inflammation in the joints . . . or something like that. . .
>
> DOCTOR: Err . . . if one looks at this question of chronic fatigue syndrome, for that's what you've come here for, because you wondered about that when you were at Rheumatology too. So we can begin by saying that at present I have some difficulty in

saying for certain that you have that diagnosis. For one thing I think we must have a little more information from other clinics about this but one can put it this way, that we doctors have all had patients who have been tired after infections and that's something we've always known that some infections entail long-lasting fatigue and patients have had difficulty in getting going as usual. Then one has internationally worked out criteria for making this diagnosis because there are no tests to do on patients or no examinations where one has been able to say for certain. One has not been able to make the diagnosis like that. So there are these criteria for making the diagnosis they're based on the patient presenting a number of symptoms and the actual course has been defined so that one can fulfill these criteria. Now, this business of fulfilling criteria is really for research. So that one can compare patients who have been examined by the doctor here with patients examined by a doctor in the USA perhaps or Australia and so on. Now, that doesn't mean that if one doesn't fulfill the criteria that one cannot have a state of fatigue as such. When you tell me that what I find like that it's that very much has actually had to do with your discomfort in the body; partly this swelling, partly the stiffness, partly the pain.

PATIENT: Yes.

DOCTOR: And of course a great deal of this means that naturally one cannot manage in the same way; one has an increased need of rest as such.

PATIENT: Mmm.

DOCTOR: And one can say, if one looks strictly at the criteria, then one can say that you don't fulfill them. But it is also the case that we know that patients with chronic fatigue vary a great deal; one can have periods with more discomfort and periods when one feels better. And I also interpret it a bit as that you have become a little better.

PATIENT: Yes.

At the beginning of the foregoing excerpt, after a number of back-and-forth questions and answers, the patient declares that she does not know whether or not she has experienced inflammation of the joints. The doctor takes this as an opportunity to present the patient's problem within a broad biomedical context. She shows great ambivalence and becomes at times quite incomprehensible. She begins by mentioning "chronic fatigue syndrome," thereby indicating what she considers it to be an appropriate framework within which to assess the patient's problem. However, she goes on to discuss the problem with CFS and mentions her difficulty in establishing this as the correct diagnosis in this particular case.

In her review of the patient's problem, the doctor moves from the everyday interpretive framework. Up to this point, the doctor has addressed different topics with the patient by asking questions and following them up. Now, however, the discourse turns into a long address that, unlike the earlier part of the consultation, contains no slots of patient response. The doctor's use of formal medical terms and her discussion of the background of CFS signals the switch from the everyday mode to the biomedical mode.

Here, it is obvious how the biomedical mode of establishing a diagnosis is based on evidence gathering. The analysis that is resulting in a diagnosis of CFS is based on data that the doctor can interpret from a medical framework. On the other hand, the woman is trying to explain and understand her situation in a performative and negotiative way that is mutable and strategic.

Later the doctor mentions that "one has internationally worked out criteria for making this diagnosis (i.e., CFS)." The indefinite pronoun "one" combined with "internationally" conveys the impression that CFS is something that is being studied both at the micro-level within the individual body and at the macro-level within the international community. Interestingly, on several occasions, the doctor refers to the existence of these international criteria without saying what these are or how they can be met, thus making it appear as though the word "criteria" functions mainly as a signal of scientific intent and authority. Finally, the doctor returns to the patient's current problem. She then harks back to "criteria" and points out that the patient does not altogether fulfill them—still without specifying what they are. She concludes by saying that if anything, the patient seems somewhat better.

Clearly, in the foregoing excerpt, the doctor presents the patient's problem within a biomedical mode, and she does so in a most vague and confusing manner. Her focus is biomedicine's international struggle to cope with bodily complaints of this particular kind and how the diagnosis in such cases is ambivalent. What stands out in this narrative despite its vagueness is a double transformation: (1) the patient's dysfunctional body is transformed into a pathological body and (2) the patient's suffering is transformed into disease. In other words, the enigmatic suffering that the patient experiences within her life and world is transformed into a more or less trivial, non-enigmatic biomedical phenomenon, and this is the resulting lack of a diagnosis that the woman is getting.

IMPLICATIONS OF THE OBJECTIFICATION OF CFS

As the consultations show, patients tend to view their bodies as part of their everyday experience, whereas doctors tend to view them as biomedical objects. Thus, the suffering body is turned into a discursive body and becomes an object for reflection, discussion, and negotiation. During the medical consultation, both patient and doctor are engaged in attempting to understand the body in terms of the criteria used to diagnose CFS. The challenge is for the doctor and patient to jointly make sense of the latter's suffering. Both have an interest in explaining bodily suffering and both do so in different ways. One of the questions with which I am concerned involves how one makes sense of suffering that lacks a biomedically established pathology, i.e., a diagnosis. How do patients feel about the biomedical interpretation of their suffering with or without the diagnostic frame? Is it real? Is it true? Is it good or is it bad for their social relations and overall life situation?

With a diagnosis of CFS, bodily experiences become medicalized; that is, they become transformed into symptoms of defects within a biological mechanism. I argue that the process of medicalizing symptoms and conducting a diagnostic discourse constitutes a sign of what Barsky refers to as "the failure of success." The success involves providing a diagnosis; the failure involves providing a diagnosis without providing either a cure or a method of treatment. Without the possibility of treatment, things come to a halt. Instead of "coming out on the other side," patients remain in a chronic state of illness and their view of their suffering may become even more complex. The dilemma posed by a diagnosis of CFS—a chronic illness that offers no demonstrable evidence of a serious physical disorder—is indeed a new problem, for both biomedicine and for the person so diagnosed.

Transforming the lived body into a medicalized body involves transforming the social into the biological. It involves disregarding the individual's life and presence in society. What does this mean for the daily life of the patient with a confirmed diagnosis of CFS? It may mean that he/she will take on a new role in relation to his/her surrounding world. The medicalized body may become "the real body," the one that determines the sorts of demands that relatives and associates may place on the sufferer.

Of the ten patients diagnosed with CFS, half seem to take on a new identity and social role. Others had already begun living lives marked by their suffering. They tended to be isolated and to have irregular daily social interactions. Because they have not been able to work or function with friends or family, these people have become depressed and lonely. Their symptoms of fatigue and pain are not perceived, either by themselves or by others, as constituting a legitimate reason to retire from an active life. For these people, a confirmed diagnosis of CFS could offer some kind of legitimacy. One of these patients explains how it feels:

> But I see it somewhat negatively that I have been diagnosed with CFS. Because I am more afraid and careful now than I was before. Because then I didn't know, you see, that there would be a reaction if I did something strenuous. Now I have this anxiety and I think that this anxiety is like a "trigger" for this illness. It becomes worse, so to speak, than what it would have been. So that is the negative side of getting a diagnosis. Well, it is almost like mourning, being like this. Before I knew that I did

things without knowing what it was and became ill but didn't understand, was just very ill. We were out paddling last summer and sometimes it was too much. And then I remember once when I was going to eat and I had to lie down on my side so that I could get the fork into my mouth—I was so weak. But I didn't know why. I thought I was just tired from the paddling. I did not understand until now that this is an illness that I have.

After having been diagnosed with CFS, the above patient became more observant of her body and she also felt more handicapped by it. The diagnosis became part of her identity and she was able to use it when family members, especially her mother-in-law, scolded her for not doing as much work as she should. Some patients, however, were relieved to receive a diagnosis of CFS because it legitimized their condition. Their associates were more inclined to understand and help them than they had been before the diagnosis. In other words, the diagnosis enabled the sufferers to be taken seriously.

Some of the issues have to do with whether diagnoses such as CFS are disabling because the label prompts people to identify with the diagnosis. At times, both physicians and patients seem to be uneasy about the possibility of a self-fulfilling prophecy that might have deleterious consequences. A diagnosis can thus contribute to identification with a legitimate sick role.

Some authors note that the diagnosis also has an enabling aspect, in that people in search of a name for and some kind of confirmation of their suffering are reassured in their relations with the surrounding world. To suffer for many years, with no explanation for one's problems and no understanding for a serious complaint of pain and fatigue, may impede a recovery.

An interest in the process of a sick role and the concept of medical impact in particular cultural settings has a long history in social science. Debates about whether giving symptoms a diagnosis is good or bad rest on implicit definitions of health and illness and on the particular health problem, as well as upon an assessment of the effectiveness of medicine and its physical, psychological, and social effects. An interest in the process has been explicit in social science at least since Parsons articulated the functional theory of illness as entailing a failure to conform to social norms and the consequent social necessity to control illness behavior (1951). The sick role simultaneously legitimizes a withdrawal from normal responsibilities, while it limits and contains the potential social disruption of illness.

According to Parsons's observations, a sick person is someone who abstains (or at least threatens to abstain) from important everyday responsibilities that he/she is expected to meet. The more serious the sickness, the greater the deviance. What distinguishes sickness from other kinds of deviant behavior are the special techniques by which society offers to exculpate, to have an excuse, for the sick person, and the fact that social accountability for his/her behavior can always be transferred onto some agency beyond the sick person's will. These agencies can be in some sense external to the sick person (a virus), within his/her own body (a physiological process of some kind) or, perhaps most often, a combination of both.

For a person to abstain from everyday responsibilities that he/she is expected to meet is never automatic. Moreover, the transfer of accountability that marks the so-called exculpation must take place under socially prescribed conditions if it is to be adequately communicated and legitimized. These special conditions are the stereotyped sets of behavior we know as diagnosis and therapy according to the Western medical model, and it is through the recontextualization of the debut narrative of the patient that this is accomplished (Burnham 2012).

While a convincing array of signs appears, as in the above case, the woman does not feel that she is allowed to pass on responsibility for producing them. In her debut narrative, she is mainly asking questions about what it is that causes her suffering. Of course, if the sufferer of such complaints produces behavior that is aberrant enough and persists in it long enough, she/he may gain exculpation anyway. Even so, the translation of the signs may not be the one she/he intended.

In recent studies, the question arises whether certain illnesses are helped by means of diagnoses where the person takes on a sick role. One of these diagnoses is chronic fatigue syndrome.

Consequently, one of the most relevant questions in this situation seems to be in what way the diagnosis can function in a positive or negative way for the patient. In its chronic state, might it be seen as a positive, a legitimate, or a marginal state? Here, the concept of liminality comes to mind, a concept discussed in classical anthropology as one of the states in rites de passage (Banks and Prior 2001; Turner 1967, 1969; van Gennep 1960).

THE DEBUT NARRATIVE AND ITS INTERPRETATION

Van Gennep defined **rites de passage** as "rites which accompany every change of place, state, social position and age." He has shown that all rites of passage or transition are marked by three phases: separation, margin (or margin, which signifies threshold in Latin), and reaggregation (on embodied liminality, see Jaye and Fitzgerald 2012).

> The liminality or the liminal people, threshold people, are necessarily ambiguous since this condition and these persons elude or slip through the network of classifications that normally locate states and positions in cultural space. Liminal entities are neither here nor there; they are "betwixt and between" (Turner 1969, 95).

The concept of rite de passage and its stages has not been used extensively in modern analysis of sickness episodes, although there is one anthropologist of medicine who has found liminality important for her interpretations of her study (Honkasalo 1999). In her study of persons in chronic pain, Honkasalo argues that they are in a state of liminality, because their situation is filled with ambiguity and paradox, i.e., it cannot be defined. For this reason, they are structurally invisible. For people with chronic pain, structural invisibility is real and factual. They are socially as invisible as the pain in their bodies.

Contrary to this study, I have found in the study of patients with CFS in Sweden that they are visible in various ways that will be described in the following. I also argue that there is a kind of "communitas" created among these people spontaneously or as a kind of refuge created by the medical institution. In some cases, they have been diagnosed with CFS, although the diagnosis does not give any hope for a cure. This means that they are classified in an ambivalent way but still feel satisfied within the CFS category. The interpretations of their debut narratives have given them a diagnosis that becomes an emblem for hope while at the same time turning their suffering into something medically and socially legitimate.

THE DISCURSIVE BODY AND MODES OF INTERPRETATION

How can we look upon the long process in CFS in terms of rites of passage? Does the ambivalence present in the diagnosis lend it to liminality where culturally prescribed actions do not suffice? Douglas (1966) argues that what cannot be clearly classified in terms of traditional criteria of classification, or falls between classificatory boundaries, is almost everywhere regarded as an anomaly. In the case of CFS, I have an impression that the people with an ambivalent suffering without disease are left during long periods of time in the darkness, alone, not totally accepted or trusted by their surroundings or by uninformed health care personnel. Until the time they come into contact with a confirmation of their suffering, they are in the dark. There are thus two different ways of looking at the CFS diagnosis and transition. I want to present some of the data in the study to discuss this situation.

What does it mean for the daily life of the patient with a confirmed chronic illness? The belief in biomedical transformations may mean, as mentioned, that people take on a new role, a new identity in relation to their surrounding world. The diagnosed body may become the real body, which can be related to in questions of responsibility and the everyday demands put on the fatigued person by spouses and other close relatives.

Out of the ten patients with diagnosed CFS, half of them seem to take on the chronic identity where the reaggregation into family life with a confirmed illness means a new accepted social role.

Others have already begun living a life totally marked by their suffering, meaning a life of isolation and irregular social contact. Not being able to work or function with friends or family has made these persons depressed and lonely. Their symptoms of fatigue and pain are not seen as a legitimate cause of retirement from life. Thus the mere naming of the illness, the confirmed diagnosis, could give quite different reactions. Depending on what?

Some patients with the diagnosis were, however, relieved, just because they could be helped to deal with their symptoms in front of others. The surrounding world met them with better understanding and helped them in new ways as it became aware of the CFS diagnosis. The patients are at least made visible in their suffering and taken seriously through the diagnosis. One man tells how he perceives being diagnosed with CFS and he gives a voice to several of the persons with the diagnosis.

> I find it great that they do not only deal with the patients but also their relatives who are invited to the clinic. I like that. Many lose their family because they don´t cope. And that is the worst that can happen in this situation. To stand alone, with all those problems. But unfortunately that is how it is for many. The other day there was one who came crying. Her husband had kicked her out, kicked her out because he could not stand it any longer. He had not been to the information for relatives that they give here.

The challenge in studies of the meaning of suffering is to identify and describe how culture works to transform painful feelings into publicly acceptable sets of symbols or, alternatively, to examine how individuals seize upon and manipulate these symbols to articulate their distress in locally meaningful terms.

DISCUSSION

Some authors who engaged in the early stage of the CFS discussions (e.g., Csordas 1990, 1994; Kirmayer 1988, 1992; Ots 1990, 1991, 1994; Scheper-Hughes and Lock 1987; and von Uexküll 1991) argued that because people are social beings, research and practice must give serious consideration to the relationship between daily social interactions and sickness. Since these authors made their statements, medicine has changed and the structural concepts and the limits of medicine they referred to are not applicable today. Greater sensitivity to bodily experience and narrated expression must be incorporated into biomedical practice as a whole, but especially where strategies for chronic care are concerned. In other words, social interactions must inform diagnostic statements. In order to describe a person as a whole being, an umbrella term that encompasses body, mind, spirit, life, experience, feelings, and complex social interactions is needed.

Under certain circumstances, the body presents itself as an object for our own and others' thoughts and communications. This occurs, for instance, when the body is in pain. It captures our attention and thus becomes an object to be considered (see Leder 1990). This is obvious in peoples' descriptions of their initial experiences of CFS (as seen in the above excerpts). However, the body-turned-object is not the same as the lived body that exists in the background of daily activities. Perceiving the body as an object involves trying to grasp it through words, categories, theories, and icons. Thus, the lived body becomes a discursive body—an object for reflection, discussion, and negotiation. Constituting the lived body as a discursive body in interactional and communicative contexts makes it possible to present it in various ways and modes (e.g., biological by the doctors; subjective, lived, and experienced by the patients).

As Good et al. (1992) argued, because serious illness disrupts the normal rhythms of life and, thereby, threatens the individual's life and world, it provokes moral questions. Causal explanations for illness, explanations that go beyond physical processes to focus on the broader context of moral life, are attempts to introduce order into disorder, to produce a meaningful context for traumatic events. In other words, one of the important functions of causal explanations is to maintain a sense of meaningfulness. When we look at the causal explanations offered to account for CFS, they appear to be arbitrary and so do not offer a morally satisfactory interpretation of the illness. To many Swedish people, it appears that those suffering from undiagnosed CFS are simply lazy or lacking in moral fiber. Being fatigued is not assigned the same moral authority as is being sick, and the sufferers of undiagnosed CFS are often relegated to a marginal (liminal) status once they are no longer able to live a normal life. As we have seen, even close family members may scold or leave them.

To patients who suffer, or suspect that they suffer, from CFS, the feelings of fatigue are of central importance. Fatigue, together with pain, is one of the main sources of their sufferings. Thus, it is important that fatigue be considered a relevant symptom of illness, a symptom that can lead to a causal explanation of the person's condition and result in him/her being given "asylum" in society. At the same time, it is crucially important that the patient not appear to be taking advantage of his/her fatigue in order to avoid having to attend to common tasks. His/her feelings of fatigue must be placed within a context of abnormality. It must under no circumstances be associated with tiredness or exhaustion due to work. In other words, the patient has to transform an everyday feeling into a symptom, and he/she must do this through the use of culturally acceptable discourses, the most obvious of which is the biomedical discourse.

From my observations, it seems clear that until CFS is understood as a particular kind of pathology, the identities of the people suffering from this disorder will be both socially and medically ambivalent. That is why I would like to sum up the discussion of the transformation of the lived body into the medicalized body by turning to medical anthropologist Gananath Obeyesekere, who stated that "the work of culture is to transform human misery into suffering and to counter sickness with healing" (1990: 23). He argues that culture, including the culture of health care and medicine, transforms various kinds of misery and suffering into symptoms that may be classified under such headings as depression, ulcers, and chronic pain, thus allowing them to be dealt with by appropriate forms of medical practice. According to Obeyesekere, in prioritizing advanced medical technology, we run the risk of allowing the structural causes of misery and suffering to persist. From my research, I conclude that Obeyesekere is correct in his view. But when it comes to CFS, the criteria are so strict that some sufferers are left undealt with, which may mean that they are left to a life "betwixt and between," i.e., undiagnosed.

NOTE

1 The Holmes et al. (1988) definition of CFS is summarized as follows: Severe fatigue that persists or relapses for more thatn six months. Classify as CFS if: Fatigue is sufficiently severe, of recent onset (i.e. not lifelong), not substantially alleviated by rest, and results in substantial reduction in previous levels of occupational, educational, social or personal activities; and four or more of the following symptoms are concurrently present for more than six months:

1. impaired memory or concentration
2. sore throat
3. tender cervical or axillary lymph nodes
4. muscle pain
5. multi-joint pain
6. new headaches
7. unrefreshing sleep
8. post-exertional malaise

Classify as idiopathic chronic fatigue if fatigue severity or symptom criteria for chronic fatigue syndrome are not met.

REFERENCES

Adelswärd, Viveka and Lisbeth Sachs. "Budbärarens Dilemma: Om Moraliska Aspekter På Information (The Messengers Dilemma: Moral Aspects in Information)." *Socialmedicinsk tidskrift (Journal of Social Medicine)* 5 (2001): 125–45.
———. "A Nurse in Preventive Work. Dilemmas of Health Information Talks." *Scandinavian Journal of Caring Science* 10 (1996): 45–52.
Banks, Jonathan, and Lindsay Prior. "Doing Things with Illness. The Micro Politics of the CFS Clinic." *Social Science and Medicine* 52 (2001): 11–23.
Barsky, Arthur J. "The Paradox of Health." *New England Journal of Medicine* 318, no. 7 (1988): 414–18.
Beard, George. "Neurasthenia, or Nervous Exhaustion." *Boston Medical Surgery Journal* 80 (1869): 217–20.
Burnham, John C. "The Death of the Sick Role." *Social History Medicine* (April 18, 2012): 761–776.
Csordas, T.J. "Embodiment as a Paradigm for Anthropology." *Ethos* 18 (1990):5-47.
Douglas, Mary. *Purity and Danger: An Analysis of Concepts of Pollution and Taboo.* London: Routledge and Kegan Paul, 1966.

Evengård, B. and Lisbeth Sachs. "Speciell Patient-läkarrelation vid Korniskt Trötthetssyndrom: Antropoolog och Läkare Söker Ny Kontaktmodell (Special Patient-doctor Relation in CFS: Anthropologist and Physician in Search of a New Contact Model)." *Läkartidningen. Swedish Medical Journal* 97 (2000): 176–81.

———. "Den Trötta Nomaden—En Modern Epidemi (The Tired Nomad—A Modern Epidemic)." *Läkartidningen (Swedish Medical Journal)* 91 (1994): 4001–5.

Evengård, B., R. S. Schacterle, and A. L. Komaroff. "Chronic Fatigue Suyndrome: New Insights and Old Ignorance." *Journal of Internal Medicine* 246 (1999): 455–69.

Fassin, Didier. *When Bodies Remember. Experiences and Politics of Aids in South Africa.* California Series in Public Anthropology. University of California Press, 2007.

Fukuda, Keiji, Stephen E. Strauss, Ian, Michael C. Sharpe, James G. Dobbines, Anthony Komaroff, and the International Chronic Fatigue Syndrome Study Group. "The Chronic Fatigue Syndrome: A Comprehensive Approach to its Definition and Study." *Annals of Internal Medicine* 121 (1994): 953–59.

Garro, Inda C. "Continuity and Change: The Interpretation of Illness in an Anishinaabe Community." *Culture, Medicine and Psychiatry* 4 (1990): 417–54.

Good, Mary-Jo D., Paul Brodwin, Bryon Good, and Arthur Kleinman. *Pain as Human Experience: An Anthropological Perspective.* Berkley: University of California Press, 1992.

Holmes, Gary P., Jonathan E. Kaplan, Nelson M. Gantz, Anthony L. Komaroff, Lawrence B. Schonberger, Stephen E. Straus, James F. Jones, Richard E. Dubois, Charlotte Cunningham-Rundles, Savita Pahwa, Giovanna Tosato, Leonard S. Zegans, David T. Purtilo, Nathaniel Brown, Robert T. Schooley, and Irena Brus. "In Response: Definition of the Chronic Fatigue Syndrome." *Annals of Internal Medicine* 109 (1988): 554–56.

Honkasalo, Marja-Liisa. "What Is Chronic Is Ambiguity—Encountering Biomedicine with Long-Lasting Pain." *Journal of the Finnish Anthropological Society* 24 (1999): 75–92.

———. "Suffering, Hope and Diagnosis: On the Negotiation of Chronic Fatigue Syndrome (CFS)." *Health* 2 (1998): 175–93.

Jackson, J. "Chronic Pain and the Tension between the Body as Subject and Object." In *Embodiment and Experience. The Existential Ground of Culture and Self*, edited by T. J. Csordas, 201–228. Cambridge: Cambridge University Press, 1994.

Jaye, Chrystal and Ruth Fitzgerald. "The Embodied Liminalities of Occupational Overuse Syndrome." *Medical Anthropology Quarterly* 26, no. 2 (2012): 201–20.

Kirmayer, Laurence J. "Mind and Body as Metaphors: Hidden Values in Biomedicine. In *Biomedicine Examined*, edited by M. Lock and D. Gordon, 57–95. Dordrecht: Kluwer Academic Publishers, 1988.

———. "The Body's Insistence on Meaning: Metophors as Presentation and Representation in Illness Experience." *Medical Anthropology Quarterly* 6, no. 4 (1992): 323–46.

Kleinman, Arthur. "Neurasthenia and Depression: A Study of Somatization and Culture in China." *Culture, Medicine and Psychiatry* 6 (1982): 117–89.

———. *Social Origins of Distress and Disease: Neurasthenia, Depression, and Pain in Modern China.* New Haven: Yale University Press, 1986.

———. *The Illness Narratives. Suffering, Healing, and the Human Condition.* New York: Basic Books, 1988.

———. *Patients and Healers in the Context of Culture.* Berkley: University of California Press, 1980.

Leder, Drew. *The Absent Body.* Chicago: Chicago University Press, 1990.

Lin, Tsung-Yi. "Neurasthenia Revisited: Ist Place in Modern Psychiatry." *Culture, Medicine and Psychiatry*, 13 (1989): 105–29.

Linell, Per. "The Dynamics of Contexts in Discourse." In *Form and Function in Language Millar* (RASK Supplement, Vol. 2), edited by S. and J. Mey, 41–67. Odense: Odense University Press, 1995.

Manderson, Lenore, and Carolyn Smith-Morris. *Chronic conditions, fluid states : chronicity and the anthropology of Illness*. New Brunswick: Rutgers University Press, 2010.

Manderson, Lenore. "Social Capital and Inclusion: Locating Wellbeing in Community." *Australian Cultural History* 28, no. 2–3 (2010): 233–52.

Mattingly, Cheryl. "Thinking with Stories: Story and Experience in a Clinical Practice." PhD thesis, Massachusetts Institute of Technology, 1989.

Mishler, Elliot G. *The Discourse of Medicine. Dialectics of Medical Interviews*. Norwood, NJ: Ablex Publishing Company, 1984.

Naraindas, Harish and Cristiana Bostos. "Healing Holidays? Itinerant Patients, Therapeutic Locales and the Quest for Health." *Anthropology and Medicine* 18, no. 1 (2011): 1–6.

Nissen, Nina and Lenore Manderson. "Researching Alternative and Complementary Therapies: Mapping the Field." *Medical Anthropology* 32, no. 1 (2013): 1–7.

Obeyesekere, Gananath. *The Work of Culture: Symboliic Transformation in Psychoanalysis and Anthropology*. Chicago: University of Chicago Press, 1990.

Ots, Thomas. "The Silenced Body—The Expressive Leib: On the Dialectic of Mind and Life in Chinese Cathartic Healing." In *Embodiment and Experience. The Existential Ground of Culture and Self*, edited by T. J. Csordas, 116–36. Cambridge: Cambridge University Press, 1994.

———. "Phenomenology of the Body: The Subject-Object Problem in Psychosomatic Medicine and Role of Traditional Medical Systems." *In Anthropologies of Medicine: A Colloquium of West European and North American Perspectives. Special Issue of Curare*, edited by B. Pflederer and G. Bibeau, 43–58. Wiesbaden: Wiesweg, 1991.

———. "The Angry Liver, the Anxious Heart and the Melancholy Spleen." *Culture, Medicine and Psychiatry* 14 (1990): 21–58.

Parsons, Talcott. *The Social System*. New York: The Free Press, 1951.

Sachs, Lisbeth. "From a Lived Body to a Medicalized Body: Diagnostic Transformation and Chronic Fatigue Syndrome." *Medical Anthropology* 19, no. 4 (2001a): 299–317.

———. "Problems of Communication in Evidence Based Medicine." *International Journal of Risk and Safety in Medicine* 14 (2001b): 107–15.

———. "The Visualization of the Invisible Body." In *Identities in Pain*, edited by Jonas Frykman, 120–132. Lund: Nordic Academic Press, 1998.

———. *Sjukdom som Oordning. (Sickness as Disorder)*. Stockholm: Gedins Förlag. Natur and Kultur, 1996, 2012.

Sachs, Lisbeth and B. Evengård. "Speciell patient-läkarrelation vid kroniskt trötthetssyndrom." *Läkartidningen* 97 (2000): 176–81.

Schepfer-Hughes, N., and M.M. Lock. "The Mindful Body: A Prologomenon to Future Work in Medical Anthropology." *Medical Anthropology Quarterly*, (1987), 1:6-41.

Turner, Victor. *The Ritual Process: Structure and Antistructure*. Chicago: Aldine, 1969.

———. *The Forrest of Symbols*. Ithaca: Cornell University Press, 1967.

Van Gennep, Arnold. *The Rites of Passage*. Chicago: University of Chicago Press, 1960.

Ware, Norma C. "Suffering and the Social Construction of Illness: The Delegitimation of Illness Experience in Chronic Fatigue Syndrome." *Medical Anthropology Quarterly* 6 (1992): 347–61.

———. "Sociosomatics and Illness in Chronic Fatigue Syndrome." *Psychosomatic Medicine* 60 (1998): 394–401.

Ware, Norma C., and Arthur Kleinman. "Culture and Somatic Experience: The Social Course of Illness in Neurasthenia and Chronic Fatigue Syndrome." *Psychosomatic Medicine* 54 (1992a): 546–60.

———. "Depression in Neurasthenia and Chronic Fatigue Syndrome." *Psychiatric Annals* 22 (1992b): 202–208.

Wessely, Simon. "Old Wine in New Bottles: Neurasthenia and ME." *Psychological Medicine* 20 (1990): 35–53.

Von Uexküll, Thure. "Are Functional Syndromes Culture-bound?" In *Anthropologies of Medicine: A Colloquium of West European and North American Perspectives. Special Issue of Curare*, edited by B. Pflederer and G. Bibeau, 13–22. Wiesbaden: Wiesweg, 1991.

6 Credibility and the Inexplicable

Parkinson's Disease and Assumed Diagnosis in Contemporary Australia

Narelle Warren and Lenore Manderson

Diagnosis is the key point of a medical encounter where some sort of sense, and an explanation of causation, is made of bodily signs and of disabling and painful conditions. Definitive diagnosis allows clinicians to map out various actions to mitigate current symptoms and delay the progression of disease and associated debility, despite some variability in even the most common health conditions (Lutfey and McKinlay 2009). Yet for some conditions, diagnosis provides neither certainty in explaining the person's embodied (and affective) experiences nor guidance in planning for treatment, remediation, and future health management. Although uncertainty has been explored within the context of mental and developmental illness (see Potter and Myers, this volume), less attention has been paid to the vagary of diagnosis for other conditions. The reason for this, as we suggest, is that physical health problems typically present in terms of their materiality—i.e., they are on, in, and of the body—whereas mental and developmental illness diagnoses rely more on self-reports from the individual or from others around them. But uncertainty characterizes conditions where the etiology remains unknown or is not fully explicated, and for conditions where there are no obvious biomarkers. Typically, the conditions that fall into this category are contested, seen as "psychosomatic" in origin: chronic pelvic and severe menstrual pain, repetitive strain injury and back pain, myalgic encephalomyelitis, and fibromyalgia are examples here (Frazier 2002; Manderson et al. 2008; Pinder 1990). Other conditions are accepted as "real" despite diagnostic uncertainty: Parkinson's disease (PD) is one of these.

PD is an incurable neurodegenerative condition that typically affects people in later life and is characterized by tremor and bradykinesia (difficulty in initiating—akinesia—or maintaining and executing movement). After dementia, it is the second most common neurodegenerative disease affecting adults in developed countries (Tanner et al. 2008), affecting at least 630,000 people in the United States (Kowal et al. 2013) and around 64,000 people in Australia (Deloitte Access Economics 2011). Yet uncertainty pervades both the lived experience of the disease and, as we discuss, the understandings of the etiology and the course of the diagnosis itself. Idiopathic in nature, it varies considerably between individuals in terms of presentation and subsequent disease course. It is thought to be the result of the reduced, and ever decreasing, production of dopamine (a neurotransmitter that governs movement) in the brain. But as the rate of dopamine loss varies from individual to individual, so too does the rate of progression and the nature of the impacts of this degeneration. Biomedical uncertainty about PD persists even at the level of etiology: although dopamine has been implicated in the jerky yet simultaneously constant movements that typify PD, questions remain as to the pathology. While it has long been understood that Parkinson's originates in the substantia nigra of the mid-brain (Olanow and Tatton 1999), an alternative hypothesis has suggested that this does not occur until the neuropathology has well progressed. Instead, it is proposed that dopamine loss is initiated in the enteric nervous system, which is located in the gastrointestinal system, the medulla (located in the brainstem), and particularly in the olfactory bulb (Braak and Braak 2000; Braak et al. 2004). This latter location explains the early loss of smell among people with PD. Despite a lack of consensus regarding its origins, the acceptability of PD as a distinct and singular condition underlies the focus in both laboratory and clinical contexts on treatment and cure. The controversies around the disease origin extend to understandings of the natural history of the condition, and these are further complicated by the existence of multiple types of the disease (Poewe 2006).

Diagnosis typically involves some level of treatment, as we discuss below. This presents a formidable and fundamental problem in clinical practice that has not been satisfactorily theorized within the social sciences (see Smith-Morris, this volume). Regardless of its manifestation (disease type), PD progression is understood in terms of stages within which degeneration varies (Kostic et al. 2002). During the pre-clinical stage, PD is thought to progress rapidly, but it remains largely unnoticed except for a series of subtle non-motor symptoms (Poewe and Wenning 1996) that only make sense in hindsight. By the time the diagnosis is made, usually during stages 1 or 2 (early-stage PD), it is estimated that about 70–80 percent of dopamine has been lost (Wu et al. 2010). Around this point in the disease course, motor symptoms, particularly those related to posture, walk (gait), or facial expression, are evident on one side of the body. As these start to affect both sides of the body, leading to greater movement limitations and "freezing" (the inability to move), mid-stage (late stage 2 and stage 3) PD is deemed to occur. Advanced Parkinson's occurs in stages 4 and 5, when people require increasing support to undertake personal care tasks and daily activities; at this stage, many are bedridden or wheelchair-bound. The course of PD is typically characterized by an exponential slowdown: as the disease advances, the rate of progression reduces (Poewe 2006). Yet the rate at which this happens is uncertain too, varying between people based on their age—younger people typically experience a slower rate of progression overall—and comorbidities (often related to age, Poewe 2006).

In this chapter, we draw on our Australian research with 32 men and women living with Parkinson's disease to elucidate the uncertainties and lived controversies around pathways to the diagnosis of PD. In doing so, we emphasize how "certaintizing" biomedical tropes regarding diagnostics—whereby diagnosis is assumed to both be certain and to provide certainty—are challenged in multiple ways. Most people diagnosed with PD are over the age of 60 years, with prevalence doubling with each decade thereafter (Tanner et al. 2008). Our sample was atypical in that about half of those who volunteered to participate had young-onset Parkinson's disease, defined not biomedically (e.g., against mean age at onset) but socially, whereby PD is diagnosed while the person is below the Australian retirement age of 65 years. Participants resided throughout the state of Victoria in urban, peri-urban, and regional areas, and were recruited through community-based support groups, personal networks, and via snowball sampling. They were also recruited through the Fox Trial Finder website, which was set up by the Michael J. Fox Foundation (Fox Trial Finder 2015) explicitly to enable people with PD to volunteer to participate in research leading towards a cure; the very existence of this website highlights the uncertainties of diagnosis and management that characterize this condition.

PATHWAYS TO DIAGNOSIS

As the natural history of the disease indicates, PD has its onset several years before any bodily signs typically first appear. These are usually indicated by the presence of a small yet pronounced unilateral tremor or stiffness that is noticed either by the affected person, or by a family member or friend. How seriously these signs are taken depends on their severity and whether any plausible alternative explanations for them can be found. Will (aged 59, diagnosed at 58) explained that his PD-related changes were so subtle and general that he initially dismissed them as signs of "stress," and as being within the range of "normal responses" to a job that required considerable travel. "I'd do a week away and I'd come back and I'd be . . . Whereas I'd normally be tired, I was, I was finding I was absolutely exhausted, like really wiped out." As a result, he was able to interpret other bodily changes—slurring his speech, clumsiness, and disrupted sleep—as fatigue-related. Like many other participants in our study, Will only started to take his symptoms seriously when others questioned his health status. At a work function, colleagues became concerned that he'd had a stroke:

> One of them comes up to me and he says, "Will, you've had a stroke, the way you're carrying your arm." He said, "That's what happened to me." I said, "Don't be [ridiculous], I haven't had a stroke." He said, "Yes you have." I said, "No I haven't." And ah, and they were commenting on the way I was carrying my arms and, just, I was slurring my speech.

Getting from the point of recognizing that something is wrong to attending an appointment with a general practitioner (GP, family physician)—who all patients in Australia must see in order to access medical specialists and begin the path of diagnosis—varies considerably. Yet GPs also have significant gaps in terms of their knowledge of PD and in their confidence to diagnose and treat the condition (Abbott et al. 2011). Most participants described how their GP either dismissed their concerns with a "wait and see" response, following up only when symptoms persisted, or referred the participant to another health professional because they had insufficient knowledge of PD to link it with the person's bodily signs. For example, Mary's (aged 77, diagnosed at 75) doctor associated her PD-related tremor to her arthritis:

> I started to tremble, very slightly at first and it was only one side. Very slightly, so I asked the doctor. I'd drop things and get really niggly (agitated), you know. And at that stage it wasn't that bad and I asked her and she said, "I think it's benign tremors." But it slowly got worse.

Part of the difficulty in diagnosing, and in making sense of the diagnosis, relates to the apparent contrariness of symptoms. It seems implausible to people with PD that a body could be constantly mobile yet simultaneously have difficulty in moving, yet this is the experience of many people with PD. Kenneth (aged 55, diagnosed in his late 30s), for example, had experienced a unilateral benign tremor since childhood, which "swapped sides" of his body due to PD, but at the same time, he "started not being able to move" and spent much of his time just "lying around." These seemingly contradictory bodily signs were a source of confusion and uncertainty for people, prompting concerns about the etiology and the accuracy of the diagnosis, particularly fear that the symptoms were related to brain tumor or stroke, or something "more sinister" (Lisa, 47, diagnosed when she was 42) that would lead to imminent death or disablement:

> I was starting to think I had a brain tumor or something like that. Um, I thought, "Oh it might be MS (multiple sclerosis)," but I didn't know what MS symptoms really are. I mean, we have friend with MS but I wasn't really sure of what the symptoms were. So I went to the doctor, I think half expecting him to say or her to say that's what it was. (Martha, 70, diagnosed at 65)

A number of GPs also originally dismissed PD as a plausible explanation of the symptoms because of the relative youth of their patients. Fay,for example, was 55 when she first saw her doctor:

> I felt a numbness in my left arm. I sort of just disregarded it and then . . . my husband noticed it before I did, while I was holding the phone

or reading a book, I had a tremor, just while I was sitting at night, just quietly. So I went to my doctor and she looked at it and she sort of said, "Look, we'll leave it go for 6 months and see how things go." And actually it got worse and then went back to her and she sent me to a physio (physical therapist). That didn't help and I went back to her again. And she said, "I think we will do a MRI," so we did that, and then she sent me to a neurologist. That was [over] a period of 18 months. (Fay, 58, diagnosed at 55)

I went from doctor to doctor saying I've got chronic fatigue (syndrome) . . . I kept telling doctors that something was wrong with me. I kept feeling it. And it comes across in a whole lot of things. There are a whole lot of different things that occur if you have PD. (Jay, 52, diagnosed at 47)

In contrast, Wayne (68, diagnosed at 62) attended a new doctor who openly admitted to him her lack of knowledge about PD:

I went to a doctor, 'cause I wasn't feeling well. I really was starting to run out of energy, I'd go to start to do something and I just couldn't do it. So I thought, that's stupid, so I went to, to see a doctor, just a GP and I said to her. I'd never seen her before, and I said, "I think I've got Parkinson's disease." And she looked at me and said, "Well I'm not qualified to, to do anything to look at that because it's more . . . observation, than anything else." So that's when she gave me a referral to a neurologist.

Such examples highlight one of the ways in which PD diagnosis contests the nature of medical authority. The public—these and other participants included—in general presume that doctors should be able to bring together any set of symptoms to produce a definitive diagnosis, either on the basis of clinical signs or as a result of various pathology tests (depending on the suspected condition, from blood tests, MRI, ultrasound, etc.). Yet, as Armstrong and Hilton (2014) found, doctors vary in their use of diagnostic tools even for common conditions, exercising discretion and often using such procedures for social rather than biomedical reasons. This is not recognized by patients, however, whose trust in medical authority is founded on the assemblages of diagnosis—tests, procedures, and tools—which all contribute to the sense of absoluteness or certainty derived from this process.

Through health education campaigns aimed at encouraging early diagnosis, through direct mail-outs encouraging people over 50 to screen for colon cancer, reminder letters to women of this age also to have a biannual mammogram, and numerous television medical documentaries and hospital drama serials, people are very familiar with the aspects of diagnosis, the technologies used to classify and provide clarity, and the etiquette of its communication.

This is not the case for PD: no screening tests or biomarkers in blood or other body fluids or tissue are available, the signs of PD vary widely from one person to another, and most signs of PD are common also across a range of other conditions. The inability of GPs to recognize or manage PD highlights the limits of biomedical, scientific, and clinical knowledge for patients seeking clarity around signs that they regard as abnormal. These limits have disrupted the traditional doctor-patient power structures within the medical encounter, eroding patient trust and confidence and leaving them to question the competence of their provider. It also has left them confused: how could so little be known about a condition with which they were already familiar?

The experiences of the individuals described above were in stark contrast to the (few) instances where the GP was able to clearly identify the nature (if not the specific reason) of the participant's complaint, which had the effect of consolidating the medical knowledge and expertise of that particular GP. Athena (51, diagnosed at 48) initially thought she had carpal tunnel syndrome due to stiffness in one arm. However, her GP suspected that this rigidity was likely to have some sort of neurological basis, and she immediately referred her to a neurologist, who then referred her to a movement disorders specialist (a subspecialty of neurology). Having opportunities to observe the person in action was clearly helpful for GPs, at least in determining the direction of their referral and so the eventual differential diagnosis and exclusion of other conditions. Will's doctor had seen him in his bathing suit at the beach, and so had observed his increasing rigidity and posture—which meant that Will typically stood with his arms perpendicular to his body (as if he was pushing a wheeled walker—rollator—or similar):

> It was only when I went to the doctor . . . it was a one minute diagnosis, you know, and he was right . . . because he'd already seen me walking and my arms, you know, when I stand in the water . . . He just said to me, "I've noticed [your symptoms] too and I was gonna tell you to come and see me."

Even when a GP was confident in his or her assessment, participants were required to attend a neurologist or, better yet, a movement disorders specialist for a formal diagnosis. The idea of a "proper diagnosis" is especially important in the context of PD, given the lack of uniform screening procedures (although screening questionnaires have been developed for specific, localized populations, Chan et al. 2000), the absence of a distinct etiology or clear natural history of the disease, and, as we describe below, the lack of clear biomarkers to definitively "prove" that the person has PD. For many participants, this was imperative in order for them to even consider accepting that they had the disease:

> I suppose at that particular point, even though he had told me that I had it (PD), and I probably deep down knew that he was 100 percent

correct, I still wanted to go through the tests and everything and sort of be properly diagnosed before I accepted that I had anything. (Will)

Diagnosis by a medical specialist as opposed to a GP was significant here for two reasons. First, it reinforced the medical authority that might otherwise be undermined by diagnostic uncertainties, by providing "the best possible" diagnosis (as described by many participants), and emphasized the idea that it takes a particular expertise to correctly identify PD. Second, this in turn reproduced biomedical tropes of "diagnosis as certainty" but more importantly, that of "certainty as diagnosis." It is to this latter point that we now turn.

DIAGNOSIS AS A PROCESS

PD diagnosis itself occurs across four phases and is based on an uncertain trajectory. First, bodily signs are considered. Then, as we outline in greater detail below, alternative explanations for these signs are excluded. Third, responsiveness to PD medication is determined, at which point a diagnosis is made: if the signs respond to the medication, then the diagnosis of PD is

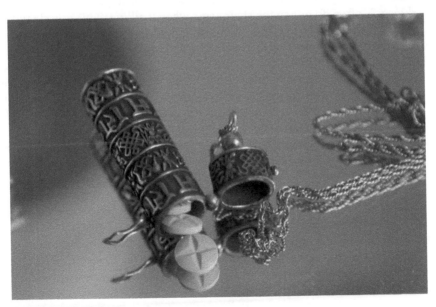

Figure 6.1   Tibetan Prayer Wheel Pillbox. Highlighting her ambivalence around the certainty of her PD diagnosis, Lisa did not disclose her diagnosis with anyone and strategically disguised her condition in multiple ways, including through the use of jewelry to hide her medication. Photo: "Lisa," photovoice project, copyright Narelle Warren

given. Fourth, a definitive diagnosis is only possible at autopsy. Each of the first three steps requires time, including the time taken to get an appointment with the specialist, and the process of diagnosis is often lengthy. For the people in our study, this took at least six months' time, with many taking at least a year to be diagnosed. Yet the process of diagnosis also continues beyond the actual moment of diagnosis—when the specialist advises the patient that he or she has PD—it is further refined through continuing tests during subsequent visits to the specialist (Jankovic et al. 2000). In this way, diagnosis operates as a type of funneling process.

Diagnosis Through Embodied Observations

Given the absence of clear biological markers or diagnostic tests, a formal diagnosis relies on the observed presence of four cardinal or main symptoms ("clinical criteria," Jankovic 2008; Litvan et al. 2003), of which at least two must be present in order for PD to be considered. *Tremor*—shaking or trembling on one side of the body when at rest—is the most readily recognized sign, yet it is not always present: Parkinson's Australia, the peak advocacy organization at the national level, suggests that up to one-third of people do not experience tremor at the time of diagnosis (2008). *Rigidity or stiffness* manifests itself in a type of resistance to movement or muscle tightness, leaving the muscles unable to relax; in consequence, people with Parkinson's often do not swing their arms when walking. This muscle tightness is also responsible for facial "masking" or *hypomimia* that is common in PD, when people show either a lack of or reduced range of expressions (Jankovic 2008). *Bradykinesia* refers to slowness in initiating (akinesia) and maintaining or performing bodily movements, which may also be a form of compensation for some of the difficulties imposed by rigidity (Phillips et al. 1994). The last cardinal sign is *postural instability*, which refers to the difficulty a person may experience in maintaining balance when performing asymmetric movements (such as reaching overhead with one hand, Morris et al. 2000); this is present in far fewer people than other signs, and is thus contested as "cardinal" (de Rijk et al. 1997). These signs are interpreted through the subjective knowledge and expertise of the treating neurologist.

PD is common enough that a popular understanding associates it almost exclusively with tremor and bradykinesia, but in fact, these can be caused by a range of things[1] and are not diagnostic. At the same time, Parkinson's is associated with a range of non-motor symptoms that appear well before any of the cardinal motor symptoms, and well before an individual with them seeks medical advice. These are mundane and common, not typically associated with PD but rather initially interpreted as related to aging, as was the case for Will:

> I'm not getting any younger. I mean I was in my late fifties [at diagnosis]. Some men in their fifties are in magnificent physical condition and,

you know, some people in their fifties are almost old and decrepit, you know. So I wasn't feeling old and decrepit, but I certainly was . . . of the belief that I was actually getting older, you know . . . more fumbling in terms of you know, making a cup of tea, or trying to get a cap off a jar or, it's sort of, as I said, things that you put down to other, to other causes . . . and even, you know, bouts of constipation, hmm . . . stuttering, the um [messy] eating . . . I wasn't consciously sort of concerned that I had anything particularly, particularly wrong.

These broad signs include reduced (hyposmia) or absent (anosmia) sense of smell, depression, pain, genitourinary problems—constipation, an overactive bladder, reduced sexual desire or inability to achieve erection/arousal or orgasm—and sleep problems (restlessness or inability to stay asleep, Chaudhuri et al. 2006; Sakakibara et al. 2010). Taken alone or in combination, many people would have these signs but would not have PD. Hence, diagnoses are made based on a confluence of common bodily signs and symptoms, such as poor mobility, tremor, and sleep problems, which vary between individuals and in the timing of their onset. Because the "symptoms" are *syndromically* considered to be *most likely* Parkinson's, PD is always a presumed diagnosis.

Diagnosis as a Method of Exclusion

Once the "fit" between the bodily signs and the cardinal markers of PD has been established, the only way to get diagnostic certainty—at least to the point that medication can be prescribed (the third step in the process)—is by excluding various other conditions. This typically involves the patient undergoing a range of tests, including blood tests, EEGs, CT scans, or MRIs, while the clinician works through possible other pathologies until all of these are excluded. At this point, the clinician reaches a point of confidence to prescribe dopamine-replacement (often, a type of *L-dopa*) medication. As potential alternative diagnoses are excluded, Parkinson's becomes increasingly likely.

The exclusionary nature of diagnostics in this context means that the diagnosis itself is rarely, if ever, made at a single clinical visit. Instead, time—both time to search for other explanations and time to observe bodily or functional changes—is an essential diagnostic component. For some participants, such as Mary and Roy (76, diagnosed at 72), temporality was employed to ascertain whether their symptoms were due to arthritis or PD, as Roy explained. He had had knee replacement surgery: "So some parts of (Parkinson's) were operating at that time . . . I can't tell the difference, I still have trouble telling the difference between what's caused by the bad knee because I still have soreness of the patella . . . That slows me through pain, whereas the Parkinson's slows me through motor organization of the body. And sometimes it's hard to tell them apart." Yet for them, the process of exclusion was fairly straightforward. Sheila (83 years), aged 79 at the time of her diagnosis, explained how she had lost power in her hands and was first referred by her GP to a geriatrician, who in turn referred her to a neurologist:

> I couldn't cut my meat. I was weak in the hand and no one was sort of taking much notice. I had trouble opening the front door sometimes with the key and that sort of thing . . . then when I said to the [geriatrician] I couldn't cut my meat, he decided, "Well we better do something," so then he . . . sent me to a, I don't know, what sort of a scan, and then he made an appointment through a specialist . . . and then he diagnosed me.

Whereas the process of exclusion to reach a diagnosis of PD was relatively straightforward for the older participants, a considerable period of time elapsed for the younger participants in our study, as their clinicians excluded first one, then another, then subsequent possibilities in the search for a potential explanation for their symptoms. Athena (51, diagnosed at 50 after one year) described how she spent several months in considerable distress thinking she had a brain tumor, before she was finally diagnosed with PD:

> It was in August 2011, just over two years ago . . . So, I went to the doctor's in January . . . and I thought, "It'll just be carpal tunnel syndrome." Didn't want to think anything else. And she said, "Oh, I think there is something wrong, and I'm not sure what it is, but I don't think it's carpal tunnel syndrome and I think I should refer you to a neurologist." So I went to see a neurologist, and that took a few months to get in to see him . . . And um, when he saw me, he actually thought that I might have had a brain tumor, which was pretty frightening. In fact it was very frightening . . . When he told me that it really rocked me, and I was actually, I mean I took it on the chin on the day, but after that I really was very worried and um, he referred me for an MRI which I couldn't get into for, I think it was a couple of weeks, and so a bit of sweating on that, you know, waiting to have the MRI . . . Then it was another week of waiting for that, and I came back to see him for the results and I found out that it wasn't a brain tumor. So that was very much a huge relief . . . and um, when he told me it was Parkinson's disease it was like, "Oh, is that all?"

Further complicating this process, GPs appeared to be reluctant to refer younger participants to specialist clinicians, and they typically searched for and excluded a range of other possibilities before they decided to refer their patient. The discretionary nature of diagnostics—and the potential influence of social factors in the GPs' decision-making—was clearly evident in these accounts (Armstrong and Hilton 2014). This was frustrating for participants, however, and, as Frida (55, recently diagnosed after 3 years) explained, it reinforced their lack of confidence in their GPs around PD:

> My GP didn't seem to follow my symptoms very well and didn't refer me to a specialist, so it took a long time to get a diagnosis . . . I developed a frozen shoulder, which is probably a classic symptom, but I thought I'd hurt myself at work . . . It was described as bursitis and I had physio (physical therapy) and cortisone injections and things like that which helped a bit but eventually it sorted itself out, and then I began to develop um stiffness in my left hand . . . and I began to have a tremor and my left leg was less strong than my right, so I began to limp a bit, so it just progressed from there . . . She thought I should have a scan, a brain scan, and I told her my mother had Parkinson's and I just felt it was MS or Parkinson's or something like that, [but] she said that [the brain scan] will solve it, and of course it (PD) doesn't show up on a scan . . . but of course I kept getting worse and eventually I went back to her, and she was a bit alarmed and sent me off to a neurologist and I got a confirmation pretty much straight away, and then [this was confirmed by] a second opinion.

The process of exclusion is a necessary part of the diagnosis of PD, precisely because of its lack of biomarkers and the possibility that the characteristic signs could be due to something more pernicious. However, the reasons for this approach—particularly to eliminate other conditions (a brain tumor, for example) for which rapid attention might be needed—were often not made clear to the patients during their interactions with the clinicians. Will described how he received no explanation of the diagnostic processes, nor what the outcomes of tests might or might not reveal:

> So [my GP] referred me to a specialist, a neurologist, and it took a long time to get in. There was a communication problem . . . in terms of understanding, he was saying, "You have the symptoms of Parkinson's, we can't give a, give a strict diagnosis, we have to monitor you over, over the next three or four months, see how you go." And he booked me in for an MRI, and the MRI came back all clear, and the way he communicated, he said, "You're all clear." But all it said, all he meant to say, was, "Your MRI is clear." And he didn't actually explain to me that they're using it to eliminate, rather than, than diagnose, you know . . . they were just eliminating that it wasn't MS or it wasn't [a] motor neuron disease . . . So I thought I was okay and then . . . I was waking up and this right hand was shaking . . . And I said, "Oh well that's it, I've gotta do something about this." I knew I was deteriorating, you know, so I managed to get into the [same] specialist pretty quickly, he'd had a cancellation, just as it turned out, that day . . . and he said, "Yes,

you've got Parkinson's." . . . And um, anyway, he sort of panicked a bit and he referred me to a [movement disorder specialist] . . . and ah, he fully diagnosed me.

Although Will felt reasonably certain after his second visit to the neurologist that he had PD, this was still not definitive: PD is always a residual or assumed diagnosis. In the context of PD and other neurodegenerative disorders, neurologists, movement disorder specialists, and GPs only have tools for exclusion, leading to an imprecise diagnosis that rests not on biomarkers or scans, but instead on a series of judgments about which they can be uncertain. In some instances, diagnostic uncertainty and the resulting lack of confidence was extended to the neurologists, despite their claim to have expertise in PD. Peach (aged 52, diagnosed at 47), for example, first sought medical advice about her symptoms at 43, but was not diagnosed with PD for another four years:

> The neurologist . . . said I could have Parkinson's disease, I could have Wilson's disease, it might be MS. They didn't even know what it was. "Go and have a brain scan." So I had a brain scan and they found, what do you call it, missing little white bits in my brain. I don't know what it was. So then I freaked out . . . They said it was nothing, basically it was fluid in my brain which was nothing to be alarmed at. So he said, "I don't know what the matter with you is. Go away and come back if it gets worse." So I went away for a year and then . . . I wasn't that much worse, but I noticed I lost my arm swing. Then I went to another doctor and another neurologist and he said, "You've got Parkinson's disease."

Because she did not understand that a differential diagnosis was not possible, Peach interpreted the failure of the first neurologist to even give her an explanation for the anomalies found on her brain scan to reflect his clinical incompetence. When her symptoms progressed, she decided to see a different neurologist.

Diagnosis therefore relies on clinical expertise and the assessment of the subjective changes noticed by individuals themselves, clinical anecdotes, and a series of assumptions, including those in relation to age. As a result, diagnostic error is high: about one-quarter of people diagnosed with Parkinson's in Canada and the UK were found to be misdiagnosed during autopsy, and UK community-based studies of people taking Parkinson's-specific medication suggest that misdiagnosis may occur in up to half of those assumed to have PD (Jankovic 2008; Tolosa et al. 2006). While the expertise of the diagnosing clinician is thought to be significant here, and movement disorder specialists are much less likely to misdiagnose than general neurologists (~8 percent, Hughes et al. 2002; Jankovic et al. 2000), these relatively high rates of error speak to the imperfectness of diagnosing PD: each misdiagnosed case represents a missed condition (i.e., the alternative explanation for the symptoms).

The exclusionary nature of different conditions in the process of PD diagnosis also highlights the importance of technologies for diagnostic certainty. Wayne, for example, had undergone a series of tests as part of the diagnosis process when he was informed that he had an elevated level of prostate-specific antigens (PSAs). As a result, he had multiple biopsies to determine whether he had prostate cancer while his clinician continued to determine whether he also had PD. The juxtaposition of the vagueness of the PD diagnosis and the certainty offered by the presence of PSA-specific biomarkers highlights why participants lose confidence in their (PD) doctor's clinical skills, and in their assessments of clinical competence. Yet, in the absence of tests, specialists rely heavily on experiential knowledge in making a judgment as to whether a patient had PD or not. Fay highlighted the simplicity of some of the PD tests, in contrast with the sophisticated technology for other conditions. She had had an MRI, which was negative (for cancer). Her doctor explained:

> With Parkinson's, there is nothing, it doesn't show at all. He then did a series of tests with me like walking. The other thing was that my husband had noticed that when I was walking I was swinging my left arm, or I would be holding it . . . So he did a series of tests where I had to walk up and down the hallway of his medical rooms and [he] looked at my gait and then, then I had my arms out and a series of tests, like make me say things backwards. And so the leg was going and the arm was going and then he said to me, "well you look like someone who probably gets on the net a bit and Googles yourself and so what do you think you've got?" And I just jokingly said, "I think I've got Parkinson's disease" and he had a stone face and he said, "look I really hate to tell you this, but that's exactly what you've got" . . . So then [he] put me on a drip start of a regime of drugs.

Treatment as Diagnosis

Over time, following multiple other tests, where no other explanation is found, a PD diagnosis becomes increasingly certain, evident by a person's responses to the drug *L-dopa* (usually prescribed under the generic name of levodopa), which promotes the production of dopamine in the nervous system. Once it is clear that a patient is responding to the dopamine, the patient is prescribed the full treatment, which involves a range of other medications in addition to levodopa. Adrian (aged 83, diagnosed at 81) was in the hospital following a bladder operation when his doctor diagnosed him with PD, seemingly out of the blue, by evaluating his response to the medication. Adrian was diagnosed only because of the treatment he was receiving for another condition. Medication may therefore "confirm" the diagnosis, although this may also occur through clinical and personal observations, as Martha explained:

> They say it's often 12–18 months until they get onto the right medica-
> tion that suits but mine was pretty good right from the start . . . At one
> stage, I thought . . . "I reckon I have been misdiagnosed, I don't have
> it at all" . . . It's just ridiculous me taking this tablets and doing all this
> when I don't really have it, so I didn't take them. I soon knew I had
> Parkinson's disease.

As is highlighted here, medication and its effects provided a type of "proof" of the PD diagnosis. Medication played a significant role in Lisa's diagnosis, for instance, although she reframed the "watch and see" approach described by Adrian as a technical approach to diagnosis: "I saw [a neurologist] and we did some tests . . . dopamine replacement tests, and I didn't do very well on any of them."

Because the onset of PD is usually at mature age, however, the effect of medication, as a pointer to diagnosis, requires careful interpretation because of the effects of other health conditions. Malcolm (aged 79, diagnosed at 72) had Crohn's disease and was unable to absorb the oral medication as he was missing part of his intestines. This presented a significant challenge during diagnosis. Although all of the other indicators pointed to PD, his failure to respond to the medication meant that the diagnosis could not be confirmed. Treatment failure is not uncommon for various reasons, and this again highlights the problematic nature of differential diagnosis. False negatives and false positives are always possible, and the ambiguity of this does little to resolve the uncertainty of diagnostics in this context.

Diagnosis as a Moment In Time

The moment of diagnosis—the point at which they were told they had Parkinson's—was salient for all of the participants in our study. For many, there were several such moments. At each visit to the specialist or GP when Wayne reported some functional or cognitive decline, the diagnosis was reinforced. "As things have gotten worse, (my neurologist) says that's telling me my original diagnosis was correct." Each visit therefore represented discrete "moments" of diagnosis. Yet this "narrowing down"—or, as we called it earlier, "certaintizing"—of the PD diagnosis can only occur within a context of functional losses, which themselves reconsolidate the authority of biomedicine (following the loss of this status earlier in the diagnostic pathway); this authority is further established in each subsequent clinical encounter. At the same time, the expertise of the individual specialist is also reinforced. The plausibility of the explanation given is central here: because diagnosis occurs via the multiple steps described above, it was sometimes met with disbelief, which led to follow-up or second-opinion consultations.

This supplementary pathway of second opinions, more tests, and the reiteration of the diagnosis was not uncommon. Because of the association between PD and aging, this was especially the case for the younger people (Baker and Graham 2004), who typically reported many more diagnostic "moments" than the older participants in our study.

Conceptualizing diagnosis as a point in time, whether it occurs at single or multiple points, is significant because it serves to resolve uncertainty, even though this may lead to new questions of treatment, etiology, heredity, prognosis, and pathways. Prior to diagnosis, there is always the possibility of "imaginitis:" almost every participant in our study reported the feeling that something "wasn't quite right," but that this was really just in their imagination. Diagnosis therefore functioned to validate the bodily (and, to a lesser extent, cognitive and emotional) symptoms of the participants, and gave these symptoms a name that suggested the possibility of manageability. Even though it led to further questions or was fleeting, diagnosis provided a moment of certainty; this was true regardless of any further uncertainties around treatment or management. For participants, being told that they had an atypical presentation was better than an admission from their neurologist that "we don't know what is wrong with you." Lisa experienced no tremors, but had extreme pain, rigidity, and stiffness; she still worked full-time in a profession that required public speaking and found that she was often tongue-tied or slurred her speech. However, because these symptoms could be attributed to other causes, she struggled with questions of legitimacy: "Because it is not so apparent in my symptoms, I feel like if I complain, I look like I'm making things up." Even though she still questioned whether she had PD, having a label to explain her symptoms was helpful in social situations when people otherwise thought she was intoxicated:

> I was at a bar once and I hadn't had a drink and I was waiting to be served and [the barman] heard me speaking to my friend next me and . . . he ignored me and he served the person behind me, and I thought, "you think I'm drunk!" . . . And when I'm really tired, my voice is worse and I can see people looking at me saying, "what is wrong with her, has she had a stroke or something."

The diagnostic label also allowed a person to interpret what they had experienced, and therefore provided some level of recovery of the past, either implicitly (as for most participants) or explicitly, as Jillian (aged 63, diagnosed at 51) exclaimed, "It was like he (the neurologist) sort of gave me back three years." A diagnosis is a vehicle of sense making. Things that happen to the body are put into perspective. Fatigue and the general slowing down of movement, for example, led to considerable confusion and consternation for participants, but made sense in light of the eventual diagnosis. For example, Fay had experienced several years of numbness and sporadic pain in different parts of her body, and had experienced constant seriously disrupted sleep: "I started acting out my dreams, and I'd be yelling and screaming and swearing, and I don't like [to] swear, and kicking and fighting [though] I would supposedly be asleep." Diagnosis brought with it a feeling of relief; it gave her a narrative structure to make sense of all of the strange bodily events that she had been experiencing. "Now that I have been diagnosed . . . it actually made me, in a way, much as I didn't like to be told that I had Parkinson's, it was like a relief. Because I actually thought I was going nuts."

This feeling of relief was reported predominantly by the younger participants in our study, who had worried that their symptoms were due to much more sinister causes, such as a brain tumor (as with Athena) or motor neuron disease (MND, also known as ALS, as with Will). Juxtaposed against this feeling of relief was a sense of disappointment. Will had thought, following his MRI, that he did not have anything seriously wrong with him; while he was relieved not to have MND or MS, his PD diagnosis was tempered by the miscommunicated reassurance from his clinician that he was "all clear:"

> The implication that I took away from it was, was that I was actually going to be okay and they were just going to monitor me, and I thought they had picked up whether I had Parkinson's or not. What had happened is that they hadn't picked up the Parkinson's.

Thus, even at the point of certainty—the moment of diagnosis—PD presents a range of conflicting responses.

The Personal Controversies of Diagnosis

The imperative to know about the reason for a related set of bodily signs (the diagnosis) is important regardless of the illness context, because it clarifies the appropriate treatments and offers an end to the pursuit of (often multiple) tests, physicians, and false starts. Diagnosis offers an opportunity, not only of certainty, but also of a new ways of life and relating with others. Many participants in our study became involved in support organizations after their diagnosis. But while diagnosis enables participants to map the actions to take in managing or living with a particular condition, it simultaneously and inevitably leads to questions about the future. The idiopathic nature—particularly the variable physical decline—of PD means that these questions often cannot be resolved to participants' satisfaction. This diagnosis is thus one of certain decline (including uncertain but increased likelihood of dementia and depression), but also of uncertain etiology, progression, controversies around medication and the range of drugs that can be used, and uncertain death. As a result, the usual moment of certainty offered by diagnosis as seen in other conditions—such as those described by Wayne—is absent. As a result, any statements about what will happen next within the illness course are always bracketed with "we don't really know, but we'll try." Some level of uncertainty or tentativeness inevitably continues.

This is particularly salient given the increasing care needs of people with PD. As they reach stages 4 and 5, participants lose independence and become increasingly reliant on others for all of their everyday needs. But future planning is limited because the point at which this occurs remains widely variable: some people are considered to have advanced PD within five years of diagnosis, whereas others will not reach this point for well over a decade. Knowing that the constellation of symptoms are Parkinson's, and not another condition, leaves each patient with "certain" knowledge of uncertainty: that the trajectory of the disease varies from individual to individual, that little can be done to intervene to alter this course, that, despite an overwhelming range of treatment strategies, the choice of medications is a matter of trial and error, and finally, that the prognosis, while negative, is unpredictable. Many chronic conditions are managed by trial and error, but the pathways available to patient and clinician are reasonably clear, and hence a diagnosis eases anxiety and provides clear direction to manage symptoms, delay progression, or to attempt to cure. A diagnosis of Parkinson's does the reverse: it confirms to patients that some states of illness and disruption are unknown, unpredictable, and intractable.

CONCLUSION

Diagnosis is a process of reading clinical signs and symptoms, interpreting pathology tests and, in some cases, assessing treatment efficacy as a diagnosis. Time is part of the diagnostic process as a means of mapping changes in signs or symptoms in order to exclude idiopathy and establish chronicity. Other conditions, including those requiring urgent attention (such as infection or a neoplasm), need to be excluded. For most diseases, especially those that are relatively common, diagnosis is sped up by the availability of serology, medical imaging, and other pathology tests. PD deviates from diagnosis as certainty because of the absence of any definitive measures. Diagnosis can only be confirmed post-mortem.

Diagnosis is a vehicle of sense making, providing an understanding as to how social lives can be managed within the context of illness. Patient confusion derives from the fact that a diagnosis is typically understood to verify or validate the felt, observed, and reported signs and symptoms as characteristics of a particular condition. Without diagnosis, these are inexplicable. People with PD are always faced with equivocation; at best, they "probably" have PD. This is usually assumed to be unproblematic or "good enough." Clinicians are not withholding a diagnosis: they don't have one. This means that the idea of a "proper diagnosis" is never fully possible. Faced with their own clinicians' uncertainty, people with PD continue to search for clarification.

The relationship of diagnostic methods to the triad of etiology, treatment, and cure dominates the biomedical literature, reflecting the interests of the research community and of advocacy organizations. Diagnosis itself is not seen as problematic; instead, it offers a gateway to this triad. Not only does the diagnostic label raise questions of etiology, but it prompts entry into a new world of treatment and generates new interest in a PD cure. Each of these are seen as worthy of research interest in their own right, as is reflected in the research strategies of the major PD-specific foundations. An industry now exists for examining the genetics of PD. The Michael J. Fox Foundation for Parkinson's Research, for example, is largely concerned with therapeutic priorities; biomarkers were only identified in late 2014 as a potentially fundable area. Similarly, the Shake It Up Australia Foundation explicitly funds research into a PD cure. Social issues—the everyday management of illness, disease, and debility and their impact on interpersonal relationships, clinical interactions and care, and quality of life—are far less imperative for researchers than a cure. GPs' lack of knowledge is combined with neurologists' lack of time and social skills in communicating their own equivocation and the ambiguities of the disease. These have profound impacts on the ways that their patients live their lives, including their decisions about disclosing their diagnosis, their ability to communicate with others about the management of existing symptoms, the emergence of new symptoms, and their prognosis. The default position is that any sign or symptom that arises after the presumed diagnosis is related to PD. This gives rise to two options. One requires vigilance both on the part of the person and their family members, with constant reporting back to clinicians to determine whether any new condition has developed. Far more common is the assumption that any new symptom—unless startlingly different—is simply another step along the PD journey.

NOTE

1 While bradykinesia is predominantly associated with neurological disorders, e.g., fibromyalgia (Heredia-Jimenez & Soto-Hermoso, 2014), dementia (Bramell-Risberg et al., 2013), Wilson's disease (Heredia-Jimenez & Soto-Hermoso, 2014), Huntington's disease (Kotschet et al., 2014), or other neurodegenerative diseases (Zhang et al., 2013), it is also caused by some infectious diseases, including spotted fever Rickettsia (Kularatne et al., 2012). In contrast, tremor is much more common and is caused by neurological or physical illness, as well as due to drug reactions, alcohol misuse, heavy metal poisoning, fatigue/exhaustion, or may be of no known cause (National Institute of Neurological Disorders and Stroke, 2014).

REFERENCES

Abbott, L. M., S. L. Naismith, and S. J.G. Lewis. "Parkinson's Disease in General Practice: Assessing Knowledge, Confidence and the Potential Role of Education."

Journal of Clinical Neuroscience 18, no. 8 (2011): 1044–47. doi: http://dx.doi.org/10.1016/j.jocn.2010.12.041.

Armstrong, Natalie and Paul Hilton. "Doing Diagnosis: Whether and How Clinicians Use a Diagnostic Tool of Uncertain Clinical Utility." *Social Science & Medicine* 120 (2014): 208–14. doi: http://dx.doi.org/10.1016/j.socscimed.2014.09.032.

Baker, Mary G., and Lizzie Graham. "The Journey: Parkinson's Disease." *BMJ* 329, no. 7466 (2004): 611–14. doi: 10.1136/bmj.329.7466.611.

Braak, H. and E. Braak. "Pathoanatomy of Parkinson's Disease." *Journal of Neurology* 247, no. 2 (2000): II3–II10. doi: 10.1007/PL00007758.

Braak, H., E. Ghebremedhin, U. Rüb, H. Bratzke, and K. Del Tredici. "Stages in the Development of Parkinson's Disease-Related Pathology." *Cell and Tissue Research* 318, no. 1 (2004): 121–34. doi: 10.1007/s00441–004–0956–9.

Bramell-Risberg, Eva, Gun-Britt Jarnlo, and Solve Elmstahl. "Older Women with Dementia Can Perform Fast Alternating Forearm Movements and Performance Is Correlated with Tests of Lower Extremity Function." *Clinical Interventions in Aging* 8 (2013): 175–84. doi: 10.2147/cia.s37733.

Chan, Daniel Kam Yin, W. T. Hung, A. Wong, E. Hu, and R. G. Beran. "Validating a Screening Questionnaire for Parkinsonism in Australia." *Journal of Neurology, Neurosurgery & Psychiatry* 69 no. 1 (2000): 117–20. doi: 10.1136/jnnp.69.1.117.

Chaudhuri, K. Ray, Daniel G. Healy, and Anthony Schapira. "Non-Motor Symptoms of Parkinson's Disease: Diagnosis and Management." *The Lancet Neurology* 5, no. 3 (2006): 235–45. doi: http://dx.doi.org/10.1016/S1474–4422(06)70373–8.

de Rijk, M. C., W. A. Rocca, D. W. Anderson, M. O. Melcon, M. M. B. Breteler, and D. M. Maraganore. "A Population Perspective on Diagnostic Criteria for Parkinson's Disease." *Neurology* 48, no. 5 (1997): 1277–81. doi: 10.1212/wnl.48.5.1277.

Deloitte Access Economics, D. *Living with Parkinson's Disease—Update*. Sydney: Parkinson's Australia, 2011.

Fox Trial Finder. *The Michael J. Fox Foundation for Parkinson's Research*. Accessed January 4, 2015. www.foxtrialfinder.org.

Frazier, Leslie D. "Stability and Change in Patterns of Coping with Parkinson's Disease." *The International Journal of Aging and Human Development* 55, no. 3 (2002): 207–31. doi: 10.2190/UA78–79LB-4GCF-8MJT.

Heredia-Jimenez, J. M., & Soto-Hermoso, V. M. "Kinematics Gait Disorder in Men with Fibromyalgia." *Rheumatology International* 34, no. 1 (2014): 63–65. doi: 10.1007/s00296–012–2651–6.

Hughes, Andrew J., Susan E. Daniel, Yoav Ben-Shlomo, and Andrew J. Lees. "The Accuracy of Diagnosis of Parkinsonian Syndromes in a Specialist Movement Disorder Service." *Brain* 125, no. 4 (2002): 861–70. doi: 10.1093/brain/awf080.

Jankovic, Joseph. "Parkinson's Disease: Clinical Features and Diagnosis." *Journal of Neurology, Neurosurgery & Psychiatry* 79, no. 4 (2008): 368–76. doi: 10.1136/jnnp.2007.131045.

Jankovic, Joseph, Ali H. Rajput, Michael P. McDermott, and Daniel Perl. "The Evolution of Diagnosis in Early Parkinson Disease." *Archives of Neurology* 57, no. 3 (2000): 369–72.

Kostic, V. S., J. Marinkovic, M. Svetel, E. Stefanova, and S. Przedborski. "The Effect of Stage of Parkinson's Disease at the Onset of Levodopa Therapy on Development of Motor Complications." *European Journal of Neurology* 9 (2002): 9–14.

Kotschet, Katya, S. Osborn, and M. K. Horne. "Automated Assessment of Bradykinesia and Chorea in Huntington's Disease." *Movement Disorders* 29 (2014): S209–S210.

Kowal, Stacy, Timothy M. Dall, Ritashree Chakrabarti, Michael V. Storm, and Anjali Jain. "The Current and Projected Economic Burden of Parkinson's Disease in the United States." *Movement Disorders* 28, no. 3 (2013): 311–18. doi: 10.1002/mds.25292.

Kularatne, S.A. M., Weerakoon, K.G.A. D., Rajapakse, R.P.V.J., Madagedara, S.C., Nanayakkara, D., and Premaratna, R. "A Case Series of Spotted Fever Rickettsiosis with Neurological Manifestations in Sri Lanka." *International Journal of Infectious Diseases* 16, no. 7 (2012): E514–E517. doi: 10.1016/j.ijid.2012.02.016.

Litvan, Irene, Kailash Bhatia, David J. Burn, Christopher G. Goetz, Anthony E. Lang, Ian McKeith, Niall Quinn, Kapil D. Sethi, Cliff Shults, and Gregor K. Wenning. "Sic Task Force Appraisal of Clinical Diagnostic Criteria for Parkinsonian Disorders." *Movement Disorders* 18, no. 5 (2003): 467–86. doi: 10.1002/mds.10459.

Lutfey, Karen E. and John B. McKinlay. "What Happens Along the Diagnostic Pathway to CHD Treatment? Qualitative Results Concerning Cognitive Processes." *Sociology of Health & Illness* 31, no. 7 (2009): 1077–92. doi: 10.1111/j.1467-9566.2009.01181.x.

Manderson, Lenore, Narelle Warren, and Milica Markovic. "Circuit Breaking: Pathways of Treatment Seeking for Women with Endometriosis in Australia." *Qualitative Health Research* 18, no. 4 (2008): 522–34. doi: 10.1177/1049732308315432.

Morris, Meg, Robert Iansek, Fiona Smithson, and Frances Huxham. "Postural Instability in Parkinson's Disease: A Comparison with and without a Concurrent Task." *Gait & Posture* 12, no. 3 (2000): 205–16. doi: http://dx.doi.org/10.1016/S0966-6362(00)00076-X.

National Institute of Neurological Disorders and N. Stroke. (July 24, 2014). *Tremor Fact Sheet.* Accessed December 17, 2014. http://www.ninds.nih.gov/disorders/tremor/detail_tremor.htm.

Olanow, C.W., and W. G. Tatton. "Etiology and Pathogenesis of Parkinson's Disease." *Annual Review of Neuroscience* 22, no. 1 (1999): 123–44. doi:10.1146/annurev.neuro.22.1.123.

Parkinson's Australia. "What is Parkinson's?", 2008. Accessed September 29, 2014. http://www.parkinsons.org.au/about-ps/whatps.html.

Phillips, James G., K. E. Martin, John L. Bradshaw, and Robert Iansek. "Could Bradykinesia in Parkinson's Disease Simply Be Compensation?" *Journal of Neurology* 241, no. 7 (1994): 439–47. doi: 10.1007/BF00900963.

Pinder, R. "What to Expect: Information and the Management of Uncertainty in Parkinson's Disease." *Disability, Handicap & Society* 5, no. 1 (1990): 77–92. doi: 10.1080/02674649066780061.

Poewe, Werner H. "The Natural History of Parkinson's Disease." *Journal of Neurology* 253, Suppl. 7 (2006): VII2–6. doi: 10.1007/s00415-006-7002-7.

Poewe, Werner H., and Gregor K. Wenning. "The Natural History of Parkinson's Disease." *Neurology* 47, 6 Suppl. 3 (1996): 146S–52S. doi: 10.1212/WNL.47.6_Suppl_3.146S.

Sakakibara, Ryuji, Tomoyuki Uchiyama, Tomonori Yamanishi, and Masahiko Kishi. "Genitourinary Dysfunction in Parkinson's Disease." *Movement Disorders* 25, no. 1 (2010): 2–12. doi: 10.1002/mds.22519.

Tanner, Caroline M., Melanie Brandabur, and E. Ray Dorsey. "Parkinson's Disease: A Global View." *Parkinson Report* (Spring 2008): 9–11.

Tolosa, Eduardo, George Wenning, and Werner H. Poewe. "The Diagnosis of Parkinson's Disease." *The Lancet Neurology* 5, no. 1 (2006): 75–86. doi: http://dx.doi.org/10.1016/S1474-4422(05)70285-4.

Wu, Y., W. Le, and J. Jankovic. "Preclinical Biomarkers of Parkinson Disease." *Archives of Neurology* 68, no. 1 (2010): 22–30. doi: 10.1001/archneurol.2010.321.

Zhang, P., Z. Gao, Y. Jiang, J. Wang, F. Zhang, S. Wang, Y. Yang, H. Xiong, Y. Zhang, X. Bao, J. Xiao, X. Wu, and Y. Wu. "Follow-up Study of 25 Chinese Children with Pla2g6-Associated Neurodegeneration." *European Journal of Neurology* 20, no. 2 (2013): 322–30. doi: 10.1111/j.1468-1331.2012.03856.x.

7 Defiance, Epistemologies of Ignorance, and Giving Uptake Properly

Nancy Nyquist Potter

Living with a mental disorder can be frightening, debilitating, and discouraging. Although the history of psychiatry has been that of containment within insane asylums—not only of the mentally ill, but also of the mentally retarded, wayward girls, and those who fail to conform to norms of society—the current face is one of helping and treating people (Shorter 1998). This chapter analyzes a particular way of thinking about the institution of psychiatry that can get in the way of accurate diagnosis. As a philosopher of psychiatry, my perspective is informed by the importance of examining assumptions in nosology and diagnosis. This chapter focuses on epistemological issues in diagnosis that are embedded in psychiatric interpretations of patient defiance. I argue that defiance can be misinterpreted and thus can lead to misdiagnosis. My primary example comes from literature on behavior interpreted as defiant in African American boys and that can lead eventually to a diagnosis of oppositional defiant disorder (ODD).

In the first section, I introduce the concept of what are called epistemologies of ignorance in philosophy and apply it to psychiatry. I then turn to the question of defiance as an activity and disposition that can be better understood by psychiatrists so as to avoid misdiagnosis or the misinterpretation of behavior. I argue that defiance sometimes is an appropriate response and should not be construed as a sign of dysfunction. The final section of the chapter highlights ways that psychiatrists can better position themselves to diagnose people who seem to be dysfunctionally defiant. This positioning involves learning to give uptake properly, a communicative ethic that I argue is a virtue.

THE INTERFACE OF PSYCHIATRY AND EPISTEMOLOGIES OF IGNORANCE

What does it mean to see and be seen, to listen and be listened to, to know and be known?

Why do well-meaning, even enlightened people fail to see that their ways of seeing, of treating them, and of constructing other persons as Other[1] can undermine the best of intentions and sometimes do harm? In this section, I place claims of not-knowing, good intentions, and best interests under scrutiny. After explaining what philosophers mean by "epistemologies of ignorance," I discuss how they might apply to psychiatry.

Epistemology is a branch of philosophy that theorizes about what can be known, what counts as knowing, and what counts as the justification for knowledge: claims as opposed to belief-claims. It standardly has been addressed as an individualist enterprise—i.e., as an achievement that each person reaches by adopting an objective, detached, and disinterested point of view. The development of social epistemology, then, which locates the individual cognizer within social groups and positionalities within hierarchies, is a welcome change (Mills 2007). Social epistemologists claim that bodies of knowledge always are created by knowers who cooperatively (but also sometimes contentiously) decide what will count as knowledge, who should be included as experts in a given field, and what those bodies of knowledge mean or are intended to mean. That is, the production of knowledge is not a mere fact-based pursuit of knowledge-claims that one pursues and others confirm or disconfirm, but a social endeavor that requires participation even as to what will count as evidence and standards for the process.

A newer development focuses on what, at first, might seem to be an oxymoron: epistemologies of ignorance. Epistemologies of ignorance are gaps in knowledge that are argued to be actively produced and sustained for the purposes of domination and exploitation (Sullivan and Tuana 2007). To say that such gaps are actively produced is to say that it takes *effort* to not know the effects of historical and persistent, systematic oppressions on others. (That is, I understand the phrase "actively produced" in connection with "for the purposes of" does not necessarily imply that such activity and purpose is conscious and deliberate, although some authors do claim that. It is my sense that it is enough to point to epistemic practices and their relationship to social groups' positions for culpability and the demand for change to be convincing. But a full discussion of these epistemic issues would require too much additional space; see Medina 2013.)

Following the ancient distinction set up by Aristotle between blameworthy and accidental ignorance, epistemologies of ignorance focus on whether or not ignorance could be avoided and what the ignorant person or group of persons does to allow or maintain that ignorance. It is not enough to avoid culpability for wrong actions by claiming that we are ignorant of the effects of our beliefs, attitudes, policies, norms, and actions. The question is: Could we have known? Can we know now? And what are we doing to not know, to maintain ignorance of structures of oppression and systematic harms? In analyzing what epistemic ignorance is in relation to racialization, Linda Alcoff states that:

> [W]hites have a *positive* interest in "seeing the world wrongly," to paraphrase Mills. Here, ignorance is not primarily understood as a *lack*—a

lack of motivation or experience as the result of social location—but as a substantive epistemological practice that differentiates the dominant group. (Alcoff 2007: 47)

Specifically, Alcoff reveals the role that dominant epistemic norms play in maintaining the belief that society is basically just, despite evidence to the contrary. She argues that cognitive norms within dominant groups have to develop that enable people to dismiss the countervailing evidence and maintain the fiction of living in a basically just world (48). An example of this is the practice of color-blindness, a practice that perpetuates racial injustice (Mills 2010). The foreclosure of alternative interpretations, analysis, and critique may result in epistemic ignorance as a kind of loss of critical rationality (53).

On this account, epistemologies of ignorance are part of training and habituating into what it means to be successful in who one is and what one does, where "being" and "doing" are social identities and actions, not merely individual ones. Epistemologies of ignorance are an ongoing task of learning to become the sort of person one is in relation to one's status, social positioning, and location in the hierarchies of power/knowledge. This education is both epistemic and moral. As Alcoff says regarding racial epistemologies of ignorance, they allow white people to believe in a just, equitable, and merit-based world and to act from those beliefs. An understanding of epistemic ignorance as structural and beneficial to the members of the dominant groups allows us to see that those benefitting from structural epistemic ignorance may have absorbed and internalized a pattern of belief-forming practices that maintain systematic ignorance and sustain its effects. Through patterns of social reward, moral development, socialization into "civility," and knowledge formation, members of dominant groups "may be actively pursuing or supporting a distorted or an otherwise inaccurate account" (Alcoff 2007: 48).

Here, I turn to apply these lessons to psychiatry and psychiatric diagnosis. Psychiatrists, too, are socialized into epistemic communities. This epistemic socialization involves an "implicit consensus about cognitive norms, it concerns what counts as a correct interpretation of the world, and what actions are right and legal in it" (Bailey 2007: 79). The *episteme* (a Greek term that has been broadened to apply to the knowledge base that shapes a given practice within a particular period of time) in psychiatry includes ontological commitments about what exists in the world: mental disorders exist; they exist as biological entities; causal explanations of mental disorders are located in brain sciences; causal explanations that refer back to spirits, ancestors, or folk magic do not. It follows from these ontological commitments that pathologies in cognition, affect, and behavior exist: people's reasoning may be distorted not just in ordinary ways but in psychotic ways; their affect may be dysregulated; their behavior may be dysfunctional.

The *DSM* is a way of organizing epistemology and grounding the ontological commitments of the psychiatric episteme. Psychiatry is charged with the identification of the lines between normal and abnormal ways of being. Psychiatrists are experts; they interpret people's presentation, body language, narratives, and behavior. They delineate and distinguish between a sick person and a well one. The psychiatric episteme grants psychiatrists the authority to decide that some people are "patients," that some people are a danger to themselves or others, and that some people are in need of containment and treatment. In situating psychiatrists with this authoritative responsibility, it prepares them through training and education to value the law or at least to work within the law and in conjunction with the law to protect the citizenry from harm, and to protect themselves from malpractice suits. It trains them to have their interpretive lens be determined by the current best practices as defined by evidence-based medicine; their lens takes in the social dimensions of a patient's life as it bears on diagnosis and treatment but brackets off most of the broader cultural and historical contexts in which persons are situated and immersed. It habituates psychiatrists to have a "detached concern"[2] for their patients. In particular, then, the episteme of psychiatry shapes diagnostic practices through enculturation into a specific ontological, evidentiary, and expertise-based way of knowing and not knowing.

This is not to say that the episteme in psychiatry contains only psychiatrists. Patients, too, are made and enacted through this episteme, but my aim is to prepare readers for a discussion of epistemologies of ignorance, specifically, which epistemologies implicate psychiatrists and the institution of psychiatry. Psychiatry holds a fundamental value of benefitting patients. Therefore, central to the episteme is a conception of psychiatry as a helping profession, with emphasis on the ideal of being helpers and healers within the bounds of biological and brain sciences. But the episteme of psychiatry *arranges* psychiatrists such that they are the authoritative body about what counts as mental health, what counts as significant deviations from mental health, and what should be done about such deviations. To accomplish such demanding tasks, it relies on a strategic epistemology of ignorance—for example, ignorance of the meaning and significance to those most affected by the historical and current context of interlocking oppression, domination, and systematic injustices—i.e., ignorance of the historical context of righteous defiance against hegemonic power. It must avert its gaze from this knowledge. There are things it must not know in order to practice the profession within its own episteme.[3]

My interest is in people who are defiant, especially as they interface with psychiatry. I argue that, for some groups of people, being defiant in the face of psychiatry may not only be reasonable, but may be a virtue. But secondly, I argue that defiance, properly understood, sometimes will affect diagnosis: a diagnosis may not be called for, if the behavior is misidentified as defiance when it is not; a diagnosis may be mistaken, if the behavior is itself an appropriate response to injustice or oppression; and a diagnosis may be mistaken, if the behavior is interpreted through a racial or gendered lens that draws upon unconscious stereotypes and biases. In order to understand these claims, a perspectival stance is called for. A shifting of perspective, what I have elsewhere described as the need for psychiatrists to decenter themselves and "world"-travel, is needed in order to open ourselves to some of the epistemic and social challenges this article raises (Potter 2003). I recognize that many members of representative institutions have good intentions and are good-hearted; yet, even so, some encounters are oppressive. That is a hard pill to swallow. Taking these challenges seriously may involve the gentle prodding of readers—and *by* readers—into examining the not-so-benign subtexts of encounters that may demand defiance in the "patient."

The next section presents my argument on the role and value of defiance, first in general terms and then in relation to psychiatry. I set this in the context of Aristotelian virtues, identifying defiance as a virtue. This discussion will help readers understand why and when a certain kind of response to defiance that I call "uptake" is needed and how the above analysis on epistemologies of ignorance is relevant.

DEFIANCE AS A VIRTUE

Although physicians, as well as teachers, government officials, law enforcement officers, and others who contribute to the functioning of society, value cooperation, compliance, and civility, sometimes being defiant is a better way to be. We value civility and compliance because they are part of the "glue" that makes social interactions run smoothly. But we do have to ask, smoothly for whom? And to what end? This section explains what I mean by claiming that defiance is sometimes a virtuous disposition to have and why I make that claim. I start with Aristotle, whose virtue ethics have been widely influential.

Aristotle's theory of flourishing, or well-being, requires that the path by which people can achieve *eudaimonia*, or flourishing, is through cultivating virtues. Virtues like justice, truth telling, friendship, and courage are good qualities of character for people to have; they are good in themselves, but they mutually benefit us socially and enhance self-sufficiency. We learn to be virtuous by doing virtuous acts that, over time, become thoughtful habits of intellect. As we have seen, a central part of cultivating virtues (and vices) involves being habituated and trained into acquiring certain dispositions that are both epistemic and moral. But Aristotle presents a world in which the background conditions for living well are ideal. Although Aristotle pays attention to power differentials, he naturalizes those differences and, instead of worrying about the negative consequences that being subordinated or subjugated entails, he endorses them.

The actual world, however, is one where many, if not most, people, live under adverse background conditions, including "the more wretched conditions present under some forms of oppression," as Lisa Tessman says

(2009: 48). According to Iris Marion Young, oppression and domination are two disabling constraints placed on certain social groups, including, women, African Americans, Hispanic Americans, Native Americans, Jews, lesbians, gay men, transgendered people, Middle Easterners, Asians, working class people, old people, and the physically and mentally disabled. By "disabling constraints," she means the systematic and group-associated injustices that take the form of exploitation, marginalization, powerlessness, cultural imperialism, and violence (Young 2011). These forms of oppression and domination are disabling because they reduce, immobilize, and shape members of affected social groups in ways that drastically hinder their ability to live well (Frye 1983a). Thus, in our non-ideal world, even being virtuous is insufficient for living well. *Eudaimonia* in an Aristotelian conception functions as an ideology that, while claiming an integral connection between being virtuous and flourishing, is unattainable for many, if not most, people.

I draw upon Tessman's proposal for a non-ideal eudaimonism in offering a virtue ethics that is practical and realistic for those living in adverse conditions. By "adverse conditions," I mean those who live with mental illnesses and also those who are racialized and gendered as inferior, subordinate, oppressed, or, as noted above, viewed as Other. "Non-ideal ethical theory must recognize flourishing as being out of reach under some conditions of oppression and must contribute to understanding moral life given this fact" (Tessman 2009: 48). In an ideal world, (privileged) moral agents are granted a capacity for practical reasoning and the ability for desires to be governed by correct reasoning. Aristotle presents moral agents (that is, the elite citizens of Greece) as interdependent in the sense that what is good for oneself also contributes to the good of others. But, as Tessman points out, such an assumption elides the real-world conditions where interdependence is replaced by relations of domination and subordination (2009: 49).

Tessman argues that:

> In a non-idealized eudaimonistic virtue ethics, one will have to assume that flourishing will be largely unattainable, in part because of moral damage, that is, damage to the virtues, and in part because of adverse external conditions. (Tessman 2009: 51)

But Tessman does believe that, even in a non-ideal world, "a trait may still qualify as a virtue when it is detrimental to an agent's well-being" (52). Her approach is to retain the concept of flourishing even when it is unattainable, while still holding that some virtues are worthy of cultivating and exercising and that flourishing is a worthy value. Tessman calls virtues that are severed from flourishing "burdened virtues;" this allows us to mark them as constitutive of the moral damage caused by trying to live out norms and expectations that keep those who live under adverse conditions occupying an inferior positionality. Burdened virtues are those that burden the moral efforts of the oppressed because of the harm done to them. She draws upon Claudia Card's idea of "moral damage," a way to characterize one of the harms done to subordinated people when they are not able to exercise the virtues (Card 1996; Tessman 2009: 51). Tessman argues that, under oppressive conditions, many people's reasoning is affected by a distorted view of acting well or virtuously and that people's desires are also distorted by a need to adapt to relations of domination and subordination (50).

Defiance can help correct for the sorts of harm that may be done to people living under adverse conditions, such as those living with mental illnesses, or even those just thought to have them, or thought to be at risk of becoming mentally ill. In this chapter, I primarily focus on *diagnosis* at the intersection of defiance and the mentally ill, keeping in mind the broader social context of oppression and domination. For all of us, our lives are embedded in the social and historical context of our lived conditions; our experiences are informed by cultural values, contested affiliations, and master narratives of normative behavior. People who have or may have mental illnesses are no exception, and so we will misunderstand acts of defiance if we decontextualize them or try to interact with people as if they are mere individuals with personal, family, and medical histories that are supposed to inform treatment in the abstract. In addition, some of the people who come from adverse backgrounds also experience encounters with psychiatrists that further exacerbate distrust, a sense of unfair treatment, and moral harm done. The intersection of living under oppressive conditions and living under adverse conditions such as mental illness is complicated by the ways that the diagnosis of mental illness historically has been used to contain and further subjugate the already oppressed (Metzl 2009; Ussher 2011). Not all those who are classified as mentally ill live under oppressive conditions, but when considering the endemic existence of racialized, classed, and gendered people, it is likely that many have. Furthermore, it is undeniable that the institution of psychiatry has not always been neutral and benign in its determinations, such that even privileged classes of people may experience their encounters with psychiatry as oppressive.[4] (This is not to imply that individual psychiatrists intentionally are doing harm to people, but that the ideology and status of psychiatry as an institution can be oppressive.) The significance of these points is that, sometimes, people who are behaving in ways that defy social norms are taken up as mentally ill when they should not be, and that even those with mental illnesses may be defiant appropriately.

Loosely placing defiance within a non-ideal eudaimonistic virtue ethics, I suggest that it is one of the dispositions worth cultivating because it does, in some significant ways, contribute to well-being. But because it can be a burdened virtue, it often is not straightforwardly beneficial. As Tessman argues, in our non-ideal world, many people who develop virtues and use them in daily life are unlikely to flourish as a result of living virtuously. Furthermore, the cost of being defiant can be high—sometimes too high.

In this sense, defiance is double-edged, as Tessman suggests: defiance can be a virtue in certain contexts, but it can also bring further harm to the person.[5] Nevertheless, as I discuss at the end of this section, good reasons exist for being defiant even with the understanding that it is a burdened virtue.

To be defiant is to express, through speech, other communication, and behavior, long-standing opposition and resistance to overwhelming pressure to buckle to the dominant norms.[6] It isn't "civilized" or domesticated. It is often, but not always, loud, angry, and "in your face." But it makes itself known and felt as a stand against injustice, or oppression, or other forms of unfairness, both interpersonal and structural. It contributes to well-being because it declares one's self-respect and self-worth in the face of pressure to submit, to comply, to accept.

A disposition to be defiant is one where a person is able to recognize a situation that calls for defiance and he/she is ready to act when such a situation arises.[7] It is not a mere knee-jerk reaction in that the person who acts defiantly has done some conscious (perhaps even consciousness-raising), psychological, and often, political background preparatory work. She/he may have engaged in self-reflection. She/he may have been part of a circle of people who, together, interrogated various ways of interpreting their worlds. Defiance as a character trait has a reasoning quality as well, but it doesn't require the rationality as it is deployed within master narratives. The point is: defiance as a virtue is not "irrational," although it is often interpreted that way within psychiatry, educational systems, and the workplace. Carving out the ways in which defiance is reasonable is difficult because it goes against the grain of ontological commitments to the ideal of the civilized, autonomous, and self-sufficient rational beings we ideally are, and it is especially difficult in the context of psychiatric diagnosis given the episteme in which psychiatrists are enculturated. My theory of defiance strikes at the heart of what counts as mental health through an investigation into the history and legacy of diagnosing disorders in psychiatry when people are strange, unruly and, by dominant cultural standards, incomprehensibly putting themselves at risk, what psychiatrists might identify as threatening people's very ability to flourish or live well. Again, this is not to say that being defiant unequivocally advances one's flourishing. If a person does have a mental health problem, then being defiant both could challenge the psychiatrist's authority in ways that could be beneficial to the person, while possibly exacerbating a mental health problem.[8] Still, we would need to ask, from what ontological and epistemological perspective is such diagnosing occurring?

When we consider how epistemologies of ignorance might play themselves out in psychiatry, we find that, in addition to its aims of helping people with mental distress to improve their functioning, psychiatry has played a central role in perpetuating dominating relations through practices of containment and control.[9] I give two examples of what I mean by this claim. First, the intersection of psychiatry and oppression is demonstrated in Metzl's (2009) historical analysis of schizophrenia in the U.S. One of the most egregious manifestations of using psychiatric means to contain and control those deemed dangerous to dominant norms and the prevailing psychiatric episteme occurred during the 1960s rise of the Black Power Movement. During this period, some psychiatrists formed a new diagnosis called "protest psychosis," a form of irrationality supposedly caused by the rhetoric and ideology of Black Power. The symptoms of this mental disorder were delusions, hallucinations, and violent impulses in black men toward white people (Metzl 2009: 100). That is, during the civil rights era in U.S. history, the increasing identification of unjust and discriminatory treatment by white people toward blacks, and the vocal, visible, and vociferous demands by black folks that white people cease and desist in their oppression and degradation of them was determined to be irrational, delusional, and demented. The diagnosis of the mental disorder of schizophrenia was a way to control the threat to white structural power and systemic violence presented by the Black Power Movement and other defiant stands taken in the demand for civil rights for all.

Oppressive and damaging psychiatry can be seen in the diagnosis and treatment of gender issues as well, as indicated above. Jane Ussher, for example, (2011) argues that understanding women's distress must be contextualized within the historical particularities of what counts as normal female behavior, desires, and relations, as well as within ways that epistemic bodies (such as medicine and, in particular, psychiatry) push women to be taken up as—and to take themselves up as—ill.[10] Norms of femininity police women, Ussher argues, to such a degree that, when they deviate from those norms, they develop "symptoms" and fall "ill." Ussher argues that a woman's presentation of distress expresses a truth about her lived experience as troubling, but that it should not be reified into pathology. But, as Ussher understands gender subordination, not only have women historically been diagnosed as mad when they deviate from prescribed gender norms that already are subordinating, but women are caught in a double bind where they cannot receive help without unconsciously being complicit in signifying their own madness. In this way, a "mental disorder" is produced that can be interpreted and addressed within the epistemic framework of psychiatry. Ussher illustrates her point with a discussion of premenstrual dysphoric disorder. I suggest that an additional double bind is also at work here: when variously positioned women defy norms of femininity, they run the risk that their behavior will be interpreted and diagnosed as symptomatic of mental disorder, while at the same time, if they do need assistance or guidance in dealing with stressors of life and exhibit compliant behavior, they may be treated with psychotropic medications that target the individual biological body and miss the larger context in which women navigate an oppressive world. Furthermore, these double binds affect women differently due to the hierarchies of privilege and oppression *within* groups of women, and psychiatric responses both to socioeconomic stressors and to defiance are far harsher for women who hold less privilege and benefits within social hierarchies. Nevertheless, I champion defiance in many situations.

My claim is that defiance is a virtue that can help correct for damages wrought upon oppressed peoples throughout North American history, policy, and practices. But being defiant can be costly to oneself and others, so the question arises: why should anyone be decisively defiant when it isn't prudent?

It is clear that many people face a double bind when they defy oppressive norms or relations. On the one hand, it is damaging to internalize—or perform as if one has internalized—an ideology where one's self is marked as inferior, damaged, or fundamentally irrational and one's rightful place in social relations is to occupy a subordinate position. Defiance would seem to be a necessary response to being taken up as and treated as flawed or diagnosed as mentally ill in order to preserve worth and value. On the other hand, defiant behavior is often responded to with punishment or proof of mental dysfunction, thus carrying risks that may be detrimental to one's well-being (Tessman 2009: 51). Still, Tessman suggests that:

> Striving in the face of the absurd permits one to maintain a claim on what one is unjustly denied (full personhood); the absurdity lies in the fact that the strivings will never attain their goal, but must be carried on nevertheless; to give up striving would be to announce one's acceptance of the injustice. (Tessman 2009: 56)

The reasons to be defiant even with the risk of retaliation are many. As Tessman says, being defiant in the face of injustice says (to oneself if to no one else) that one will not stand for injustice. It preserves integrity; it claims one's self-worth and dignity in the face of people who view one as inferior, or dysfunctional, or sick. It affirms self-respect at those junctions where it might be threatened.

> The powerless but self-respecting person will declare his self-respect. He will protest. His protest affirms that he has rights. More important, it tells everyone that he believes he has rights and that he therefore claims self-respect. When he has to endure wrongs he cannot repel and feels his self-respect threatened, he will publicly claim it in order to reassure himself that he has it. His reassurance does not come from persuading others that he has self-respect. It comes from using his claim to self-respect as a challenge. (Boxill 1995: 102)

Finally, defiance signals to others that we have not agreed to give up our moral rights (Hill 1995). Defiance indicates—without any appeal to moral rights or the assertion of our basic worth—that some ways of behaving are simply beneath us (Hill 1995: 119). In a non-ideal eudaimonistic theory of virtue, defiance is a good, and a good way to be, not because it furthers flourishing, but because it allows us to survive well in an imperfect world.

DIAGNOSIS AND DISCUSSION

In this section, I present a case and discussion in which I suggest that defiant behavior within a psychiatric setting, when understood within a broader historical context, is an expression of a virtue. I then expand the discussion to look at how a diagnosis of oppositional defiant disorder may present challenges to good diagnostic practices.

Vignette

> Jewell, a coffee-colored woman in her early twenties, is brought in to meet with the psychiatric team because she has been kicked out of the halfway house she has been living in. She reports that she has left there voluntarily because she hates it, it is "crazy unreasonable" and that "no one should have to follow that many rules." She appears distressed and agitated. When members of the psychiatric team ask her to explain what is wrong with the place she came from, she becomes angry, saying "I. Already. Told. You." Psychiatrists and others explain that they want her to consider going back there and that she will need to abide by those rules, but that they are "good rules." She stands up and starts pacing back and forth, "There's too many rules! I can't live that way!" When the psychiatric team explains that they believe it is the right place for her and that it will be better for her to learn to follow rules, she shouts, "You people don't understand." Upon being asked to take a seat so this can be discussed calmly and reasonably, she leaves the room, slamming the door.

Members of the team discuss what would be the best thing to do for this patient. But all of them see her as displaying tendencies of personality disorder and other symptoms of mental disorder, which impede the patient's ability to follow rules. The discussion centered on tendencies toward antisocial behavior. She was diagnosed tentatively with "personality disorder, not otherwise specified."

Discussion

What was not discussed was the fact that, except for the coffee-colored woman, all of the other people in the room were white.

Norms for compliant behavior for patients in psychiatry include that the patient does not exhibit defiant or threatening behavior. Standing up abruptly, shouting, interrupting, gesturing at the psychiatric team can be read as both defiant and threatening. But two intersecting issues exist if that lens is used to interpret and diagnose Jewell's behavior. One is that for Jewell, as for other patients, psychiatry is ontologically committed to mental disorders as occurring in individuals. This commitment means that, although the *DSM 5* gives more credence to sociocultural contexts than do earlier versions of the *DSM*, the ontology that undergirds psychiatry is individualistic and increasingly biologically oriented. Jewell, then, is viewed primarily as an individual—more specifically—as a generic individual—whose race and gender are only incidental to understanding her behavior. And the entailment of this approach to patients is that the broader historical context in which each of us is situated is overlooked, ignored, or erased. This is not to say that Jewell could not be exhibiting symptoms of mental health problems that may undergird her defiant behavior. My point is that, as long as her experiences and background social group identity as simultaneously racialized and gendered are overlooked or bracketed off—including as a strategy of epistemologies of ignorance—psychiatrists face an extremely complex task of identifying which behaviors are symptomatic and in need of psychiatric diagnosis and intervention, which behaviors are appropriately defiant but misinterpreted or misdiagnosed, and which behaviors are both.

Oppositional Defiant Disorder

One of the issues that arises when considering the case of Jewell in the above vignette is that a racialized patient may be diagnosed with defiant, antisocial behavior without taking into account two things: first, how racialization affects the development of the person she is now, and second, how an epistemology of ignorance may prevent the psychiatrist from properly situating the person's behavior in the context of that racialized background, development, and experience.

Let's look at the diagnosis of defiant behavior through this lens: a recent report issued by the U.S. Department of Education Office for Civil Rights found that minority children—including preschoolers—are disproportionately likely to be suspended, referred to law enforcement, physically restrained, and placed in seclusion (U.S. Department of Education 2014). This report exposes the beginnings of what Young (2011) calls "disabling constraints" through the singling out of minority children as disruptive, defiant, and in need of control. The disproportionality is a sign that social and racial injustice continues well into the 21st century and that it begins at an early age.

I have argued elsewhere (2012) that the culturally inflected behaviors seen in some African American boys in the school system are interpreted by teachers as defiant according to mainstream norms for school behavior; students viewed as defiant of the authority of teachers and the school structures are viewed as troublemakers, sent to punishment rooms, and set on a trajectory of being constructed as "bad." And the worry is that some of these young African American boys eventually may be diagnosed with oppositional defiant disorder (Potter 2012). Research suggests that, at least for some African American groups, the cultural norms for interacting with adults and authority figures are different than white cultural norms. This difference is crucial to take into account when authority figures disproportionately judge African American boys to be defiant and thus in need of some form of expulsion. This way of "marking" young boys as troublemakers has a developmental effect in that these boys may internalize a "bad boy" identity that haunts and informs their behavior later in life. While I am not arguing that it is impossible that African American boys' defiance—if it is that—could be a sign of mental distress, I am arguing that the potential for misinterpretation and misdiagnosis of ODD is racialized and that this is a reason to disentangle the relationship between cultural ways of answering to authority, which are read as defiance and sometimes characterized as *being* defiant, and the move toward diagnosing those behaviors, a strategy that serves to control the racialized Other through an epistemology of ignorance.

Despite the enormous risks involved in being defiant—as manifested in the case of Jewell and more generally, in the diagnosis of ODD in African American boys—it sometimes is the appropriate response when facing authoritative bodies, such as the schools and psychiatry. Jewell, for instance, may be responding defiantly to norms and expectations from the health care team that she sit quietly, civilly, and circumspectly, and that she ultimately agree to return to the halfway house. Jewell may perceive rightly that the roomful of white folks trained into the psychiatric episteme are imposing standards for behavior that fail to account for her experiences as an oppressed, racialized woman who is constantly expected to conform to the dominant norms for behavior. Jewell may be defiant because she has reached a breaking point for demands that she subordinate herself; she may need to preserve her self-worth *on her terms*. Again, this is not to dismiss the possibility that she may also be dealing with mental distress that needs intervention. My aim is for readers to consider why Jewell might be acting defiantly from her own point of view and within her frame of reference as a racialized woman and to not close off the possibility that her defiance may not be symptomatic and diagnostic. Similar points would be made about African American boys who are seemingly defiant in the schools: is their behavior more a sign of a cultural difference and therefore not indicative of bad behavior? Is their behavior an appropriate response to the perceived unjust treatment of African Americans in school?

If my argument is on the right track, then how should psychiatrists respond when faced with (apparently) defiant patients? And what might make it difficult for psychiatrists to respond appropriately? The psychiatric episteme can powerfully impede an accurate understanding of an oppressed person where an historical legacy interacts with current systemic oppressions. But it is from *within that context* that defiant behavior can be more accurately understood.

THE VIRTUE OF GIVING UPTAKE

I have argued that defiance sometimes is an appropriate response to the disabling constraints of oppression and domination. But an appropriate response exists to defiance, as well, and it is to interact with a defiant person and, sometimes, a patient, in a way that does not exacerbate the relations of domination and subordination. As Tessman argues (2005: ch. 3), domination is a vice, and so people habituated into epistemologies of ignorance need to work on their character as well.

Psychiatric ethics require that all members of a psychiatric health care team, including medical students, residents, social workers, chemical dependency counselors, nurses, security personnel, and staff follow ethical principles of treating patients with justice, fairness, benevolence, and respect. People are expected to approach patients with an attitude of equality. Psychiatric training instills in students the importance of holding good will and respectful engagement toward patients.[11] In this chapter, I have argued that values such as equality, justice, benevolence, and respect are not the experience of most peoples who historically and contemporarily encounter structures of power and oppression; therefore, I suggest that assumptions about the place of liberal values need to be examined. Furthermore, training also develops in practice, not just theory, and students absorb mixed messages. For example, research shows that patients diagnosed with borderline personality disorder, 75 percent of which are women, are viewed as deliberately manipulative, treated with less empathy, and actively disliked by psychiatrists and staff (Potter 2009). In general, formal and informal training tend toward a discourse of surface liberal values that simultaneously perpetuates institutionalized relations of domination and subordination and maintains systemically produced adverse living conditions. A key strategy of such perpetuation is through epistemologies of ignorance as they apply to psychiatry. Those who occupy privileged positions socioeconomically, politically, or professionally ought to avoid domination and work to change unjust structures and disciplines. Yet it is difficult to see how psychiatrists can make such changes.

My suggestion is to cultivate virtues that are epistemologically, politically, and ethically *responsive* to attempts to assert one's worth—or autonomy, or to challenge the status quo—through a virtue such as defiance. For the sake of brevity, I will discuss one virtue for those whose positions of psychiatric authority are vulnerable to a failure to respond properly to defiance—but who consciously do not want to collude in structural harms to patients—and that only in sketch: giving uptake (Potter 2000, 2009, ch. 5 for a full treatment of this virtue.) I introduce the concept of uptake by beginning with Marilyn Frye's analysis of women's anger (1983b). Frye, in discussing the trivialization, ridicule, and ignoring of women's anger, says that women's anger is not given uptake (Frye 1983b). Uptake is a speech convention that, as introduced by Austin, is necessary in order for certain speech acts to "come off." For example, one cannot be said to have made a promise if the listener doesn't recognize it as a promise. Elsewhere, I have argued that, because many of our conventions in communication are constitutive of hegemonic relations, we need to be vigilant about how we receive the communications from subordinated others (Potter 2000). Those in positions of privilege, including those in authority ranging from parents to teachers to worker/boss relations to psychiatrists, need to give uptake to those in subordinated positions.

> Cultivating a disposition to give uptake rightly is necessary for the full flourishing of individuals and of society, as it provides the means for genuine communication in a variety of kinds of social settings. It facilitates democratic practices, as it enhances the possibilities of understanding what justice is and when we have gotten it wrong. (Potter 2002: 152)

I apply this idea to those on the receiving end of defiance. By giving uptake, I say: you can count on me to take you seriously according to your idea of seriousness and not mine alone, and you can expect me to treat your picture of the world seriously and take your defiance seriously. To take defiance seriously is to recognize the claim another is making to you, norms that you are enforcing, practices that benefit you but not the defier. Taking defiance seriously means that you are willing to consider the possibility that you are implicated in systemic, harmful relations and oppressive regimes. It indicates that you recognize the historically and experientially grounded effects of oppression on the communicator. You shift your epistemic authority by decentering yourself and learning to suspend or bracket off your own worldview in favor of moving into the worldview of the communicator. You do not assume the defiant one has a mental disorder—but you also do not assume he/she does not have one. Developing a disposition to give uptake rightly means that, when confronted with defiant behavior, you reflect not on their behavior, but your own. Yet, such shifts, suspensions, and epistemic movements can be very challenging, as my analysis has shown. It asks of psychiatrists that they are willing to accept that they may come to psychiatric encounters with strategies of distorted knowing.

For a significant part of the population in North America, the institution of psychiatry is so embedded in the ontology, ideology, and lives of people that the interface of mental distress with psychiatric interventions is unavoidable. Some people have severe mental disorders, while others are at risk of being predicted to develop mental disorders. And even then, patients sometimes are defiant in ways that proclaim their self-worth in the face of adversity and unfairness. Within a matrix of psychiatry, systematic disabling constraints, and virtuous defiance, how should psychiatrists give uptake rightly?

CONCLUSION

If we are to listen properly, in a way that genuinely gives uptake to the communicator, it is not enough to encounter with good will the person as an individual with a mental disorder or as someone who is defying dominant norms by "acting out." I suggest five things that clinicians can do as they determine whether a diagnosis is appropriate and, if so, which diagnosis to make. First, the clinician should situate the person/potential patient within his/her social and historical context, a context that will often include oppressive conditions. Second, the clinician should situate himself/herself socially and historically, including as an authority and expert on mental health and mental illness and what that authority means in the context of systematic relations of domination and oppression. Third, the clinician needs to know enough about interlocking oppressions critically to engage with them structurally as well as within the patient/psychiatrist encounter. Fourth, the clinician needs to educate himself/herself about what epistemologies of ignorance are and how they work to maintain hegemonic relations. Finally, the clinician can counter-strategize her or his own epistemology so as to combat the gaps in ignorance that benefit dominant structures.

The first point, that of situating the person within her or his social context, is acknowledged to be relevant in the new *DSM-5*. Under "Other Conditions That May Be a Focus of Clinical Attention," the *DSM* includes diagnostic classification numbers for "Other Problems Related to the Social Environment" such as "acculturation difficulty" and "target of (perceived) adverse discrimination or persecution" (*DSM-5* 2013: 724). The introductory discussion in this section makes clear that these conditions are not to be considered mental disorders but instead as additional information in making diagnoses, treatment plans, and in justifying the ordering of particular tests. But the space devoted to each of these social background factors is minimal; for example, under "acculturation difficulty," one sentence is written and the assumption that the problem is unidirectional goes unquestioned. Furthermore, because the nosological structure is founded firmly in a biologically based and individualist construct of psychopathology, recognition of the social context does nothing to shift those ontological commitments. It is left to psychiatric education to teach residents the value, significance, and ontological assumptions behind social factors.

Beyond that, numbers two through five above are left to the morally and politically committed to do on their own, meaning without the cooperation of the institution of psychiatry. But engagement with others is necessary for, as many of us saw in the consciousness-raising practices during the Civil

Rights Movement in the United States, unlearning what we think we know and understand and value, and producing a more epistemically and morally responsible knowledge base, requires that we place ourselves willingly in positions where we will be challenged, critiqued, and treated with distrust (Lugones and Spelman 1983). Both activist and academic strategies of resistance—perhaps psychiatrists' own form of defiance—are available and accessible at every turn, if people are serious about it.

Listening well—giving uptake properly—is not just a characteristic needed at the point of determining which treatments, and perhaps medications, would be best to suggest to the patient; giving uptake is a crucial element in proper diagnostic reasoning. Ethical qualities in the clinician, such as listening with empathy and attending to relational aspects of the patient/psychiatrist encounter, are integral to the ways of knowing that psychiatrists must draw upon when making diagnoses. This chapter highlights the fact that diagnostic skills are not merely a matter of gathering information during an intake interview, information that provides some of the evidence for making a proper diagnosis; diagnostic skills necessarily call upon the qualities of connection and attention—ethical qualities—that psychiatrists bring to the encounter. These skills especially are necessary given the issues my analysis has brought to light, such as problems in epistemologies of ignorance that trouble the lives of the privileged and powerful. Thus, ethics and epistemology are integrally bound up together in the process of diagnosis itself, and giving uptake properly is one of the central features of good diagnostic reasoning. The development and employment of deep and critical engagement with the problems identified in this chapter will bring clinicians that much closer to a reliable and just practice of diagnosis for people whose distress or problems in living call for diagnosis and to avoid misdiagnosis.

ACKNOWLEDGMENTS

Lisa Tessman, David Owen, Philosophy Phi Sigma Tau students, and Carolyn Smith-Morris.

NOTES

1   "The Other" is a way of referring to the process of positioning members of minority groups as strange, alien, incomprehensible, or inferior. It often relies on and recreates harmful stereotypes. See Johnson et al. 2004.
2   This phrase is taken from the title of Jodi Halpern's book, *From Detached Concern to Empathy: Humanizing Medical Practice*, 2001.
3   Mills emphasizes that any understanding of epistemologies of ignorance must be placed in an historical context (2007), but that discussion is beyond the scope of this essay.

4 For example, see Elyn Saks' memoir, *The Center Cannot Hold*, a memoir that contains many examples of this. Saks 2007.
5 Communication with Tessman.
6 A full discussion of defiance, and of virtue, is more than I can provide here. For instance, it needs to be distinguished from civil disobedience and the unconscious resistance identified in psychoanalytic theories. I develop these ideas in my current work-in-progress, a monograph called *The Virtue of Defiance and Psychiatric Engagement: Psychiatry and Norms for Compliance*.
7 I am describing the mean for defiance. On a roughly Aristotelian framework, the deficiency would be submission of, or resignation to, the norms that structure one's social position as subordinate and inferior. The excess would be physical violence, relational aggression within other subordinate groups (horizontal violence), and law breaking that serves one's own interests at the expense of others within one's own community and other groups with whom one shares some commonalities of oppression.
8 Communication with Tessman.
9 Michel Foucault (1999) gives a history of the disciplines of psychiatric containment that begins much earlier than my examples do, but a fair representation of Foucault's contribution to this point is beyond the scope of this chapter.
10 Some of this discussion is taken from Potter 2015.
11 A more thorough sketch of psychiatric ethics is beyond the scope of this chapter; however, I refer readers to *Psychiatric Ethics*, 4th ed. (Block & Green 2009); *The Virtuous Psychiatrist Character Ethics in Psychiatric Practice* (Radden & Sadler 2010); and *The Oxford Handbook of Psychiatric Ethics*, (Sadler, Van Staden, and Fulford, editors, 2015).

REFERENCES

Alcoff, Linda. "Epistemologies of Ignorance: Three Types." *Race and Epistemologies of Ignorance*, edited by Sullivan and Tuana, 39–57. Albany, NY: State University of New York Press, 2007.
Aristotle. *Nicomachean Ethics*. 2nd ed. Translated by Terence Irwin. Indianapolis: Hackett, 1985.
Bailey, Alison. "Strategic Ignorance." In *Race and Epistemologies of Ignorance*, edited by Sullivan and Tuana, 77–94. Albany, NY: State University of New York Press, 2007.
Block, Sidney, and Green, Stephen. *Psychiatric Ethics*. 4th ed. Oxford: Oxford University Press, 2009.
Boxill, Bernard. "Self-respect and Protest." In *Dignity, Character, and Self-Respect*, edited by Dillon, 93–104. New York, NY: Routledge, 1995.
Card, Claudia. *The Unnatural Lottery: Character and Moral Luck*. Philadelphia: Temple University Press, 1996.
Frye, Marilyn. *The Politics of Reality: Essays in Feminist Philosophy*. Freedom, CA: Crossing Press, 1983a.
———. "A Note on Anger." In *The Politics of Reality: Essays in Feminist Philosophy*, 84–94. Freedom, CA: Crossing Press, 1983b.
Foucault, Michel. *Civilization and Madness: A History of Insanity in the Age of Reason*. London: Routledge, 1999.
Halpern, Jodi. *From Detached Concern to Empathy: Humanizing Medical Practice*. Oxford: Oxford University Press, 2001.

Hill, Thomas. "Servility and Self-respect." In *Dignity, Character, and Self-Respect*, edited by Dillon, 76–92. New York, NY: Routledge, 1995.

Johnson Joy L., Joan L. Bottorff, Annette J. Browne, Sukhdev Grewal, Ann Hilton, and Heather Clarke. "Othering and Being Othered in the Context of Health Care Services." *Health Communication* 16, no. 2 (2004): 255–71.

Lugones Maria and Elizabeth Spelman. "Have We Got a Theory for You! Feminist Theory, Cultural Imperialism, and the Demand for 'The Woman's Voice.' " *Women's Studies International Forum* 6, no. 6 (1983): 573–81.

Medina, José. *The Epistemology of Ignorance: Gender and Racial Oppression, Epistemic Injustice, and Resistant Imaginations*. Oxford: Oxford University Press, 2013.

Metzl, Jonathan. *The Protest Psychosis: How Schizophrenia Became a Black Disease*. Beacon Press, 2009.

Mills, Charles. "White Ignorance." *Race and Epistemologies of Ignorance*, edited by Sullivan and Tuana, 13–38. Albany, NY: State University of New York Press, 2007.

———. "Blacks and Social Justice: A Quarter-Century Later." *Journal of Social Philosophy* 41, no. 3 (2010): 354–69.

Potter, Nancy Nyquist. "Feminist Psychiatric Ethics in the 21st Century and the Social Context of Suffering." *Oxford Handbook of Psychiatric Ethics*, edited by KWM Fulford, Martin Davies, Richard Gipps, George Graham, John Sadler, Giovanni Stanghellini, and Tim Thornton. Oxford University Press, 2015: 293–306.

———. "Oppositional Defiant Disorder: Cultural Factors that Influence Interpretations of Defiant Behavior and Their Social and Scientific Consequences." *Classifying Psychopathology: Mental Kinds and Natural Kinds*. MIT Press, 2014b: 175–194.

———. "Mad, Bad, or Virtuous? The Moral, Cultural, and Pathologizing Features of Defiance." *Theory & Psychology* 22, no. 1 (2012):23–45.

———. *Mapping the Edges and the In-Between: A Critical Analysis of Borderline Personality Disorder*. Oxford: Oxford University Press, 2009.

———. "Moral Tourists and World-travelers: Some Epistemological Considerations for Understanding Patients' Worlds." *Philosophy, Psychiatry, and Psychology* 10, no. 3 (2003): 209–223.

———. "Giving Uptake." *Social Theory and Practice* 26, no. 3 (2000): 479–508.

Radden, Jennifer and John Sadler. *The Virtuous Psychiatrist Character Ethics in Psychiatric Practice*. Oxford: Oxford University Press, 2010.

Sadler, John Z., C. W. Van Staden, and K. W. M. Fulford, editors. *The Oxford Handbook of Psychiatric Ethics*. Oxford: Oxford University Press, 2015.

Saks, Elyn. *The Center Cannot Hold: My Journal Through Madness*. New York: Hyperion, 2007.

Shorter, Edward. *A History of Psychiatry: From the Era of the Asylum to the Age of Prozac*. Indianapolis, IN: Wiley, 1998.

Sullivan, Shannon and Nancy Tuana, editors. *Race and Epistemologies of Ignorance*, Albany, NY: State University of New York Press, 2007.

Tessman, Lisa. "Feminist Eudaimonism: Eudaimonism as Non-Ideal Theory." *Feminist Ethics and Social and Political Philosophy: Theorizing the Non-ideal*, edited by L. Tessman, 47–58. New York, NY: Springer, 2009.

———. *Burdened Virtues: Virtue Ethics for Liberatory Struggles*. Oxford: Oxford University Press, 2005.

U.S. Department of Education. "Civil Rights Data Collection. Data Snapshot: School Discipline." 2014a. Accessed April 26, 2014. http://www2.ed.gov/about/offices/list/ocr/docs/crdc-discipline-snapshot.pdf.

————. "Expansive Survey of America's Public Schools Reveals Troubling Ra-
cial Disparities: Lack of Access to Pre-School, Greater Suspensions Cited,"
2014b. Accessed January 20, 2015. http://www.ed.gov/news/press-releases/
expansive-survey-americas-public-schools-reveals-troubling-racial-disparities.
Ussher, Jane. *The Madness of Women: Myth and Experience*. London:
Routledge, 2011.
Young, Iris Marion. *Justice and the Politics of Difference*. Princeton, NJ: Princeton
University Press, 2011.

Part III

Diagnosis in a Global Community

8 Supervirus
The Framing of a Doomsday Diagnosis

Johanna Crane

Ever since effective HIV treatment was first developed in the mid-1990s, the question of who should have access to these life-extending drugs has been a topic of debate among physicians, policy makers, researchers, patients, and activists. Enthusiasm over the drugs' ability to seemingly rescue AIDS patients from the brink of death (dubbed the "Lazarus effect" by the press) was quickly tempered by anxieties over the long-term implications of anti-retroviral treatment for both individuals and the greater public health. The diagnosis of drug-resistant HIV—when viral strains mutate and render the drugs no longer effective—emerged as a salient concern.

For individuals with HIV, a diagnosis of drug resistance often means a change to a more complicated and/or toxic drug regimen and eventually, a worsening of their disease as viable treatment options run out. This diagnosis—not of disease but of drug resistance—is simultaneously a moral burden, a paradox, and a contested event. In terms of public health, the rise of drug-resistant strains of the virus has posed the threat of a secondary epidemic of difficult-to-treat HIV, as these strains can be passed from person to person—meaning that even a newly infected individual who has never taken antiretroviral (ARV) drugs before can be infected with a virus that is already unresponsive to medications. And this process has introduced a new diagnostic controversy over whether and how HIV has become a "supervirus."

Fears about the development and spread of a potential drug-resistant "supervirus" have impacted access to ARVs both at the micro-level of clinical practice and the macro-level of international health policy (Crane 2013). Because drug resistance has been linked to poor medication adherence ("compliance"), patient populations seen as more likely to miss doses or take medication improperly have been framed as risky candidates for antiretroviral treatment, due to speculation that they would foster drug-resistant strains of the virus. Most often, these "risky" populations have been groups marked by race and poverty: poor, often African American, patients in the U.S., as well as patients in the low-income sub-Saharan African countries that have been hit hardest by the global epidemic. The debates over drug resistance reached their political apex in the early 2000s, when some researchers and health officials cautioned against expanding access to HIV drugs in Africa, warning that treatment could lead to "antiretroviral anarchy" (Harries 2001), and turn developing countries into a "veritable 'petri dish' of drug-resistant strains" (Popp and Fisher 2002). In part due to these beliefs, HIV in Africa went largely untreated for the first full decade of the treatment era. This lack of treatment may have prevented the development of a resistant virus, but it also enabled millions of deaths from untreated AIDS.[1] Fears and uncertainties about HIV drug resistance—although not solely responsible for this outcome—were significant in that they provided "scientific" support for global health policies that discouraged ARV access on the African continent.

While claims that both the U.S. urban poor and patients in Africa would be poorly adherent to ARVs were subsequently deflated by studies showing the contrary (McNeil 2003; Bangsberg et al. 2000), the question of HIV drug resistance—what it is, how it is diagnosed, and how it came to be such a powerful idea—remains largely unexamined. In fact, the diagnosis of "resistant" HIV is much more complicated and less straightforward than is often apparent in public scientific debates. Medical historian Charles Rosenberg uses the term "framing disease" to describe how we come to know a disease through processes of diagnosis, prognosis, and illness experience, as well as our social, political, and institutional responses to it. "In some ways," Rosenberg writes, "disease does not exist until we have agreed that it does, by perceiving, naming, and responding to it" (Rosenberg 1992: xiii).

In this chapter, I use ethnographic research and interviews conducted with HIV scientists to explore the "framing" of HIV drug resistance as a stand-alone diagnosis. In doing so, I track how drug resistant HIV has been *made* (or constructed) as both a scientific and a political object, and show how the diagnosis of "resistant" HIV is, in fact, much more complicated and less straightforward than has often been apparent in public debates over HIV treatment.[2] The carving out of this separate diagnostic category, or version, of HIV creates a particular type of space in both the medical and political worlds. And it reveals how the act of diagnosis itself is harnessed for humanitarian, economic, and moralistic ends.

In applying a constructivist approach to the diagnosis of drug resistance, I have sometimes encountered skepticism from HIV researchers, who—when told I was interested in the production of knowledge about antiretroviral resistance—feared I was implying that drug resistance does not, in fact, exist. As I explained to them, and as I elaborate below, my goal in interrogating the science of HIV drug resistance is not to argue that resistance does not exist, but rather to describe the challenges (both biological and social) to its concise definition and diagnosis. The difficulty of defining drug resistance is important precisely because the term "resistant" is so often taken for granted in public discussions about the virus and its dangers. Taking resistance for granted is, in fact, crucial to maintaining the framing of drug-resistant HIV as a cause for a major public health alarm—in other words, its framing as a potential supervirus. By exploring the complexity of

HIV drug resistance as it manifests in the laboratory and clinical practice, alternative and more complex framings may emerge.

I undertake this examination in three parts. I begin by providing some historical background to the problem of diagnostic uncertainty and HIV drug resistance. I track how initial assumptions that a diagnosis of resistance would not be consequential were transformed into panic about the possibility that a dangerous, multi-drug-resistant supervirus might emerge. These fears, in turn, rendered certain groups of patients morally suspect and impacted their ability to access treatment. In the second part of the paper, I examine controversies within the scientific profession over the diagnosis, causes, and consequences of HIV drug resistance, focusing on challenges to the conventional wisdom regarding medication adherence and resistance, as well as evidence that a diagnosis of drug resistance may paradoxically have some clinical benefits. These findings, I show, trouble the framing of drug-resistant HIV as a "supervirus" and upset the moral calculus that labels poorly adherent patients as threats to public safety.

Lastly, I describe ongoing challenges to diagnostic certainty by highlighting the differences between laboratory and clinical diagnoses of HIV drug resistance. I outline the ways in which HIV drug resistance is measured in the laboratory and argue that HIV "drug resistance" is not the self-evident diagnosis that it so often appears to be in public debates about the virus and its dangers. In fact, there are multiple ways of defining resistance and ongoing debates about the ability of molecular laboratory tests to adequately represent the clinical and public health consequences of drug resistance. I conclude by considering the tension between in vitro and in vivo diagnoses of HIV drug resistance, and the implications of the molecularization of HIV medicine for patients and doctors in different parts of the world.

FIRST FRAMINGS

Dr. Ron Pajaro saw his first AIDS patients shortly after finishing his medical residency. At that time, in the early 1980s, the virus itself had not yet been identified. Over the next twenty years, he would make a name for himself in AIDS medicine, balancing continuous work attending to patients in the clinic with a prominent research career studying HIV drug resistance. By the time I met him in 2005, he was a nationally recognized expert in the field. When we spoke, he surprised me by telling me that during the early years of the epidemic, there was "huge skepticism" that HIV drug resistance would have any clinical relevance—in other words, that it would have any negative impact on patients. At that time, the predominant view in medicine was that viruses, once they developed drug-resistant mutations, became too weak to replicate in the body and were thus unable to cause disease. This belief was based on clinical experience treating the herpes virus with the drug acyclovir. Dr. Pajaro explained,

It was common to find acyclovir-resistant virus, but acyclovir would still usually work. It was only in the rare case when it wouldn't work. And the reason for that, it was learned after a while, was that the acyclovir-resistant viruses didn't grow very well in the body. They didn't really replicate well enough for it to cause any disease. And so that was the expectation for HIV resistance.

Pajaro wanted to test this expectation, and made his mark in the field by putting together a group of doctors and virologists to study the impact of HIV drug resistance on patients. The team he organized analyzed the results of a large clinical trial of AZT (zidovudine), the principal antiretroviral drug available at the time. Their findings showed that drug-resistant HIV was in fact quite different from drug-resistant herpes. AZT-resistant HIV remained able to reproduce itself inside the body, and rendered AZT useless in a matter of months:

> So we did this big analysis of a large clinical trial, and basically we and subsequently many others showed that in fact people who had an AZT-resistant virus didn't respond to AZT and they didn't even respond all that well to related drugs. And all of our presentations were met with skepticism. I remember at the time, the guy who had just resigned from being the chair of the AIDS Clinical Trials Group, this big national research organization, challenged us when we presented our findings and said, "Well, this is just confounding. Everybody knows that drug resistance in viruses is meaningless. Go back and reanalyze your data. You've made a mistake somewhere." And we all said to him, "No, we did it right! This is it!" And subsequently, we were proven right.

As it would turn out, Pajaro's findings would coincide with historical events that rapidly caused the pendulum of scientific opinion about HIV drug resistance to swing from dismissal to fear—demonstrating Shapin and Shaffer's observation that the vindication of what is scientifically "right" is not inevitable, but rather an outcome contingent upon historical and social context (Shapin and Shaffer 1987).

The realization by Dr. Pajaro and others that drug resistance could undermine any benefits offered by AZT and other early antiretroviral drugs came in the early 1990s, sharp on the heels of a well-publicized epidemic of multi-drug-resistant tuberculosis (MDR-TB) in New York City. This outbreak was to have profound consequences for the framing of HIV drug resistance, as it set the stage for the diagnosis of drug-resistant HIV to be understood through the lens of MDR-TB. Using this lens, the clinical diagnosis of "drug resistant" became inseparable from the behavioral diagnosis of "poorly adherent," which in turn came with problematic associations about risk, race, and class.

In the late 1980s and early 1990s, tuberculosis rates in the U.S. began to climb at an alarming rate, spurred on by Reagan-era cuts to anti-TB programs and rising cases of HIV (which made infected individuals more susceptible to TB by weakening their immune systems). Significantly, however, TB was relatively rare among the gay, white, middle-class patients who were the most public faces of AIDS in the U.S. at the time. Instead, TB appeared most commonly among HIV-positive Haitians (who were more likely to have been exposed to the disease in Haiti, where TB prevalence was high) and HIV-positive homeless people or prison inmates, as the overcrowding and poor ventilation common in both shelters and prisons facilitated TB transmission (Rosenthal 1990). The jump in tuberculosis was particularly acute in New York City, where the TB rate in 1991 topped 4,000 for the first time since 1967 (Specter 1992). In addition, many more of these TB cases were drug resistant than ever before, making the disease more difficult to treat successfully and more likely to result in death. In 1991, an outbreak of MDR-TB killed 13 inmates in New York prisons (McFadden 1991). Tuberculosis experts quoted in the press argued that resistant TB was on the rise because many patients were failing to complete the months-long regimen of antibiotics required to cure active tuberculosis, often because of mental illness, drug abuse, and/or homelessness.

Understandably, health officials were alarmed at the possibility of a growing epidemic of a microbe that was difficult to treat, easy to spread, and potentially lethal. As a result, the city began to impose enforced hospitalization on tuberculosis patients who repeatedly failed to complete their treatment. These modern-day Typhoid Marys were most often African Americans from the most marginal fringes of society—the addicted, the mentally ill, and the homeless.[3]

Similar issues arose in other U.S. cities as they confronted their own growing rates of tuberculosis. Health officials justified the medical detention of non-adherent patients as necessary for public safety. One Denver professor of medicine put it this way: "Say I'm totally drug resistant and I still like going to movies and I like going to restaurants and I like getting in buses and I like teaching in schools," he told a *New York Times* reporter. "If I had a gun and I waved it around in all those places you would lock me up. This is no different than a loaded gun" (Belkin 1991).

The timing of the TB outbreak and the public health alarm that it caused shifted the lens through which a diagnosis of drug-resistant HIV was viewed. Rather than comparing HIV to drug-resistant herpes, experts likened it to multi-drug-resistant TB, which was potentially lethal and carried with it a particular image of danger marked by race and class (Bangsberg et al. 2004). "HIV drug resistance frighteningly recapitulates the history of antimicrobial drug resistance in bacteria with a pernicious twist," wrote one prominent HIV researcher in 2004. "HIV is not curable and drug-resistant variants are archived within each patient for life" (Richman 2004: 1398). Following the TB publicity, Pajaro told me, the discourse "was very much the broad brushstroke that resistant HIV is not going to respond to anything." He was circumspect about this shift, laughing as he told me that

"that's the pattern for much of HIV research. It's always from one extreme to the opposite extreme."

The coding of incomplete adherence as a threat to not only one's own health but to the general public, as well as the public image of the poorly adherent patient as poor and African American, would play a significant role in the subsequent controversies over the diagnosis of drug-resistant HIV. Like TB, successful HIV treatment required patients to take a combination of several drugs over an extended period of time. Understandably, adhering to such regimens was challenging for many patients—especially given that the treatment for HIV was indefinite, with no endpoint in sight. Having witnessed the recent upsurge of MDR-TB, many AIDS doctors feared the development of drug-resistant strains of HIV among their poorly adherent patients. Some doctors went so far as to withhold ARVs from homeless or drug-using patients who they believed would be unable to adhere (Bangsberg et al. 1998; Collins 1996; Sontag and Richardson 1997).[4] A spirited debate ensued as to whether this practice was a breach of the Hippocratic oath, or a professional obligation necessary to protect the public's health (Baxter 1997; Bayer and Stryker 1997; Lerner et al. 1998; Senak 1997; Sollitto et al. 2001). Once pressure began to mount for antiretroviral treatment in Africa, similar fears resurfaced with a new international slant. While experts who cautioned against global treatment access did not make direct comparisons between the U.S. urban poor and patients in Africa, it seems noteworthy—as one American epidemiologist told me, with intentional irony—that the targets of fear remained "poor black people." In this way, the emerging diagnostic controversy over HIV drug resistance became inseparable from social, political, and moral controversies over race, class, and access to treatment.

CHALLENGING THE CONVENTIONAL WISDOM

As research on HIV treatment evolved, scientists and clinicians grappled with rising uncertainty and controversy over the diagnosis of drug resistance *and* the diagnosis of non-adherence, as well as the relationship between the two. Challenges arose to two key pieces of conventional wisdom within HIV medicine: first, the belief that poor adherence inevitably caused drug resistance; and second, that a diagnosis of drug resistance signaled the end of drug efficacy and a rapid decline in patients' health.

Sociologist of science Dorothy Nelkin has argued that although scientific controversies typically take the form of debates over technical issues, they are at heart of debates over moral and political questions (Nelkin 1995). This has certainly been the case with HIV drug resistance, where diagnostic debates over viral mutations and pharmaceutical chemistry have never been far from moral and political controversies over treatment access. The diagnostic framing of a drug-resistant virus as a superbug akin to MDR-TB (with similar racial and class overtones) is an example of how the political question of who gets treatment and the moral question of who is deemed "deserving" of it were often articulated through the technical, expert language of epidemiology and public health. However, it was also from within these more technical domains that the frame of the "supervirus" later confronted some of its biggest challenges. This happened when HIV researchers began to question both the causes and the consequences of a drug resistance diagnosis.

Based on previous experience with tuberculosis treatment, the belief that missed medication doses would lead to drug resistance was widely accepted from early on in the field of AIDS medicine. In both the research literature and published treatment guidelines, the importance of assuring patient adherence was stressed as a key tool for warding off the development of a drug-resistant virus (see, for example, U.S. DHHS 2003). Experts believed that patients needed to take between 80 and 95 percent of their antiretrovirals as prescribed in order to benefit from antiretroviral treatment (Chesney 2003). However, research suggested that the typical adherence rates were closer to 70 percent (Golin et al. 2002). In a 2003 article reviewing the literature on antiretroviral adherence, a leading AIDS prevention researcher argued that the prevention of HIV drug resistance required "near perfect" adherence, in the range of 95 percent or higher (Chesney 2003).

However, in 2002, a team of researchers at the University of California, San Francisco (UCSF) began to challenge the conventional wisdom, posing the provocative question, "Is average adherence to HIV antiretroviral therapy enough?" (Bangsberg and Deeks 2002). These researchers argued that the association between poor adherence and resistance to ARVs was based on inadequate research, and that their research suggested a more complex—and sometimes paradoxical—relationship between adherence and resistance. In a study of antiretroviral treatment among U.S. HIV patients, the researchers found that drug resistance was most commonly diagnosed among *highly* adherent patients—those who took nearly all of their doses as prescribed (Bangsberg et al. 2003). Patients with the worst adherence (under 65 percent) had little drug resistance, though they also had little clinical benefit from treatment. The researchers explained this surprising finding by arguing that the relationship between poor adherence and drug resistance was different for different types, or classes, of HIV drugs.

At the time, there were three different classes of antiretroviral drugs in use in the United States: NRTIs (nucleotide reverse transcriptase inhibitors, or "nukes"), such as AZT, NNRTIs (non-nucleoside reverse transcriptase inhibitors, or "non-nukes"), and protease inhibitors. Most regimens paired two "nukes" with either an NNRTI or a protease inhibitor. For NNRTI-based regimens, the conventional wisdom did hold, and poor adherence led unequivocally to drug resistance. But for protease inhibitor-based regimens, the relationship was more complex, and resistance appeared primarily in patients with near-perfect adherence to the medications. Though

initially counter-intuitive, the researchers explained these results as a factor of different drug-specific "genetic barriers" to resistance: HIV can often
become resistant to an NNRTI by undergoing a single mutation. However, it
must mutate many times in order to become resistant to a protease inhibitor.
Patients who look less than 65 percent of a protease inhibitor-based regimen
simply did not maintain high enough levels of the medication in their bodies
to force the virus to undergo the multiple mutations necessary to become
drug resistant.[5] Given the common belief that it was poor adherence that
caused drug resistance and "near perfect" adherence that prevented it, these
findings were provocative. In addition to upsetting the conventional wisdom
in HIV medicine, they also complicated the moral calculus established during the MDR-TB outbreak that linked a diagnosis of drug resistance to poor
adherence to "recalcitrant" (even "dangerous") patients. Paradoxically, it
was the "model" patients who were developing drug resistance.

Challenges to the conventional wisdom regarding the *causes* of antiretroviral resistance coincided with the emergence of disagreements regarding the
consequences of a drug resistance diagnosis. In the early 2000s, physicians
studying the management of U.S. patients with resistance to multiple HIV
drugs began publishing data showing that many patients diagnosed with
drug resistance continued to do well clinically (Deeks et al. 2000). These
patients' CD4 counts remained stable—meaning their immune systems continued to function—and the level of the virus in their blood remained relatively low. In other words, even though diagnostic testing showed them to
be "resistant" to the drugs they were on, the medicines were continuing preserve their health. These results troubled the common-sense view that drug
resistance by definition rendered antiretrovirals ineffective and led rapidly
to progression towards AIDS.

The reason behind these paradoxical findings, researchers argued, was
that resistance mutations weakened the virus. As a result, resistant viruses
were less able to replicate efficiently, which ended up keeping their numbers
at bay and preserving the health of the patient (Barbour et al. 2002). Furthermore, these weaker viruses appeared to be more difficult to transmit to
others (Leigh Brown et al. 2003; Booth and Geretti 2007), suggesting that
drug-resistant HIV might also be less of a public health threat than had been
initially thought. This reduced "replicative capacity" or "viral fitness" was
an unexpected benefit of many drug resistance mutations—a sort of a silver
lining to an otherwise dark cloud. To recall Dr. Pajaro's comparison, the findings suggested that drug-resistant HIV perhaps bore closer resemblance to
drug-resistant herpes than to drug-resistant TB after all. Jim Greene, one of
the senior researchers who contributed to these findings, made a similar comparison when we spoke. "The way I think about it is: is HIV like MDR-TB or
is it like drug-resistant herpes?" he told me. "Clearly [HIV lies] somewhere
in between. The latest news suggests that it's more toward the herpes side.
I think more data is needed, but I think that it's more toward the herpes side."

Although these findings are now widely accepted, the research was very
controversial when first presented at scientific meetings. David Capelli, a

young PhD involved in the research on viral fitness, told me of scientific conference sessions that ended up in "shouting matches" over their data:

> I think people were very concerned about what the message of our work could be. . . . We were—I think "accused" is the right word—of saying that we thought it was okay for people to have drug resistance. And that maybe it was even good news. You know, and I think even though we tried to very carefully deliver our message onto the broadest stages in the field, I think there was still active misinterpretation of that message. We were never trying to suggest that we thought drug resistance was okay.

Dr. Capelli's account of the controversy suggests that the debate over this research was moral as much as it was scientific. The implication that drug resistance might be "okay" was volatile. Just as the controversial findings about adherence and resistance had upset the moral equation of "bad" (non-adherent) patients equating to a "bad" (drug-resistant) virus, the studies on viral fitness further complicated this calculus by suggesting that drug resistance might actually have some clinical benefits. For years, scientists, clinicians, and patients had been trained to view a diagnosis of antiretroviral resistance with dread. The discovery that, in certain cases, this diagnosis might be "okay" was initially treated as a form of blasphemy.

These scientific controversies over the causes and consequences of HIV drug resistance entered the public arena in a rather dramatic fashion in the winter of 2005, when the New York City Department of Health and Mental Hygiene held a press conference to announce the discovery of a man who appeared to have been infected by a form of HIV that was both highly drug resistant and extremely aggressive. The patient, a gay man and methamphetamine user in his 40s, was described as resistant to all three major classes of antiretrovirals even though he had only recently tested HIV positive and had never taken any antiretroviral drugs previously. Furthermore, his CD4 count was quite low and he had been diagnosed with advanced AIDS even though he had been infected only a few months earlier.[6] In the press release, New York City's Health Commissioner, Dr. Thomas Frieden, described the man's virus in ominous terms, as "a strain of HIV that is difficult or impossible to treat and which appears to progress rapidly to AIDS" and warned that the case should serve as a "wake up call to men who have sex with men, particularly those who may use crystal methamphetamine" (NY DOHMH 2005). The Department also issued an alert to clinicians and hospitals, asking them to screen their HIV-positive patients for evidence of the resistant virus. This alarm was echoed in a case study of the infection that was published a month later in the medical journal the *Lancet*, in which a group of doctors at New York's prestigious Aaron Diamond AIDS Research Center asserted that the case had "great public health ramifications" (Markowitz et al. 2005).

The news media jumped on the story, producing multiple articles about the arrival of the potential "AIDS superbug" (Edozien 2005; Honigsbaum 2005; Perez-Pena 2005; Santora and Altman 2005a). In typical tabloid fashion, the February 12, 2005 cover of the *New York Post* posted a nearly full-page headline warning of the discovery of a "nightmare strain" of HIV in New York City. At a major scientific AIDS conference that was held (coincidentally) just two weeks after news of the infection was made public, last-minute changes were made to the conference schedule in order to devote an entire session to discussion of the virus (Conference on Retroviruses and Opportunistic Infections 2005).

However, challenges to the "superbug" characterization soon surfaced, and it rapidly became clear that scientific opinions were divided over whether the decision to publicize the case had been necessary to protect the public's health, or ill-informed fear mongering. Commissioner Frieden came under fire both from gay activists—who objected to the portrayal of gay men "as crazed drug addicts . . . wantonly spreading a killer bug"—and from fellow AIDS experts, who felt that the alarm over the case was overly hasty (Santora and Altman 2005b). Dr. David Ho, a scientist famous for developing the protease inhibitor class of ARVs, defended Frieden with the assertions that "there's no case like this," and "this is not a wimpy virus," arguing that the New York City virus was unique and deserved special scrutiny and public health attention (Cohen 2005). But other equally prominent AIDS experts declared nearly the opposite, describing the case as "not a discovery," "not a surprise," "hardly unique," "not a novel finding," and "common" (Brower 2005; Cohen 2005; Smith 2005; Piller 2005; Volberding 2005). "It would, in fact, be strange," a representative of an AIDS advocacy think tank opined, "if this did not occur" (Jeffreys 2005). A number of experts noted that similar cases of HIV had been documented in Vancouver in 2003, and that these viruses had not been passed on to others, suggesting that they were not highly transmissible (Chan et al. 2003). They argued that the New York City health department's decision to issue a public warning about the drug-resistant virus implicitly minimized the everyday dangers posed by the "regular virus" (Montaner, in Brower 2005). "Dr. Frieden's call for increased vigilance against drug resistant HIV implies that regular, old-fashioned HIV infection is not horrific enough," argued one commentary in the scientific journal *Retrovirology* (Smith 2005).

In the end, some of the key assertions in the New York City DOHMH's press release proved to be overstated. Although the virus was in fact multi-drug resistant, it was not accurate—as the press release had reported—that it "did not respond to three classes of anti-retroviral medication." In fact, several months later, the patient was reported to be doing well with therapy, though his treatment consisted of a combination of six drugs rather than a more typical three- or four-drug regimen. In addition, the DOHMH's claim that the patient seemed to have progressed rapidly to AIDS—perhaps as "within two to three months" of becoming infected—was rejected by many experts, who thought it was more likely that he was infected closer to 20 months earlier, shortly after last testing HIV negative in May 2003 (Volberding 2005). This was still comparatively rapid, but not unprecedented and still within the normal limits of HIV disease progression. Some experts suggested that the patient's rapid clinical decline might have little to do with the virus itself, and could instead be the result of what they called "host factors"—in other words, characteristics of the patient's immune system, as well as his addiction—rather than a particularly aggressive virus. Furthermore, a number of researchers expressed doubt that the virus was highly transmissible, and argued that even if it were to be transmitted to others, it would likely behave differently in different patients or "hosts." When I asked one prominent drug resistance researcher about the case four months after the initial publicity, he told me the scientific consensus was that the initial reaction to the infection had been "hyperbole." In his opinion, most experts agreed that "this was worrisome and needed investigation, but it's a single case and not yet an epidemic." Dr. Paul Volberding, director of UCSF's Center for AIDS Research and a senior scientist in the field, was more blunt, telling the *New York Times*: "This is a non-story" (Santora and Altman 2005b).

Given that public anxieties about HIV drug resistance had until this point been largely targeted at Africa, the emergence of a candidate "killer bug" in the United States serves as an important reminder that it is wealthy countries, where treatment is abundant, that actually pose the greatest risk for cultivating drug-resistant strains of HIV.[7] In addition, the panic over the New York City "supervirus" as well as its subsequent dismissal as hyperbole highlights the significant scientific uncertainties that surround the causes, consequences, and precise diagnosis of HIV drug resistance. These uncertainties are perhaps most evident in the paradoxical relationship between drug resistance and viral fitness: as in the New York City case, mutations that theoretically make a virus resistant to drugs (and thus difficult to treat) end up weakening its ability to replicate and to infect others. In other words, the very thing that was supposed to turn the virus into a "superbug" rendered it, in the end, a "non-story."

Significantly, the finding that drug resistance could sometimes weaken the HIV virus was meaningful not only to researchers and clinicians, but also to drug manufacturers, as it provided an alternative, positive spin for mutations that would otherwise be seen as a strike against their product. For example, one clinician I interviewed described being visited by a representative from GlaxoSmithKline, the manufacturer of the common NNRTI called 3TC (lamivudine). This drug is known to cause a common resistance mutation called M184V.[8] In addition to causing 3TC resistance, the M184V mutation also significantly weakens the virus, impairing its ability to reproduce. The Glaxo representative, unaware that the clinician he was speaking with was also a leading drug resistance researcher, showed him some drug product information listing only the beneficial (virus-weakening) effects of the mutation and not the fact that it also caused resistance. This was in contradiction to guidelines issued by the International AIDS Society-USA (IAS-USA), an independent body of experts, which listed M184V as a resistance mutation. Because this clinician was an expert on resistance, he recognized the omission. However, though the IAS-USA guidelines are widely used and respected, there is no single standardized list of resistance mutations, making it easy for different bodies to compile lists that reflect their own interests.[9] In this case, the drug company successfully marketed an alternative interpretation of the mutation directly to doctors. As this clinician told me in 2005:

> Three or four years ago, it was very common for doctors to believe that if you were on this drug and you developed this one particular resistance mutation, you didn't really need to stop the drug. You could keep the drug going. In vitro, it would look like the virus was resistant to the drug. But the drug was still providing benefit. . . . There may be some truth to it, but the reality is that you know it's a good way to sell the drug. You never have to stop using it. Just always keep using it. And so the drug company very early on recognized this as a good marketing tactic and very aggressively marketed the decreased fitness of the mutant [virus].

In actuality, both interpretations of M184V are true—the mutation both reduces the drug's effectiveness *and* weakens the virus—but the company was seeking to highlight the latter while obscuring the former, essentially using the mutation as a selling point.[10] Thus, in this example, we see how pharmaceutical manufacturers can also use diagnostic uncertainty for strategic marketing purposes.

"MY PATIENT IS NOT A LAB" (CLINICAL DIAGNOSIS IN THE AGE OF MOLECULAR MEDICINE)

Given the scientific uncertainties over the causes and consequences of drug resistance, it seems important to dig deeper and examine what drug resistance, in fact, *is* in practice. What constitutes antiretroviral resistance, and how is it defined? These are, in many ways, evolving questions. The diagnosis of resistance varies according to the specific antiretroviral medication in question and the tools used to measure it. Scientific and clinical understandings of drug-resistant HIV have been shaped in particular by the development of two different diagnostic laboratory tests: the genotype and phenotype resistance assays. In many ways, these technologies act as "inscription devices," tools to transform otherwise chaotic information into concise, legible data that can be used by scientists and doctors (Latour and Woolgar 1986). Diagnostic technologies in particular, writes Keith Wailoo, "do not *define* diseases so much as they stand in some relation to disease phenomena, framing and giving a particular coherence to lived experience, labeling sets of symptoms, and directing social policy" (Wailoo 1997: 2). As such, these scientific tools and the knowledge they generate "co-construct" one another (Clarke and Fujimura 1992), making understandings of drug resistance inseparable from the particular technologies used to measure it. It follows, then, that genotyping and phenotyping imply somewhat different framings of what constitutes drug resistance. In addition, both of these framings challenge the simplistic portrayals of drug-resistant HIV as an ominous "AIDS superbug."

Most frequently, HIV drug resistance is described as resulting from genetic mutations in the virus. In this framing, HIV undergoes genetic changes that allow it to evade the suppressive effects of antiretroviral medications. Genotype resistance testing works by producing a genetic sequence or "map" of the virus's RNA that can then be examined for resistance mutations. HIV is a highly diverse virus, and as a result, any given HIV-positive individual carries millions of copies of the virus that are each slightly genetically different from one another—a "population" of viruses, rather than identical copies of a single virus. Genotype assays are useful because they are able to take the assemblage of diverse viruses carried by any one patient and generate from it a single, aggregate list of drug resistance mutations that are most common. For this reason, they have proven very useful both to researchers and to clinicians, who often rely upon these diagnostic tests to ascertain which drugs a patient will respond to best. This is particularly important in the case of patients who have been on antiretrovirals for a long time and may have developed resistance to several drugs, and for patients infected with drug-resistant variants, such as the New York City man described earlier.

However, not all mutations result in drug resistance, and scientific consensus about which mutations are considered resistance mutations is constantly evolving as new drugs and new studies of resistance emerge. Experts disagree about the meaning of certain mutations, and there is no single, standardized list of resistance mutations that is shared by all scientists and clinicians. Commercially produced genotype assays often rely upon a list provided by the manufacturer. Many researchers refer to the mutation lists published by the IAS-USA or the similar European body. Still others consider a list put out by a group at Stanford University to be the "gold standard." Furthermore, genotype tests typically sequence only limited sections of the HIV genome, and thus do not account for the possibility that mutations elsewhere in the virus might impact drug susceptibility. Thus, while a useful tool, genotype resistance assays present only a partial and uncertain picture of resistant HIV.

Genotyping is an indirect measure of resistance that uses genetic markers as a proxy for viral behavior in the presence of drugs. Phenotyping, in contrast, provides a more direct measure of resistance by examining how a patient's virus reacts upon actual exposure to drugs in the laboratory. If a drug stops the virus in its tracks, the virus is fully susceptible. But if the virus continues to reproduce despite the presence of an antiretroviral, it is resistant to that drug. Often, the result is somewhere in between, meaning the virus is only partially resistant.

Because phenotype assays measure resistance along a continuum, doctors and scientists must decide which points along this continuum constitute the line between "susceptible," "partially susceptible," and "resistant." These points, called "cut-offs," vary depending on which criteria are used. Initially, a *technical* cut-off was used, where the virus being tested was compared to a commonly used laboratory reference strain of HIV. However, the lack of commensurability between laboratory strains of HIV and those most commonly found in patients made this technical cut-off limited in applicability outside the laboratory (see Crane 2011). A move was made to use *biological* cut-offs, which defined resistance in comparison to viruses taken from patients never treated with ARVs ("treatment-naïve" patients). Still, this comparison was based on how these viruses reacted to drugs in a petri dish, not in the human body, and—as one California physician told me— "Clinicians are saying, 'Yeah, that's great, that's what happens in the lab. But my patient's not a lab. What happens when I give it to my patient?'"

Most recently, there has been a push in HIV medicine to develop *clinical* cut-offs for both "intermediate" and "full" resistance. These cut-offs are the points at which a drug's efficacy begins to decline (intermediate resistance) and at which a drug provides no benefit at all (full resistance) to patients undergoing antiretroviral treatment. The development of clinical cut-offs is labor-intensive because they can only be determined by collecting large amounts of clinical trial data from patients receiving treatment. In addition, each antiretroviral drug has its own cut-off, in other words, a different point at which it ceases to be effective. Because it is ineffective (and thus unethical) to treat an HIV patient with less than three drugs, teasing out the different cut-offs of each drug in a three-drug combination from clinical trial data is a tricky and labor-intensive endeavor.

In comparing HIV genotype and phenotype testing, it is evident that drug resistance is not a stable, fixed entity, but rather an idea with multiple, variable meanings, some of which overlap. Resistance can be defined in molecular terms, as an attribute of mutations in the viral genome, or in more traditional laboratory terms, as the virus's ability to reproduce when exposed to drugs in a petri dish. Both of these definitions may or may not correlate with a patient's clinical decline, depending in part on whether resistance mutations have impaired the capacity of the virus to replicate. This complexity can lead to the paradoxical situation described earlier, in which patients who show resistance mutations nonetheless continue to benefit from their antiretroviral drugs. The New York City case is a good example of the trickiness of pinpointing drug resistance, and the gaps that may exist between genetic resistance (genotype), resistance measured in vitro (phenotype), and clinical resistance (the patient's health). Genotype testing showed the New York patient to be "broadly resistant" to all three major classes of antiretrovirals in common use at the time (NRTIs, NNRTIS, and protease inhibitors). But phenotypic testing found that his virus responded normally to a number of these drugs. He was successfully treated with a combination of NRTIs, an NNRTI, and a drug called Fuzeon (enfurvitide), the first of a newer class of antiretrovirals called entry inhibitors.

To be sure, this was a more complex and intensive antiretroviral regimen than would normally be prescribed for a newly infected patient. But it worked, and the fact that it included both NRTIs and an NNRTI troubles the characterization of his virus as "broadly resistant" to these classes of drugs. This does not mean that this characterization was false; rather, it reflects the gaps between genomic, laboratory, and clinical framings of antiretroviral resistance. It is these gaps that allowed the New York City patient's virus to be constructed as a potential superbug according to genotype results, and yet resisted as such by the patient's positive clinical response to treatment.

CONCLUSION: TREATMENT HISTORIES AND FUTURES

Although the clinical applicability of HIV resistance testing was initially uncertain, in recent years, the use of resistance assays (and particularly genotyping) has become integrated into HIV patient care in wealthy countries. Once reserved primarily for research purposes, genotype testing is now recommended for patients initiating or switching HIV treatments in order to prevent the prescription of any drugs to which the patient might already be resistant (Hirsch et al. 2003; DHHS 2013). As a result, HIV drug resistance testing has emerged as one of the few clinically applicable techniques to emerge from the much-touted field of pharmacogenomics or "personalized" medicine. By using molecular diagnostic technologies to create optimized antiretroviral regimens, HIV resistance testing has succeeded in delivering on personalized medicine's promise of high-tech therapies tailored to individual biologies. Indeed, the HIV phenotyping company formerly called ViroLogic changed its name to Monogram Biosciences in the mid-2000s, and described itself as dedicated to "advancing individualized medicine." On its website, the company posited, "[T]he goal of individualized medicine is to move from a 'one drug suits all' approach to providing the right treatment to the right patient at the right time."

It is the clinical application of HIV resistance testing that best exemplifies the promise of personalized medicine: medication regimens individually tailored to a patient's disease. Yet, as I hope my discussion of genotyping and phenotyping exemplified, there is often a gap between diagnostic specificity in vitro and medicine in vivo—in other words, between a molecular and a clinical diagnosis. The drug resistance mutations detected by genotype assays do not always reflect clinical resistance (Flexner 2000; Tamalet 2000), and the cut-offs used to demarcate phenotypic resistance are only rough estimates of when a patient might stop benefiting from a drug.

This tension between "objective" genetic measures and "subjective" clinical indicators of resistance reflects a larger shift in the relationship of the laboratory to the clinic. Laboratory methods are increasingly being adopted into diagnosis, resulting in a "culture of clinical experimentation" that links spaces of patient care to molecular and virology labs, and ultimately to processes of pharmaceutical production (Löwy 2000: 68). In the current era of molecular medicine, the ability to integrate molecular measures into patient diagnosis and care is increasingly central to "the art of medicine," as one American HIV clinician and drug resistance researcher I spoke with phrased it. In turn, molecular information collected through clinical care may also feed back into laboratory research and into industry. For example, the companies that make and sell genotype and phenotype assays have built valuable databases of resistant HIV sequences to which they sell access—often to drug companies, who use the information in their drug development process. The sequences in these databases are culled from the clinical samples sent to them by doctors and hospitals for drug resistance testing.

However, this feedback loop between clinic, lab, and industry is profoundly shaped by geography. In many areas of sub-Saharan Africa, doctors have a very limited choice of antiretrovirals, often struggle to access monitoring tests like CD4 counts and viral loads, and almost never have access to genotyping, except in a few very rare research contexts. By contrast, in the U.S., doctors can choose from nearly thirty drugs and all available diagnostics, including new tests designed to detect resistance to new classes of ARVs. Outside wealthy, industrialized nations, HIV medicine is much less molecularized and personalized. In fact, while individually *tailored* diagnostics based on genotype profiling have become the norm in the U.S., discussions in international health focus on the development of *standardized* HIV regimens for use in low-income settings (Weidle 2002)—in other words, "one drug suits all."

Though the gap between in vitro and in vivo results is nothing new in medical science, the rise of molecular HIV medicine may raise new questions for this age-old quandary. What is gained from the molecular diagnostics of this disease, and what is lost? Do differences at the molecular level really matter at the clinical level? What are the political and economic implications of the molecularization of HIV diagnosis? In conceiving of the body as a space of interaction between genes and highly commercialized pharmaceutical and diagnostic products, "molecular," "pharmacogenomics," and "individualized" medicine imply a particular relationship between biologies and markets. In the global AIDS epidemic, what practices and discourses determine whose bodies and which biologies will constitute this marketplace?

NOTES

1   Researchers have estimated that HIV treatment saved over 3 million years of human life in the United States between 1989 and 2003 (Walensky et al. 2006), a finding that suggests that many millions more years of life were lost

during this period in Africa, where infection rates were much higher and treatment access much lower. Indeed, one study estimated that the lack of access to antiretrovirals in South Africa alone was responsible for the loss of 3.8 million person-years of life in that country between 2000 and 2005 (Chigwedere et al. 2008). (This was not only due to pharmaceutical pricing, but also due to former South African President Thabo Mbeki's controversial embracing of "dissident" or "denialist" AIDS science, and his skepticism over whether HIV was the cause of AIDS; see Fassin 2007; Mahajan 2006).

2 The argument presented here is based on ethnographic research conducted among American and Ugandan doctors and HIV researchers in 2004 and 2005, when I was a doctoral candidate in medical anthropology at the University of California, San Francisco. In order to protect the participants' privacy, all interviewees are identified by pseudonyms.

3 Of the 33 tuberculosis patients detained by the NYC Public Health Department between January of 1988 and April of 1991, 79 percent were black, 79 percent were drug users, 49 percent were homeless, and 61 percent were men (Navarro 1993). Many were also mentally ill, and had been hospitalized for TB several times previously. Seventy-three percent had drug-resistant tuberculosis (Navarro 1992). The law under which tuberculosis patients were forcibly hospitalized dates from the era of Mary Mallon—"Typhoid Mary"—who was believed to have infected 50 people with typhoid fever prior to 1915 (Barbanel 1991).

4 Studies later showed that clinicians' estimates of who would and would not be adherent were no more accurate than random guessing (Tchetgen et. al. 2001; Paterson et. al. 2000).

5 Mutation only occurs when the virus is replicating. Ideally, perfect adherence keeps drug levels in the blood high enough to prevent the virus from reproducing, thus also stopping it from mutating. However, when drug levels drop—perhaps due to missed doses—the virus may begin to replicate again. When HIV replicates in the presence of an antiretroviral drug—or under what scientists call "drug pressure"—the mutations that develop are likely to be resistance mutations, as it is these genetic changes that give the virus the ability to "escape" the drug. In the study, patients who took less than 65 percent of their protease inhibitors had levels of medication in their blood that were simply too low to push the virus to undergo the numerous mutations needed to develop resistance. For these patients, it was essentially as if they were taking no medication at all. But in patients who were highly—but not quite perfectly—adherent to protease inhibitors, drug levels dipped low enough to allow viral replication but stayed high enough to force the virus to mutate in order to do so, creating a perfect pharmacokinetic storm for the development of drug resistance.

6 Often the time between infection with the HIV virus and the development of the AIDS syndrome is as long as a decade.

7 For example, one study of San Diego patients reported that nearly half of those receiving treatment had developed some degree of drug resistance during the late 1990s (Garrett 2001; Richman et al. 2004). Research also indicated that these drug-resistant viral strains were being transmitted to others. Although exact numbers are difficult to come by, a 2004 review showed that anywhere from 8 to 27 percent of newly infected (and never-treated) patients in the United States carried a virus with at least one drug-resistant mutation, and that 10 percent of people newly diagnosed with HIV in Europe showed some drug resistance (Tang and Pillay 2004). In contrast, the review included only one study of drug resistance in Africa, conducted in Cote

d'Ivoire between 1997 and 2000, which found no evidence of transmitted ARV resistance.

8   The notation used to refer to viral mutations describes the location on the genome where the mutation occurred and the substitution of one amino acid for another. Thus, M187V refers to the substitution of valine ("V") for methionine ("M") at location 187.

9   In fact, the clinician explained to me, the IAS-USA list of resistance mutations was developed as an attempt to generate an objective list in the face of pressure from pharmaceutical interests. "Everybody recognized that there were different tables and lists out there," he told me. "Some of them were being promoted heavily by some of the drug companies to say that, you know, 'oh, this mutation that's selected by my drug is really not a bad mutation, and it doesn't confer resistance.' So that was what really drove having an objective, standardized listing so physicians would be able to counter the drug detail men and say, 'Well, no. Here's what the IAS-USA says. You're wrong.'"

10 Companies use drug resistance as a marketing tool in other ways as well—for example, by arguing that their drug causes less resistance than that of a competitor. This practice is facilitated by FDA regulations allowing drug companies to withhold their drug resistance data from the public as "proprietary" information (Shafer 2005, letter to FDA).

REFERENCES

Bangsberg, David R., and S.G. Deeks. "Paradoxes of Adherence and Drug Resistance to HIV Antiretroviral Therapy." *The Journal of Antimicrobial Chemotherapy* 53, no. 5 (May 2004): 696–99.

———. "Is Average Adherence to HIV Antiretroviral Therapy enough?" *Journal of General Internal Medicine: Official Journal of the Society for Research and Education in Primary Care Internal Medicine* 17, no. 10 (October 2002): 812–13.

Bangsberg, D. R., F. M. Hecht, E. D. Charlebois, A. R. Zolopa, M. Holodniy, L. Sheiner, J. D. Bamberger, M. A. Chesney, and A. Moss. "Adherence to protease inhibitors, HIV-1 viral load, and development of drug resistance in an indigent population." *AIDS (London, England)* 14, no. 4 (Mar 10, 2000): 357-66.

Bangsberg, David R., M. Robertson, E.D. Charlebois, J. Tulsky, F.M. Hecht, J.D. Bamberger, and A. Moss. "Protease Inhibitors (PI) in the HIV+ Homeless and Marginally Housed (H/M): Good Adherence but Rarely Prescribed." Oral presentation #389/32406, International AIDS Conference, Geneva, Switzerland, 1998.

Bangsberg, David R., E.D. Charlebois, R.M. Grant, M. Holodniy, S.G. Deeks, S. Perry, K.N. Conroy, et al. "High Levels of Adherence Do Not Prevent Accumulation of HIV Drug Resistance Mutations." *AIDS (London, England)* 17, no. 13 (September 5, 2003): 1925–32.

Barbanel, Josh. "Rise in tuberculosis forces review of dated methods." *New York Times* (July 7, 1991).

Barbour, J.D., T. Wrin, R.M. Grant, J.N. Martin, M.R. Segal, C.J. Petropoulos, and S.G. Deeks. "Evolution of Phenotypic Drug Susceptibility and Viral Replication Capacity during Long-Term Virologic Failure of Protease Inhibitor Therapy in Human Immunodeficiency Virus-Infected Adults." *Journal of Virology* 76, no. 21 (November 2002): 11104–12.

Baxter, Daniel. "Casting Off the 'Unreliable' AIDS Patient." *New York Times*, March 6, 1997, sec. Op-Ed.

Bayer, R. and J. Stryker. "Ethical Challenges Posed by Clinical Progress in AIDS." *American Journal of Public Health* 87, no. 10 (October 1997): 1599–602.

Belkin, Lisa. "Top TB Peril: Not Taking the Medicine." *New York Times*, November 18, 1991, A1..

Booth, C.L. and A. M. Geretti. "Prevalence and Determinants of Transmitted Antiretroviral Drug Resistance in HIV-1 Infection." *The Journal of Antimicrobial Chemotherapy* 59, no. 6 (June 2007): 1047–56.

Brower, V. "New superbug or tempest in a teapot?" *EMBO Reports* 6, no. 6 (June, 2005): 502-4.

Chan, K.C., R.A. Galli, J.S. Montaner, and P.R. Harrigan. "Prolonged Retention of Drug Resistance Mutations and Rapid Disease Progression in the Absence of Therapy After Primary HIV Infection." *AIDS (London, England)* 17, no. 8 (May 23, 2003): 1256–8.

Chesney, M. "Adherence to HAART Regimens." *AIDS Patient Care and STDs* 17, no. 4 (April 2003): 169–77.

Chigwedere, P., G.R. Seage 3rd, S. Gruskin, T.H. Lee, and M. Essex. "Estimating the Lost Benefits of Antiretroviral Drug use in South Africa." *Journal of Acquired Immune Deficiency Syndromes* 49, no. 4 (December 1, 2008): 410–5.

Clarke, Adele and Joan Fujimura. "What Tools? Which Jobs? Why Right?" In *The Right Tools for the Job: At Work in the 20th Century Life Sciences*, edited by Adele Clarke and Joan Fujimura, 3–46. Princeton: Princeton University Press, 1992.

Cohen, J. "HIV/AIDS. Experts Question Danger of 'AIDS Superbug'." *Science (New York, NY)* 307, no. 5713 (February 25, 2005): 1185.

Collins, Huntly. "Among the Poor, Battling the Odds: The Rigid Regimen of the New Drugs Requires More Discipline Than Many Can Muster." *Philadelphia Inquirer* (December 30, 1996): http://articles.philly.com/1996-12-30/news/25640234_1_protease-inhibitors-aids-drugs-aids-patients. Retrieved June 7, 2015.

Conference on Retroviruses and Opportunistic Infections (CROI). "Special Symposium: Transmitted HIV-1 Drug Resistance and Rapid Disease Progression." Boston, MA, February 24, 2005.

Crane, Johanna Tayloe. *Scrambling for Africa: AIDS, Expertise, and the Rise of American Global Health Science. Expertise: Cultures and Technologies of Knowledge*, edited by Dominic Boyer. Ithaca, NY: Cornell University Press, 2013.

———. "Viral Cartographies: Mapping the Molecular Politics of Global HIV." *Biosocieties* 6, no. 2 (2011): 142–66.

Deeks, S.G., J.D. Barbour, J.N. Martin, M.S. Swanson, and R.M. Grant. "Sustained CD4+ T Cell Response After Virologic Failure of Protease Inhibitor-Based Regimens in Patients with Human Immunodeficiency Virus Infection." *The Journal of Infectious Diseases* 181, no. 3 (March 2000): 946–53.

Edozien, Frankie. "New AIDS Super Bug—Nightmare Strain shows Up in City." *New York Post*, 2005.

Fassin, Didier. "The Embodiment of Inequality. AIDS as a Social Condition and the Historical Experience in South Africa." *EMBO Reports* 4 Spec No, (June 2003): S4–9.

———. *When Bodies Remember: Experiences and Politics of AIDS in South Africa*. Berkeley: University of California Press, 2007.

Flexner, C. "HIV Genotype and Phenotype—Arresting Resistance?" *JAMA: The Journal of the American Medical Association* 283, no. 18 (May 10, 2000): 2442–44.

Garrett, Laurie. "HIV Drugs Losing Power for Many." *San Francisco Chronicle*, December 18, 2001.

Golin, C.E., H. Liu, R.D. Hays, L.G. Miller, C.K. Beck, J. Ickovics, A.H. Kaplan, and N.S. Wenger. "A Prospective Study of Predictors of Adherence to Combination Antiretroviral Medication." *Journal of General Internal Medicine* 17, no. 10 (October 2002): 756–65.

Harries, A. D., D. S. Nyangulu, N. J. Hargreaves, O. Kaluwa, and F. M. Salani-poni. "Preventing Antiretroviral Anarchy in Sub-Saharan Africa." *Lancet* 358, no. 9279 (August 4, 2001): 410–4.

Hirsch, M. S., F. Brun-Vezinet, B. Clotet, B. Conway, D. R. Kuritzkes, R. T. D'Aquila, L. M. Demeter, et al. "Antiretroviral Drug Resistance Testing in Adults Infected with Human Immunodeficiency Virus Type 1: 2003 Recommendations of an International AIDS Society-USA Panel." *Clinical Infectious Diseases: An Official Publication of the Infectious Diseases Society of America* 37, no. 1 (July 1, 2003): 113–28.

Honigsbaum, Mark. "West Side Story: A Tale of Unprotected Sex which could be Link to New HIV Superbug." *The Guardian*, 2005, http://www.theguardian.com/world/2005/mar/26/aids.usa. Retrieved June 7, 2015.

Jefferys, R. "Multidrug-Resistant, Dual-Tropic HIV-1 and Rapid Progression." *Lancet* 365, no. 9475 (June 4–10, 2005): 1923; author reply 1924.

Latour, Bruno and Steve Woolgar. *Laboratory Life: The Construction of Scientific Facts*. Princeton, NJ: Princeton University Press, 1979.

Leigh Brown, A. J., S. D. Frost, W. C. Mathews, K. Dawson, N. S. Hellmann, E. S. Daar, D. D. Richman, and S. J. Little. "Transmission Fitness of Drug-Resistant Human Immunodeficiency Virus and the Prevalence of Resistance in the Antiretroviral-Treated Population." *The Journal of Infectious Diseases* 187, no. 4 (February 15, 2003): 683–86.

Lerner, B. H., R. M. Gulick, and N. N. Dubler. "Rethinking Nonadherence: Historical Perspectives on Triple-Drug Therapy for HIV Disease." *Annals of Internal Medicine* 129, no. 7 (October 1, 1998): 573–8.

Löwy, Ilana. "Trustworthy Knowledge and Desperate Patients: Clinical Tests for New Drugs from Cancer to AIDS." In *Living and Working with the New Medical Technologies: Intersections of Inquiry*, edited by Margaret Lock, Allen Young and Alberto Cambrosio, 49–81. Cambridge, UK: Cambridge University Press, 2000.

Mahajan, Manjari. "Right to Certainty: AIDS Activism in South Africa." Annual Meeting of the Society for the Social Study of Science, Vancouver, BC, November 4, 2006.

Markowitz, M., H. Mohri, S. Mehandru, A. Shet, L. Berry, R. Kalyanaraman, A. Kim, et al. "Infection with Multidrug Resistant, Dual-Tropic HIV-1 and Rapid Progression to AIDS: A Case Report." *Lancet* 365, no. 9464 (March 19–25, 2005): 1031–8.

McFadden, Robert. "A Drug-Resistant TB Results in 13 Deaths in New York Prisons." *New York Times*, November 16, 1991, 22.

McNeil, Donald. "Africans Outdo U.S. in Following AIDS Therapy." *New York Times*, September 3, 2003.

Nelkin, Dorothy. "Science Controversies: The Dynamics of Public Disputes in the United States." In *Handbook of Science and Technology Studies*, edited by Sheila Jasanoff, Gerald Markle, James Petersen and Trevor Pinch, 444–56. Thousand Oaks, CA: Sage Publications, 1995.

New York City Department of Health and Mental Hygiene. "New York City Resident Diagnosed with Rare Strain of Multi-Drug Resistant HIV that Rapidly Progresses to AIDS." 2005. (Accessed January 15, 2015). http://www.nyc.gov/html/doh/html/pr/pr016–05.shtml.

Paterson, D. L., S. Swindells, J. Mohr, M. Brester, E. N. Vergis, C. Squier, M. M. Wagener, and N. Singh. "Adherence to protease inhibitor therapy and outcomes in patients with HIV infection." *Annals of Internal Medicine* 133 no. 1 (Jul 4,2000): 21-30.

Perez-Pena, Richard. "Chilled by Findings, Investigators Dreaded the Mounting Evidence." *New York Times*, February 12, 2005, http://www.nytimes.com/2005/02/12/health/chilled-by-findings-investigators-dreaded-the-mounting-evidence.html. Retrieved June 7, 2015.

Piller, Charles. "AIDS Experts Awaken to a False Alarm." *Los Angeles Times*, Jun 5, 2005, http://articles.latimes.com/2005/jun/05/science/sci-aids5. Retrieved June 7, 2015..

Popp, D. and J.D. Fisher. "First, Do No Harm: A Call for Emphasizing Adherence and HIV Prevention Interventions in Active Antiretroviral Therapy Programs in the Developing World." *AIDS (London, England)* 16, no. 4 (March 8, 2002): 676–8.

Richman, D.D., S.C. Morton, T. Wrin, N. Hellmann, S. Berry, M.F. Shapiro, and S.A. Bozzette. "The Prevalence of Antiretroviral Drug Resistance in the United States." *AIDS (London, England)* 18, no. 10 (July 2, 2004): 1393–401.

———. "The Prevalence of Antiretroviral Drug Resistance in the US." 41st Interscience Conference on Antimicrobial Agents and Chemotherapy. Chicago, IL, 2001. Abstract LB-17.

Rosenberg, Charles. "Framing Disease: Illness, Society, and History." In *Framing Disease: Studies in Cultural History*, edited by Charles Rosenberg and Janet Golden, xiii. New Brunswick, NJ: Rutgers University Press, 1992.

Rosenthal, Elizabeth. "The Return of TB: A Special Report." *New York Times*, July 15, 1990, http://www.nytimes.com/1990/07/15/us/return-tb-special-report-tuberculosis-germ-resurging-risk-public-health.html. Retrieved June 7, 2015.

Santora, Mark and Lawrence Altman. "Rare and Aggressive HIV Reported in New York." *New York Times*, February 12, 2005a.

———. "Alarm Over Single AIDS Case Is Challenged by Questioners." *New York Times*, February 21, 2005b.

Senak, M. "Predicting Antiviral Compliance: Physicians' Responsibilities vs. Patients' Rights." *Journal of the International Association of Physicians in AIDS Care* 3, no. 6 (June 1997): 45–48.

Shafer, Robert. "Re: Comments and Suggestions Regarding the Draft Guidance Document Entitled 'Guidance for Industry Role of HIV Drug Resistance Testing in Antiretroviral Drug Development' (Docket Number 2004D-0484)." 2005. http://hivdb.stanford.edu/pages/news/letter_to_FDA_2005_02_25.html.

Shapin, Steven and Simon Schaffer. *Leviathan and the Air Pump: Hobbes, Boyle, and the Experimental Life*. Princeton, NJ: Princeton University Press, 1987.

Smith, S.M. "New York City HIV Superbug: Fear Or Fear Not?" *Retrovirology* 2 (March 2, 2005): 14.

Sollitto, S., M. Mehlman, S. Youngner, and M.M. Lederman. "Should Physicians Withhold Highly Active Antiretroviral Therapies from HIV-AIDS Patients Who Are Thought to be Poorly Adherent to Treatment?" *AIDS (London, England)* 15, no. 2 (January 26, 2001): 153–59.

Sontag, Deborah and Lynda Richardson. "Doctors Withhold H.I.V. Pill Regimen from Some." *New York Times*, March 2, 1997, http://www.nytimes.com/1997/03/02/nyregion/doctors-withhold-hiv-pill-regimen-from-some.html. Retrieved June 7, 2015..

Specter, Michael. "Neglected for Years, TB Is Back with Strains that are Deadlier." *New York Times*, October 11, 1992, http://www.nytimes.com/1992/10/11/nyregion/neglected-for-years-tb-is-back-with-strains-that-are-deadlier.html. Retrieved June 7, 2015..

Tamalet, C., C. Pasquier, N. Yahi, P. Colson, I. Poizot-Martin, G. Lepeu, H. Gallais, P. Massip, J. Puel, and J. Izopet. "Prevalence of Drug Resistant Mutants and Virological Response to Combination Therapy in Patients with Primary HIV-1 Infection." *Journal of Medical Virology* 61, no. 2 (June 2000): 181–6.

Tchetgen, E., E.H. Kaplan, and G.H. Friedland. "Public health consequences of screening patients for adherence to highly active antiretroviral therapy." *Journal of Acquired Immune Deficiency Syndromes (1999)* 26, no. 2 (Feb 1, 2001): 118-29.

USDHHS (U.S. Department of Health and Human Services). "Guidelines for the Use of Antiretroviral Agents in HIV-1-Infected Adults and Adolescents." 2013.

————. "Guidelines for the Use of Antiretroviral Agents in HIV-1 Infected Adults and Adolescents." Department of Health and Human Services, 2003.

Volberding, P. A. "The New York Case: Lessons Being Learned." *Annals of Internal Medicine* 142, no. 10 (May 17, 2005): 866–8.

Wailoo, Keith. *Drawing Blood: Technology and Disease Identity in Twentieth-Century America.* Baltimore: Johns Hopkins University Press, 1997.

Walensky, R. P., A. D. Paltiel, E. Losina, L. M. Mercincavage, B. R. Schackman, P. E. Sax, M. C. Weinstein, and K. A. Freedberg. "The Survival Benefits of AIDS Treatment in the United States." *The Journal of Infectious Diseases* 194, no. 1 (July 1, 2006): 11–19.

Weidle, P. J., T. D. Mastro, A. D. Grant, J. Nkengasong, and D. Macharia. "HIV/ AIDS Treatment and HIV Vaccines for Africa." *Lancet* 359, no. 9325 (June 29, 2002): 2261–7.

9 Diagnosing Psychosis
Scientific Uncertainty, Locally and Globally

Neely Myers

INTRODUCTION

Perhaps one of the greatest medical controversies of the modern era is how to interpret, diagnose, and treat experiences of madness.[1] This debate is far from over. But in a recent bold move by Thomas Insel, the Director of the National Institute of Mental Health (NIMH), the debate has made a paradigmatic shift. In 2013, Insel posted an unprecedented blog post that sparked spirited debates. In a post on the Director's Blog, Insel asked that research scientists move away from the "folk psychology" of the consensually defined, imprecise diagnostic categories enshrined by the *Diagnostic and Statistical Manual (DSM)* "dictionary," and focus instead on a novel "clinical neuroscience" approach (Insel 2013: 1). The new approach would involve "mapping the cognitive, circuit, and genetic aspects of mental disorders" to "yield new and better targets for treatment" (Insel 2013: 1).

To promote and define this approach, the NIMH has launched its flagship Research Domain Criteria (RDoC) project. RDoC is a diagnostic grid (see Figure 1) that clinical neuroscientists are being asked to "fill in" with imaging, physiological, and cognitive data related to specific neural circuits in people who are healthy and in people who have been diagnosed with various mental disorders. Completing RDoCs has been compared to mapping the ocean floor, and the co-founder of RDoC (psychophysiologist Bruce Cuthbert) has casually suggested that it may take a century (Voosen 2013). However, this information is presumed necessary to understand how neural circuits become "dysregulated" in various psychiatric disorders so that they can be targeted in the development of future treatments (Cuthbert and Insel 2010). In short, RDoC is expected to generate greater certainty in psychiatric diagnosis. Whether the new diagnostic strategies proposed by Insel will lead to a greater or lesser capacity of mental health diagnosis to capture the vast array of human experience currently associated with psychotic disorders—largely considered to be the most serious form of mental disorder—is the subject of this chapter.

Using a case study from three years of ethnographic fieldwork in the United States, this chapter considers the future of mental diagnoses in the recently heralded era of "clinical neuroscience." At the root of this discussion is how psychiatric diagnosis is approached: from the top-down, through the continual refinement of broad (and at times overreaching), consensus-based diagnostic categories; or from the molecular level upwards, using biological and pharmacological specificity to identify "dysregulation" in the brain. Psychiatric diagnoses have always been reliant on subjective interpretations of symptoms even though they are thought of as *not* scientific. Clinicians must rely on patients' self-descriptions to diagnose. Their expertise is built on a good faith assumption that clinicians have successfully lumped together constellations of symptoms to identify disorders that can then be traced to specific neural substrates. Through RDoC, self-reported symptom checklists can ideally be replaced with information about neural systems, how they become dysregulated to propagate symptoms of mental disorders, and how we can intervene to prevent those malfunctionings (Ford et al. 2014). The RDoC approach demands that diagnoses indicate the "real" disease behind the symptom. This may be optimistic given that in the past 20–30 years, there have been almost no positive achievements in biological or pharmaceutical treatments for serious psychiatric disorders. Disappointed laboratory-based "bench" scientists suspect that the absence of genetic biomarkers for any specific psychiatric disorder, for example, is due to clinical inaccuracies—inaccurate diagnoses and clumsy diagnostic categories that cannot accurately sort people into haves and have-nots.

This particular chapter focuses on the complex discussions surrounding the diagnosis of what is widely considered to be the most puzzling mental disorder, psychosis. Psychosis is best known as a symptom of "schizophrenia," and is defined as a complete break with reality (Compton and Broussard 2009). Whether what we call "schizophrenia" is a sign of one specific, identifiable disease entity or a constellation of symptoms that appear in a range of similar disorders remains unclear. The symptoms of schizophrenia are diverse, some argue, and may not be so much a sign of underlying disease, but rather a collection of phenomena bundled together (using *DSM* diagnostic strategies)—perhaps erroneously—as indicative of one basic problem. Loosening the diagnostic rigidity around schizophrenia and looking instead at "domains" may be helpful for people seeking care for their symptoms, as well as for researchers trying to develop a more precise sense of what may be changing in any one person's brain over the course of life.

SHIFTING DIAGNOSES IN THE AMERICAN HEARTLAND (STEPH)

"You name it, I've had it," Steph told me during our initial interview. Her list of diagnoses included bipolar disorder, schizophrenia, schizoaffective disorder, and borderline personality disorder. Steph and I met as part of a three-year ethnographic project I undertook in a psychiatric rehabilitation clinic for people with serious mental illnesses in the American Midwest.

I never asked people about their diagnoses, but many people described themselves in diagnostic terms, anyways, as it had framed many aspects of their everyday experiences.

Steph also told me about the psychiatric treatment she had received for these various conditions. These included a wide range of antipsychotics, anxiolytics, antidepressants, mood stabilizers, and prescription sleep aids, such as hypnotics. She told me that her appearance had changed dramatically since she had begun taking psychiatric medications a decade earlier. As with so many people I have met in psychiatric treatment facilities over the past decade, Steph spent years trying to identify a cocktail of medications that reliably controlled her symptoms. Her medications all had powerful side effects. She no longer menstruated and had gained about sixty pounds. Her most notable issue, though, was the frozen position of her neck. Her head was twisted slightly askew and did not move freely, so that she had to look sideways at people.

Steph's troubles began when she went to college. She developed a growing sense that there were messages in billboards meant for her, which was distracting. She began to hear people whispering about her, laughing at her, mocking her. She found herself spending hours staring at the ceiling as her voices argued with one another. She forgot to bathe, to get out of bed, to eat.

When she failed her first semester at school, her parents were shocked. They sent her back in the spring, but Steph did not attend class. Her parents asked for a medical leave, and then hid her in the house, hoping the neighbors would not notice. Her father was the director of a prominent community organization, Steph explained, "What would people think if his daughter was losing her mind?"

It was okay, though, Steph said, because she did not want to talk to anyone. She felt very antisocial. The medications made her drool. Her feet shuffled. She could not gather her thoughts. It was easier to be alone.

Things continued to go terribly wrong. Steph tried and failed another semester of college. Instead of worrying about college, spring break, internships, and relationship building, Steph was trying to find medications that stopped the voices, bouncing between a variety of psychoanalysts, therapists, spiritual advisors, and psychiatrists. All this time she also shifted between many provisional housing situations—her parent's home, shelters, group homes, psychiatric hospitals, subsidized apartments—in three states. Steph tried to explain her parents' confusion, the sleepless nights spent roaming city streets, and then the final straw: her arrest.

At that time, Steph was too impaired to work. Her parents—who were middle-class and lived far away—helped pay her rent. Her everyday life was very isolated, but she loved to stroll through a local garden. And then, one day, Steph noticed new signs posted along the way to the garden. "Smith for City Council," they said, and she knew those signs had been left for her.

Steph told me that she had then mapped the location of the signs carefully until she could decipher the code. Smith's signs, she realized, were meant to communicate his secret passion for her. She began to follow him, his wife, and his children. She could hear him talking to her, describing all of the erotic things he would do for her if she killed his wife.

Then, she was arrested. With a record of ten years of mental health-related hospitalizations, she had a strong insanity plea. At her hearing, she explained, the judge placed a restraining order on her to keep her from disrupting Smith's family, and then sentenced her to outpatient commitment. Steph was now required to attend the mental health program where we met for "treatment" every day.

When Smith won the election, Steph knew it was because of her. His voice told her so. I asked her how she felt her diagnoses and mental health treatment had affected her. She said the diagnoses had never helped; they had just shifted the ways people responded to her, which often meant more medications, more restraints, more hospitalizations, more weight gain, and now the irreversibly stiff neck—and without menstruation, she added, with a flicker of sorrow, no children. As Warren and Manderson mention (see Warren and Manderson, this volume), her experiences of diagnoses had been a "funneling process," which had included her in specific kinds of lifestyles and excluded her from others.

DEFINING PSYCHOSIS

The reason we even use diagnostic categories like schizophrenia is because it has long been assumed that a proper diagnosis would indicate the best treatment. A diagnosis justifies certain kinds of medical and legal interventions, including forced treatments (Brodwin 2012). For Steph, this included multiple unwanted impairments—a stiff neck, the absence of menstruation—and no relief from her primary symptom of hearing distressing voices. Despite their power, psychiatric diagnoses have always been based on self-report and clinical intuition rather than objective "signs." Many people in high-income countries (HICs), like Steph, received multiple diagnoses as various clinicians evaluated the meaning of their symptoms in different ways and struggled to find a medication that worked.

Hearing distressing voices—a very serious part of Steph's own experience of madness—occurs across multiple diagnoses with a variety of outcomes, including bipolar disorder, major depression, borderline personality disorder, posttraumatic stress disorder, and temporal lobe epilepsy (Ford et al. 2014). Psychotic experiences like hearing voices are *not*, on their own, indicative of an underlying pathology (DeVylder et al. 2014). About 0.2 percent of the population hears regular voices speaking in sentences and does not meet the criteria for a diagnosis of a psychotic disorder (Johns et al. 2002), which confirms that hearing voices does not always signal a diagnosable pathology. Others who are not in treatment but claim to hear voices, known as nonclinical voice-hearers, can be found in 4–7 percent of the general population (Kelleher and Cannon 2010), making a stronger case that people can hear voices without being "ill" according to the *DSM* or even society's designations.[2]

Many people like Steph who hear voices and find them to be impairing are diagnosed with a psychotic disorder such as schizophrenia. Around 70 percent of people diagnosed with schizophrenia have reported hearing distressing voices talking to them (Sartorius et al. 1986). In a recent study, 88 percent of the people whose voices said negative things to them were identified as having a psychotic disorder, most often schizophrenia (Daalman et al. 2011).

In the early 20th century, Eugene Bleuler developed the term "schizophrenia" (Bleuler 1911) to index people with the worst prognosis (Bleuler 1974). The diagnosis of schizophrenia has appeared in every edition of the *DSM* for mental disorders since its first edition in 1958. In earlier versions, it was described as a "schizophrenic reaction" to adverse social situations, such as childhood abuse. By the time the *DSM-III* was published, the symptoms of schizophrenia had to be experienced for at least six months before the diagnostic label could be applied (Robins and Guze 1970). The purpose of this restriction was to demarcate people with a brief psychotic disorder (a more transient, non-recurring form of psychosis) or other forms of a psychotic-like illness (e.g., depression with psychotic features) from people with a chronic deteriorating course prior to applying the rather grim label of schizophrenia. As with Steph, when it comes to living with a diagnosis of schizophrenia, the treatments available for it, the societal stigma associated with it, and the ramifications of having this diagnosis assigned to one's legal and medical records have profoundly shaped the lives of people so diagnosed.

According to the *DSM-IV* (American Psychiatric Association 2000), the last version of the *DSM* that the NIMH recognized as legitimate, a person with "schizophrenia" must have experienced at least one "positive" and one "negative" symptom for at least one month continuously, with some symptoms enduring for at least six months (APA 2000: 298). "Positive" symptoms refer to hallucinations, disordered thoughts, and delusions. The most common "negative" symptoms affect the emotions, such as an inability to experience pleasure (anhedonia) or an inability to express emotions (affective flattening) (APA 2000: 298–301).

Importantly, positive and negative symptoms must also disrupt one's life before the label may be applied—more evidence for the centrality of the social context in this diagnosis. It is a diagnosable disorder only if it affects a person's ability to manage life tasks, such as interpersonal relationships, work or education, and self-care, to a level that is "clearly below what might have been achieved" (APA 2000: 302). Men tend to fall ill in their late teens and twenties and women in their late twenties and thirties (Robins and Regier 1991)—years when people typically build their careers and relationships—leading to a potentially serious disruption of a person's life plans (Millon et al. 1999; Warner 1994). Many people end up seriously disabled—as with Steph—but it is not clear if that disability is a result of the way people diagnosed with schizophrenia are treated after their diagnosis, if it is part of some disease process, or a result of both.

DIAGNOSIS-BY-TREATMENT

Psychiatrists have been treating people demonstrating symptoms of a psychotic disorder like Steph with antipsychotic medications ever since Thorazine became available in 1955 and initiated a "pharmacological revolution" in psychiatry (Shorter 1997). Later, psychiatrist Nancy Andreasen put forth her model of "the broken brain." She posited that schizophrenia is a product of a "chemical imbalance" in the brain rather than a product of upbringing or social context (Andreasen 1984).

For decades now, the "truth" of this diagnosis has relied on the false impression of a "chemical imbalance in the brain" and the presumed efficacy of antipsychotic medications for treating that imbalance. Many believe that pharmaceutical treatments reduce the level of disability experienced by people with a psychotic disorder, and that if people would just take their medications and restore a chemical balance in their brain, they would be fine. These are assumptions, and they do not always hold true. Antipsychotic medications only eradicate voices, for example, about 1/3 of the time; they eliminate or reduce voices another 1/3 of the time, and they do not work at all for 1/3 of the people who hear voices (Shergill et al. 1998).

Moreover, it is not clear that long-term use has any advantages. In a 13-year-long follow-up study, people on continuous antipsychotic medication relapsed more frequently and had worse outcomes than those on low-dose or no antipsychotic medication at all, including: being less likely to achieve symptom remission (59.4 percent versus 85.3 percent), being more functionally impaired (21.7 percent versus 55.9 percent), and being less likely to achieve full recovery (17.4 percent versus 52.9 percent) (Harrow and Jobe 2013). People who take antipsychotic medications also die, on average, 25 years earlier than their peers, in part because the use of antipsychotics also has profound negative effects on people's cardiovascular and metabolic systems (Newcomer 2007). Psychiatrist McGorry (2013: 898) states, "[M]any would now contend that much of the poor outcome in psychosis is an artifact of late detection, crude and reactive pharmacotherapy, sparse psychosocial care, and social neglect." Insel (2009: 700) has similarly suggested, "For too many people, antipsychotics and antidepressants are not effective, and even when they are helpful, they reduce symptoms without eliciting recovery."

Prescribing antipsychotics in very low doses or time-limited doses at the time of acute symptoms (for the first six months after a diagnosis) may lead people towards recovery more quickly than the long-term prescription of antipsychotics or "maintenance therapy" that has long been a gold standard practice in psychiatry (Wunderink, et al. 2013). A "less is more" attitude towards antipsychotic medications is now being promoted (McGorry et al. 2013).

Where does this leave psychiatry in the 21st century? And where does this leave people like Steph, the "patients" who so often had little say in their own treatment and who, having been diagnosed by what is now seen as a faulty system, are highly vulnerable to public mental health regulations and recommendations capable of forcing involuntary medication-based treatment of their behavior? Despite clear evidence of the harmful potential of long-term antipsychotic medication and the lack of evidence that they work, antipsychotics and antidepressants remain the third and fourth most purchased drugs in the United States, representing $25 billion in market value (IMS Health Inc. 2007). Kirmayer and Gold (2012) suspect that much of the push to believe that pharmaceuticals can target specific aspects of psychiatric disorder and their presumed underlying neurological targets arose from the powerful pharmaceutical companies invested in promoting this concept. Pharmaceutical companies have profited from implanting the false concept of a "chemical imbalance" in what anthropologist Janis Jenkins aptly called the "pharmaceutical imaginary" (Jenkins 2010). In the pharmaceutical imaginary, pharmaceutical drugs bring us closer to our imagined potentials. One could be even better "if only" one had more energy, or could pay better attention, or had an easier time feeling happy, or was always rational, or was perhaps more chemically in balance. This was all part of a broader "medical imaginary" that renders people "susceptible to hope engendered by the cultural power of the medical imagination" (Good 2001: 397).

It would seem that people with a psychotic disorder—people who have been told to be hopeless by psychiatry—are highly beholden to this medical imaginary. Steph is an exemplar of madness in HICs because she came of age at a time when forced medication was normative. We now know that this diagnosis-by-treatment approach may have destroyed both her long-term mental health and her physiological maturation. She will never know whether her distraught and disabled condition is the product of a terrible decline in mental function, a complex set of long-term medication side effects, or both.

Upon close examination, it may be clear that Steph's diagnoses shift *as* medications take hold, or fail to, and over time (as in Warren and Manderson, this volume). It is not only this tenuous relationship of experience with named diagnosis and medication that is disconcerting; it is also the enormous potential for harm that inhabits people in HICs' experiences when they enter a range of abnormal experiences. Whether by well-meaning professionals using any available pharmaceutical, or by social pressures aimed at the control of unruly behaviors through a medical imaginary, abnormality seems to be a transgression that the broader public believes can be fixed pharmaceutically, despite their limited success in promoting recovery.

TOP-DOWN OR BOTTOM-UP DIAGNOSIS?

It is unlikely that much of this information has escaped the attention of the NIMH, which funds 85 percent of global clinical research (Miller 2010). On April 29, 2013, Insel publicly declared that "patients with mental disorders deserve better" than the *DSM* (now in its 5th edition)—and, by proxy, the more internationally used *International Classification of Disorders* (now in its 10th edition). Insel's team proposed investigating domains of psycho-neural structures that cluster together in the performance of patterned functions. These "domains" were described for the lay public as neural circuits responsible for the following: "one for keeping the brain up and running; one for social processes; one for storing and using information; one for moving toward positive rewards, like food and shelter; and one for avoiding harm" (Voosen 2013). The most exciting part of the focus on domains is their presumed malleability. If there are malleable domains of neural functioning, and we can understand what makes them "dysregulate" (assuming they do), then we may also be able to fix them with targeted pharmaceuticals and non-pharmaceutical interventions like cognitive behavioral therapies, activated peer support, and community-based interventions that build on local knowledge and resources.

In this formulation, spectrums of symptoms become possible, in which clinicians and researchers can account for symptom severity, as in the autism spectrum, although they are not expected to map onto any single specific circuit and are not envisioned as diagnostic tool. These spectrums might strengthen linkages between healthy and "dysregulated" people to reduce people's sense that people are "abnormal." Quoting RDoC founder Bruce Cuthbert, "[T]he defining image of RDoC, then, is not two buckets, one full of the healthy, the other the ill. It is a grid. Down the side run the domains and their dimensions. Across the top go the means of probing them: through genes, molecules, cells, circuits, physiology, behavior, self-reports, and 'paradigms'" (Voosen 2013). These efforts turn us away from identifying healthy/unhealthy individuals, and toward a more molecular focus thought to enable people to see more similarities across the human condition. Moreover, it can help us *prevent* dysregulation, at least in theory, and assuming this is desired.

Here is how the RDoC architects imagine this will work. Neuroimaging and psychiatric biomarkers will easily identify early stages of psychosis, just as plasma lipids (blood tests) for cholesterol and cardiac imaging identify heart disease. And just as statins can then be prescribed to reduce one's risk of heart attack, psychoactive drugs can be prescribed to prevent changes in the neural circuits that lead to the heart attack of the mind—namely, a psychotic break. Insel (2009) argues that "developing the 'statins' that will preempt the psychosis of schizophrenia or bipolar illness may well be the next frontier." Notably, the current research suggests that statins for cardiovascular disease only perpetuate around a 25–35 percent reduction in risk when used daily for one's entire life.

Clinicians who appreciated the consensus-based diagnoses in the *DSM-IV* in everyday practice are concerned. Jablensky et al. (2014: 43–44) wrote, "[T]here is a knowledge gap between RDoCs and the clinic." Insel (2013: 1) acknowledged this: "[S]ome will see RDoC as an academic exercise divorced from clinical practice." However, this is all part of his longstanding vision to realign psychiatry with neurology to form a new discipline of "clinical neuroscience" (Insel 2009).[3] Insel claims RDoCs moves the field beyond a rigid "chemical imbalance" theory to a more fluid neural systems theory. "Many psychiatric disorders can be understood as dysfunctions within brain circuits" and RDoC will aim to reveal the underlying psycho-neural mechanisms of the symptoms central to the previous diagnostic strategies (Insel 2009: 702).

One view of Insel's controversial approach is that the *DSM* is being cast aside in favor of a more precise science, which has proven to be expensive—and not so useful—to date. For example, millions of research dollars have been spent on genetic studies of "mental illnesses." However, nearly all of the genetic correlates identified thus far are merely that: correlates that confer risk for—but do not explain—multiple disorders, from schizophrenia to unipolar depression, substance abuse, and epilepsy (Brandon et al. 2009; Cook and Scherer 2008; International Schizophrenia Consortium 2009). Some have blamed the *DSM*. If all research started from arbitrarily assigned but invalid diagnostic categories, then what kinds of "real" correlations could the data suggest? Some advocated that researchers should drop the preconceived top-down diagnostic categories in research endeavors and start fresh with new classifications. These would be drawn from the bottom up, grounded in knowledge of the ways "normal" neural circuits operate and become "dysregulated" (Insel 2009).

There are also contextual reasons for a negative reaction to the RDoC model. Many labs and institutes are built around the study of specific disorders as designated by the *DSM*. Entire research careers have been built around the investigation of one diagnosis, rather than cross-cutting domains.

Moreover, the existing *DSM* categories drive pharmaceutical development, as with other controversial diagnoses discussed in this volume (see Smith-Morris, Hardon, and Rohden, this volume). When people bring drugs to the Food and Drug Administration (FDA) for approval, they must be designated for a specific disorder and FDA clinical trials must then test the drug on people with that precise diagnosis. Even so, not a single novel drug (mechanistically) has hit the pharmaceutical market in 30 years (Fibiger 2012). Drug companies have shut down their research program on antipsychotic medications (Miller 2010). RDoC, if clinical neuroscience findings are strong, may rekindle interest. But at the moment, the lack of linkages between drug development and the new *DSM-V* will be a challenge.

Many also expressed concern that the abandonment of the *DSM* could push many of the clinical and financial institutions now reliant on that diagnostic "dictionary" into chaos. *DSM* categories are used in the exercise of various kinds of biopower. In the United States, entire insurance billing and reimbursement systems are built on the codes supplied by the *DSM*, which determine whether or not a condition warrants the costs of (often expensive) biomedical care (pharmaceuticals) and psychiatric disability benefits. The stagnating impact of this larger self-referential diagnostic system was acknowledged by Cuthbert, the co-founder of RDoCs, when he wrote, "[T]he system has served so well for clinical, services, administrative and legal purposes that any changes are now fraught, and may impact eligibility for mental health services, insurance, prevalence rates, health care costs, research using these categories, and so on" (Cuthbert 2014: 29).

Departure from the *DSM* has some promise. The *DSM* never carved nature at its joints into natural kinds (Plato 1925), and seems to have assigned people into loaded categories. These categories, embraced by the authoritative and market-dominant structures of biomedicine, gained unwarranted traction and perpetuated disability by mobilizing stigmatizing discourses: in the case of schizophrenia, ideas of genetic dangerousness (for relatives and offspring), a chronically deteriorating course, a propensity for violence (Choe et al. 2008), an inability to work (Cook 2006), and more. Even when people feel better and enter a state of recovery, they are still deeply troubled by this diagnosis and its implications, which they find additionally disabling (Jenkins and Carpenter-Song 2008).

To minimize social stigma and corresponding disability, people in low-and middle-income countries (LMICs), such as India and China, deliberately avoid using the term "schizophrenia" on behalf of their ill relatives (Marrow and Luhrmann 2012; Yang et al. 2009). People in sub-Saharan Africa prefer to attribute symptoms of psychosis to malevolent spirits—ghosts, demons, and witches—rather than to biological events (McGruder 2004; Patel 1995). Perhaps they are (actively? indirectly?) avoiding what much research in HICs has shown—that the label of schizophrenia can have profoundly deleterious effects on one's sense of self (Estroff 1993). In fact, in one HIC, Japan, people have relabeled schizophrenia from "mind-split disease" to "integration disorder," with some positive effects (Sato 2006; Takahashi et al. 2009).

If the departure from the *DSM* diagnostic categories (at least for clinical neuroscience research) is a good thing, it is also a serious game changer. If biomedical treatments and care have been offered based on diagnoses that the NIMH Director (Insel 2013: 1) now claims lacked validity, and constituted some kind of "folk psychology," and their treatments are generally ineffective, we must ask where that leaves people experiencing madness, their families, and even caregivers—patients and healers in a variety of cultural contexts, struggling against very serious, disruptive, symptoms. The message from the NIMH seems to be that everyone should wait twenty more years until we can get a better handle on this, and please practice care as usual until then.

"RUNNING CRAZY:" CARE AS USUAL IN TANZANIA

And what of the situation in low- and middle-income countries? How might waiting twenty more years for care to catch up to precision medicine affect them? Nearly a decade after I interviewed Steph, I interviewed 60 women in three regions of Tanzania about their everyday lives and well-being. Part of the project took part in a Maasai community where many lived communally in a *boma*, or a group of huts positioned in a circle to protect livestock (which are kept in the center) from predators. Often, a *boma* included one man and his co-wives and children. The huts were constructed of sticks, dried cow dung, and mud. The *bomas* I visited had no electricity or running water.

Rachel, my guide, helped me visit several *bomas* where she thought that the women might be willing to speak with me about their lives. One morning, we approached a *boma* where the oldest woman present agreed that we could talk to her, and then offered to let us speak with a young wife first. The men had gone out to herd the livestock. The women were busy doing their "duties." Two tiny wooden stools were brought out, and Rachel and I sat under the only tree in sight on a bright, hot day.

The young wife's name was Sarah.[4] While we sat on the stools, she sat in the dirt, nursing her son. After obtaining Sarah's informed consent, I set out my iPad to record our conversation. A small band of goats came over and kicked plumes of dust in our direction. We had stolen their shade.

I asked Sarah to tell us about her life; Rachel translated, and Sarah began. Sarah told us that she was 19, and that she had been married when she was around the age of 12, she thought, but it was hard to know, she explained, because there were no birth records. She had two children—one three-year-old boy and one nursing infant. Her husband had another wife, but she had passed away, so Sarah began taking care of her son (only five years her junior) at a very young age.

She said that as a young girl, she was doing well in school, but her father, she claimed, wanted her to fail so that he could marry her and collect more. Not doing well in school justified early marriage to many people, Sarah explained. Sarah said her father took her to a traditional healer who did something that then made it difficult for her to concentrate, much like the practices traditional healers use to stop the rain. She could not pass her exams and was married to a middle-aged man who lived far from her home. The man gave her father two cows.

All of her dreams were smashed, she said in a hushed voice. Her husband was a drunkard, and did not help. Sarah was now in charge of three children.

When asked if she ever heard voices or knew someone who had, she said yes, that she heard voices. She heard someone calling her name and responded, but then there was no one there. She said, "I've heard it—and when you go outside, there's no one there. You come back and you ask yourself—who was calling me?" She added, "You begin to fear in your heart," indicating that she found these voices to be distressing.

> SARAH said that she would not talk to anyone about the voices be-
> cause no one knew what it was, and when it happened peo-
> ple would say that "you're crazy."
> RACHEL added, "If you go around asking people, someone's call-
> ing me, people will say you are 'running crazy nowadays.
> You're about to run mental, crazy.'"
> RACHEL then asked Sarah what she did about the voices, and she
> said she would say "*shindwa*," which meant, "be defeated."
> This is what local people said to demons to ask them to go
> away, Rachel explained.

I then asked what happens to people who are "running crazy."

> SARAH: If they bring problems, I tell someone from their place to
> take them away, because I don't want problems.

Sarah was indicating how families are often the first point of care for people experiencing serious emotional distress in LMICs, just as they are in HICs. As the conversation continued, the options for care that families had in this extremely low-income setting became more clear—and included physical restraint, beatings, and visits to a traditional healer.

> RACHEL: This crazy person—a person overcome with craziness—if
> they're harassing people, what do you do?
> SARAH: You beat them. They're beaten, so they get some sense. Be-
> cause there are others who have plans to do bad things.

Here, Sarah is indicating how people in Tanzania with serious emotional distress are socially vulnerable, just as people in the United States are much more likely to be victims of rape and violent crime (Choe et al. 2008; Teplin et al. 2005).

> RACHEL: Those who didn't do things intentionally?
> SARAH: Those ones you tie with rope.

This option of restraining people is one that families in the United States, at least in my experience, never describe. On the other hand, as soon as a psychiatric patient arrives in the emergency room in the United States, they are often restrained and given a sedative. In Tanzania, where medications were scarce and hospitals few and far between, tying a person up was one of the only options they had for a person who was agitated.

> RACHEL: So, if they're tied up, will they be healed?
> SARAH: No, but they might be taken to the traditional healer (*laibon*).
> ME: No hospital?
> RACHEL: Will they go to the hospital?
> SARAH: No.

Again, here Sarah described a trend reported in multiple interviews during my time in Tanzania. People preferred to use a traditional healer rather than going to the hospital. They did not perceive the hospital as a useful resource for dealing with serious emotional distress.

While my research in Tanzania was preliminary, this interview with Sarah and Rachel provides an excellent example of the global diversity of experiences of madness and the influences of the social context of care. In sharp contrast to HICs, people in LMICs rarely have the opportunity to go to the hospital, whether for optional or mandatory treatment. First of all, the hospitals are not always easy to access from rural areas and can be a great expenditure for impoverished families. The situation in the hospitals, for the people who do arrive there, is often very grim. Primary care providers in East Africa have no training in specialty mental health (World Health Organization 2011), and often have stigmatizing attitudes towards people with mental health concerns (Ndetei et al. 2011). Instead, many people initially visit "nonspecialists" for mental health care, such as community-based traditional healers (Ngoma et al. 2003). Traditional healers appeal to people as a source of care in sub-Saharan Africa because they are thought to be more trustworthy and accessible, they often share their client's supernatural belief system, and people believe that a visit to a traditional healer invites less stigma than visiting a hospital (Chadda et al. 2001).

It would seem that more communal and nonspecialized care that utilizes community health workers, traditional healers, peer providers, and so forth, may be the least stigmatizing, and the most promising, for the restoration of mental health in the presence of serious emotional distress. That 85 percent of the world's mental health research funding does not flow in this direction is testimony to the pharmaco-centric diagnostic system we now have. Moreover, what remains unclear is whether RDoC and neural psychiatry will improve or exacerbate this dilemma.

DIAGNOSIS IN CONTEXT, DIAGNOSIS AS CONTEXT (SARAH)

Sarah's story highlights some of the pressing complications of trying to identify and treat potentially serious mental health concerns in LMICs. An estimated 80 percent of the world's population lives in LMICs (Saxena et al. 2006). Based on ICD-9 definitions of psychosis, psychotic disorders are among the top five contributors to the global disease burden and have the worst impact in LMICs (Collins et al. 2011). Of course, this assumes that people labeled as people with psychotic disorders were accurately represented in the data. More than 75 percent of people with serious psychiatric disabilities in LMICs do not receive any organized psychosocial or pharmacological treatment (Becker and Kleinman 2013).

But even if the classificatory system and data collection was not perfect, mental health concerns in LMICs are an urgent concern. Poverty is a risk factor for mental disorders, as is traumatic stress (Jenkins et al. 2010). In LMICs, where the prevalence of poverty and traumatic stress is high, people may be even more in need of care than they are in HICs. However, in these same places, we find a striking lack of mental health care options. Tanzania, for example, has one psychiatric hospital and five psychiatric units in general hospitals, three of which are tertiary care. There are an estimated 20 psychiatrists for over 47 million people (WHO 2011). There is a huge gap between what is needed and the help available, which we need to reduce the disease burden of psychosis on individuals, families, and communities. Without some knowledge about serious emotional distress and how it might best be managed, there is a great deal of room for (and documentation of) inadvertent abuse at the hands of desperate family members and local healers, and even in the hospitals. This is a very grim picture in terms of care for people with serious mental health concerns in LMICs, and it is my hope that we can do more to strengthen community systems of care by helping to educate and empower families, peer groups, and healers.

Under these circumstances, in LMICs, where biomedical testing may be inaccessible, stigmatized, and misunderstood, how can a clinical neuroscience-based psychiatry possibly be of use? Even if there is a set of biomarkers for psychosis, and more people can be identified early, what kinds of treatments would be available, and how accessible will they be? New pharmacotherapies may be proposed to address issues in neural circuits, introducing Western norms at the neural level to further global pharmaceutical imperialism (Ford et al. 2014), but this is unlikely to help most families struggling on the ground. Families cannot afford the psychiatric medications available now. When primary care physicians with minimal training in mental health care are rare, and few people receive prescriptions even now, the likelihood of making RDoC achievements relevant is unlikely.

Moreover, the technology for neural circuitry mapping is not portable, and sparsely available even inside Western countries. This elite technology may never be used to account for differences across the many ethnicities, life experiences, and exposures to Western psychopharmaceuticals. For settings where pharmaco-centric treatment has not taken hold, can lessons be learned from LMIC settings that will improve RDoC's ability to create alternate views of schizophrenia, psychotic experiences, and futures for those who struggle?

It seems that most of the research for RDoC is going to take place in HICs without any targeted effort towards addressing human variation in terms of pathophysiology, environment, culture, or diversity, or finding people whose brains have not been affected by psychopharmaceuticals. Yet these are the very samples that will help science to escape its own self-referencing trap. This calls the accuracy of supposedly unbiased findings about the "normal" and "dysregulated" brain and the treatments that stem from these findings into question before the data collection has even begun. Diagnosis will, once again, be a reflection of what is at stake for people in HICs, rather than taking on a more diverse perspective.

CONCLUDING REMARKS: COLLABORATIONS FOR A MORE PRECISE MEDICINE

It seems that the NIMH, in its quest for scientific "precision" in diagnosis, is moving in the opposite direction from LMICs. Most LMICs are seeking ways to use local resources in sustainable ways to provide people with the moral support they need to seek their own recovery. These efforts have recently been widely celebrated by the scientific community, even as Insel's call for a clinical neuroscience begins to dominate research funding streams. For example, there are solutions offered by nonspecialized interventions that are not contingent on diagnostic specificity per se (e.g., a neural-level diagnosis), such as those offered by traditional healers, community health workers, peer providers and potentially religious professionals, which seem to be working in a variety of settings where mental health care is limited—namely, most of the world.

To offer people a fair shot at recovery, we must address some of the staggering structural inequalities that impact people with madness—so often present among the most vulnerable (Estroff et al. 1997; Hopper 2007b; Jenkins and Carpenter-Song 2008; Metzl and Hansen 2014). Some have argued that even in the face of knowledge about genetic or neurodevelopmental trajectories of mental illness, it is social context, and not precise diagnosis, that we are most able to control, and social context that should be the target of public health interventions (Kirkbride et al. 2010), such as funding programs that help keep people with mental illnesses in prisons out of solitary confinement. Even as RDoC moves the research focus towards a diagnosis-focused biological model, many of the most influential treatment innovations in recent times have emerged from the psychosocial realm. These innovations include the successful use of peer-provided mental health services (Lloyd-Evans et al. 2014), the use of voice dialogues (including the very exciting use of avatar therapy) (Leff et al. 2013; Romme et al. 2009), cognitive behavioral therapy (Chadwick and Birchwood 1994), and mindfulness meditation practices for people experiencing symptoms of psychosis (Abba et al. 2008; Chadwick et al. 2009), to name a few.

These innovations are decidedly *not* a part of the touted neural psychiatry because their positive effects have not yet been identified and proven on the neural level that the RDoC paradigm demands. Therefore, the efficacy of these interventions cannot be trusted. In the future, it would seem, interventions that cannot show some effect on neural circuits will be discounted—self-report that some treatment is working well for people with potentially invalid diagnoses will no longer suffice as a *scientific enough* form of evidence. It thus remains to be seen how psychosocial approaches and the importance of consensual diagnoses will fare under the RDoC paradigm. It is not that they cannot be done under the new paradigm, it is that they are unlikely to be prioritized, funded, and tested enough to inform the evidence base and secure more funding from policy makers. In the push for diagnostic specificity, we may be distracted by what is really helpful in mental health and healing.

In a recent *Nature* article, neuroscientist David Lewis stated that the knowledge we have about schizophrenia is best understood through the old parable of blind men trying separately to describe the nature of an elephant. At the moment, researchers are gaining "a bit more synchrony" in their findings so that maybe one part of the elephant is starting to be described in the same way (Dobbs 2010). But how will the RDoC approach advance diagnostic practice from here? What is being gained, and what is being lost, in our turn to this new approach?

RDoC was motivated by the absence of any improvements in trajectory or outcomes for psychiatric patients over thirty years, despite high expenditures in genetic and pharmaceutical research. This approach seems more of the same—just much, much more of it (i.e., mapping the ocean floor). This chapter has argued that some of the most interesting advances in knowledge about what contributes to psychosis, and how we may best help people address everyday challenges, comes from studying how people make sense of their experiences/perceptions in diverse social contexts. To be fair, the creators of RDoC insist that social context has a role in the new construct. As Cuthbert (2014: 30) has written, RDoC is about "developing a more mechanistic understanding of how such factors as life events and the social environment interact with development to produce a range of observed outcomes."

The idea of a "mechanistic" understanding of lived social context and its effects on the brain is of concern. Most of what we know about culture and environment only translates into risk, and risk does not translate into disorder. Risk is not causation. Lumping together such a diversity of experience, perception, and neural development amounts to an over-biologization of mental distress. RDoC's anti-progressive biological determinism may ultimately be deployed to say that madness is not sociopolitical, but rather a matter of inferior biology. All of our data about social context and its influences on experiences show that this is not true. Fitzgerald et al. (2014) suggests, and I agree, that we may need to set such questions aside to examine the "mutually constitutive relationships between biology, embodiment and social suffering." In other words, we need more ethnography to flesh out and remedy—as best as possible—scientific uncertainties.

The NIMH will have to fund more than clinical neuroscience. We will also need to know more about psychosocial factors (Morgan et al. 2008), placebos (Moerman and Jonas 2002), healing rituals (Teuton et al. 2007), the possible value of dissociative states (Seligman 2010), the cultivation of flexible minds (Lewis 2013), and so forth, and their effect on mental health. These may speak to the nature of diagnoses, as well—what we label as dysfunctional, and the strengths and errors of those labels.

In the meantime, what is happening to the patients? As Snyder and Mitchell (2006) have written, people who try to help people with disabilities, such as family members and clinicians, often inadvertently subjugate the very population they are trying to help. Anthropologists have long shown apprehension about the tyrannical march of biomedicine towards the seeming eradication of human variation—especially in terms of the mind (Benedict 1959; Kleinman 1988; Martin 2007). A variety of social scientists, for example, have questioned the chemical approach to molecular difference in psychiatry (Martin 2007), voicing suspicion of pharmaceutical claims about specificity and precision targeting (Kirmayer and Gold 2012).

This is all part of a broader "medical imaginary" in American popular culture, which is "enamored with the biology of hope," instead of, perhaps, the power of hope that arises from intimate connections between people (Good 2001: 407). The hope engendered by the medical imaginary of a "chemical imbalance" originated from good intentions, but it misconstrued the evidence at hand. While this rhetoric may have liberated families from feeling at fault for a loved one's problems, Jenkins (2012) argued, it did little to solve the existential problems of agency, kinship, and morality that mattered most to people with psychiatric disabilities.

Another danger has been in our search for a neuro-circuit imbalance, some flaw fatale that renders the most troubling among us comprehensible, and finally wrings the truth out of madness. The terminology of "brain disorders" could continue to have negative effects on so many, against which so many have fought. We know that calling serious emotional distress a "brain disorder" propagates stigma cross-culturally (Sartorius 2010). Is this the dreaded scenario Biehl (2007: 11) warns about, in which "the demoralization of everyday experience via scientific categories such as depression and post-traumatic stress disorder . . . remake people as objects of technological manipulation without allowing for the possibility of remorse, regret, or repentance"? Or is it the moment of "collaboration," which Rose et al. proposed would be needed to finally unpack the relationships between suffering, embodiment, and experience? In mental health, I would argue, the scanning and re-rendering of our own personal biologies should not trump the importance of our stories and subjectivities, which are historically situated and politically and economically bound.

It is possible to offer some kind of ethnographic corrective to clinical neuroscience. Some invitations for ethnographic-type corrections have come from clinical neuroscientists. Some have acknowledged a key construct of anthropological thought: that research needs to be longitudinal. The functional magnetic resonance imaging scan, despite its popularity, does not image reality; it captures one brain state at one (rather unpredictable) point in time (Weinberger and Goldberg 2014). If the work of RDoC is isolated to brain scans at one point in time, much will be lost, as time is not typically incorporated into cross-sectional studies. Moreover, it is an important corrective because mental health and its neural correlates are developed, as anthropologists have observed: "one continually learns and relearns to live with as much as through one's body, in its various states of health and illness, youth and old age, boredom and trauma, routine and instability" (Biehl et al. 2007: 10).

In addition, an assumption of the field—that high activation on brain scans indicates disorder—is also false, as in the case of grief (more active) versus dyslexia or mild depression (less active, but more impairing) (Wakefield 2014). Matching narratives to brain scans and long-term ethnographic engagement to longitudinal investigations of small groups of people who are at risk for a disorder may help correct for these kinds of errors and provide a focused look at psychosis. In a high-risk family, with neural images available from early life and across generations, who goes on to develop psychosis and who does not? Who develops a psychotic disorder? These kinds of questions are undoubtedly compelling, and suggest the potential for a strong partnership between neuroscience and longitudinal anthropology, that some have begun to call neuroanthropology (Lende and Downey 2012; Myers 2012).

In the end, focusing research funds on pinning down diagnoses is probably not the best plan. We would be better served to embrace scientific uncertainty of the cause or precise diagnostic boundaries of mental events, and instead increase research on the roles, rules, and relationships in diverse social contexts that ultimately matter in healing from serious emotional distress. In an ethnography of therapeutic options in Zaire, anthropologist Janzen (1978: 68) writes, "[W]hat the prophet-seer and healer provided here—assurance, definition in the midst of despair, hopeful action—will either have to be accommodated as it presently exists in customary therapy beyond the doors of the ward, or it will have to be presided in the ward." RDoCs both brings us closer to this possibility by loosening the rigidity of psychiatric thought (diversifying, for example, perceptions of normal and abnormal), but it may be distracting (demanding that we somehow neutrally justify our mental health care interventions) and also deepen the structural inequalities in care between HICs and LMICs.

Regardless, this makes for an exciting (albeit, confusing) time to be a psychiatrist, a neuroscientist, or an anthropologist committed to serving people with serious emotional distress. "A good psychiatrist," a psychiatrist has recently written, "[gains] empathic understanding of each patient's story, and then offers a tailored range of interventions to ease the suffering, whether it represents a disorder or is part of normal life" (Pierre 2014). In the future, a good clinical neuroscientist will need to do the same. And to do so, they will surely benefit from the presence of a good psychiatric anthropologist. Diagnoses communicate much more about bodies, minds, and histories than neural dysregulation, and they should represent and invite a broad range of experiences. Subjective experience and clinical expertise should be no less valued in this new paradigm, and need not be excluded. Strong ethnographers focused on documenting the experience, understanding, and treatment of serious emotional distress around the globe can help. As so many papers in this volume have argued well, diagnoses both come from and create a social context that neuroscientists cannot ignore if they hope to find the best ways to understand and treat madness in the future.

NOTES

1 While madness has been a contested term, informants who began to read what "we" anthropologists, sociologists, and psychologists, etc., were writing about them selected madness as a way to describe their experiences in a nonclinical way, and its usage is meant to at least signal this preference (Brettell 1993).

2 In fact, some argue that the existence of a "nonclinical" population of people who hear voices suggests that psychotic behavior lies along a proneness-persistence-impairment continuum, which, if studied, may begin to indicate how a person progresses from fleeting psychotic-like symptoms, such as magical ideas, to symptoms that are "persistent" and "impairing," such as a full-blown psychotic disorder like schizophrenia (Van Os et al. 2009). These new conceptualizations of psychosis offer a radical departure from earlier diagnostic rigidity because they look at how everyday life and neural development intertwine over the life course, which may both push a person towards developing a psychotic disorder or even hinder its progression in vulnerable people (Myers, 2012).

3 Even so, the discrediting of a century of clinical wisdom antagonized many in the scientific community. Cuthbert, Insel's director of the RDoC program, then softened these claims by publicly describing RDoC as more of a framework for conducting research than a clinical tool (Cuthbert 2014). This semi-retreat signaled how serious the pushback was from the community of psychiatrists that consensually produced the *DSM* based on 100 years of clinical experience.

4 This name has been changed from a traditional Maasai name to conceal her identity.

REFERENCES CITED

Abba, Nicola, Paul Chadwick, and Chris Stevenson. "Responding Mindfully to Distressing Psychosis: A Grounded Theory Analysis." *Psychotherapy Research* 18, no. 1 (2008):77–87.

American Psychiatric Association, editor. *Diagnostic and Statistical Manual of Mental Disorders: DSM-IV-TR.* Washington, DC: American Psychiatric Association, 2000.

Becker, Anne E. and Arthur Kleinman. "Mental Health and the Global Agenda." *New England Journal of Medicine* 369, no. 1 (2013): 66–73.

Benedict, Ruth. "Anthropology and the Abnormal." In *An Anthropologist at Work: Writings of Ruth Benedict*, edited by Margaret Mead, 262–283. Boston: Houghton Mifflin, 1959.

Biehl, Joao, Byron Good, and Arthur Kleinman, eds. *Subjectivity: Ethnographic Investigations.* Berkeley: University of California Press, 2007.

Bleuler, M., & Bleuler, R. "Dementia praecox oder die Gruppe der Schizophrenien: Eugen Bleuler." *The British Journal of Psychiatry* 149, (1986): 661-2.

.Bleuler, Mandred. "The Long-Term Course of the Schizophrenic Psychoses." *Psychological Medicine* 4 (1974): 244–54.

Brandon, Nicholas, J. Kirsty Millar, Carsten Korth, Hazel Sive, Karun K. Singh, and Akira Sawa. "Understanding the Role of DISC1 in Psychiatric Disease and During Normal Development." *The Journal of Neuroscience* 29, no. 41 (2009): 12768–75.

Brettell, Caroline. *When They Read What We Write: The Politics of Ethnography.* Wesport, CT: Bergin and Garvey, 1993.

Brodwin, Paul. *Everyday Ethics: Voices from the Front Line of Community Psychiatry.* University of California Press, 2012.

Chadda, RK, Vivek Agarwai, Megha Chandra Singh, and Deepak Raheja. "Help Seeking Behaviour of Psychiatric Patients Before Seeking Care at a Mental Hospital." *International Journal of Social Psychiatry* 47, no. 4 (2001): 71–78.

Chadwick, Paul and Max Birchwood. "The Omnipotence of Voices: A Cognitive Approach to Auditory Hallucinations." *British Journal of Psychiatry* 164 (1994): 190–201.

Chadwick, Paul, Stephanie Hughes, Daphne Russell, Ian Russell, and Dave Dagnan. "Mindfulness Groups for Distressing Voices and Paranoia: A Replication and Randomized Feasibility Trial." *Behavioural and Cognitive Psychotherapy* 37, no. 4 (2009): 403–12.

Choe, Jeanne Y., Linda A. Teplin, and Karen M. Abram. "Perpetration of Violence, Violent Victimization, and Severe Mental Illness: Balancing Public Health Concerns." *Psychiatric Services* 59, no. 2 (2008): 153–64.

Collins, Pamela Y., Vikram Patelk, Sarah S. Joesti, Dana March, Thomas R. Insel, Abdalah S. Daar, Isabel A. Bordin, E. Jane Costello, Maureen Durkin, Christopher Fairburn, Roger I. Glass, Wayne Hall, Yueqin Huang, Steven E. Hyman, Kay Jamison, Sylvia Kaaya, Shitij Kapur, Arthur Kleinman, Adesola Ogunniyi, Angel Otero-Ojeda, Mu-Ming Poo, Vijayalakshmi Ravindranath, Barbara J. Sahakian, Shekar Saxena, Peter A. Singer, Dan K. Stein, Warwick Anderson, Muhammad A Dhansay, Wendy Ewart, Anthony Phillips, Susan Shurin and Mark Walport. "Grand Challenges in Global Mental Health." *Nature* 475 (July 7, 2011): 27–30.

Compton, Michael T., and Beth Broussard. *The First Episode of Psychosis: A Guide for Patients and Their Families.* New York: Oxford University Press, 2009.

Consortium, International Schizophrenia. "Common Polygenic Variation Contributes to Risk of Schizophrenia and Bipolar Disorder." *Nature* 460, no. 7265 (2009): 748–52.

Cook Jr., Edwin H. and Stephen W. Scherer. "Copy-number Variations Associated with Neuropsychiatric Conditions." *Nature* 455, no. 7215 (2008): 919–23.

Cook, Judith A. "Employment Barriers for Persons with Psychiatric Disabilities: A Report for the President's New Freedom Commission." *Psychiatric Services* 57 (2006): 1391–405.

Cuthbert, Bruce N. "The RDoC Framework: Facilitating Transition from ICD/DSM to Dimensional Approaches that Integrate Neuroscience and Psychopathology." *World Psychiatry* 13, no. 1 (2014): 28–35.

Cuthbert, Bruce N. and Thomas R. Insel. "Toward New Approaches to Psychotic Disorders: The NIMH Research Domain Criteria project." *Schizophrenia Bulletin* 36, no. 6 (2010):1061–2.

Daalman, Kirstin, Marco P. M. Boks, Kelly M. J. Diederen, Antoin D. de Weijer, Jan Dirk Blom, and Rene S. Kahn. "The Same or Different? A Phenomenological Comparison of Auditory Verbal Hallucinations in Healthy and Psychotic Individuals." *Journal of Clinical Psychiatry* 72, no. 3 (2011): 320–5.

DeVylder, J. E., Burnette, D., & Yang, L. H. "Co-occurrence of psychotic experiences and common mental health conditions across four racially and ethnically diverse population samples." *Psychological medicine* 44, no.16, (2014): 3503-3513.Estroff, Sue E. "Identity, Disability, and Schizophrenia: The Problem of Chronicity." In *Knowledge, Power and Practice: The Anthropology of Medicine in Everyday Life*, edited by S. Lindenbaum and M. Lock, 247–86. Los Angeles: University of California Press, 1993.

Estroff, Sue E., D. L. Patrick, C. R. Zimmer, and W. Lachicotte, Jr. "Pathways to Disability Income among Persons with Severe, Persistent Psychiatric Disorders." *The Milbank Quarterly* 74, no. 4 (1997): 495–532.

Fibiger, H. Christian. "Psychiatry, the Pharmaceutical Industry, and the Road to Better Therapeutics." *Schizophrenia Bulletin* 38, no. 4 (2012): 649–50.

Fitzgerald, Des, Nikolas Rose, and Ilina Singh. "Urgan Life and Mental Health: Re-Visiting Politics, Society and Biology." Blog post. 2014. Accessed April 15, 2014. http://discoversociety.org/2014/02/15/urban-life-and-mental-health-re-visiting-politics-society-and-biology/.

Ford, J. M., Morris, S. E., Hoffman, R. E., Sommer, I., Waters, F., McCarthy-Jones, S. . . . & Cuthbert, B. N. (2014). "Studying hallucinations within the NIMH RDoC framework." *Schizophrenia bulletin*, sbu011.

Good, M. J. "The biotechnical embrace." *Culture, medicine and psychiatry*, 25 no. 4 (2001): 395-410.

Harrow, Martin and Thomas H. Jobe. "Does Long-Term Treatment of Schizophrenia with Antipsychotic Medications Facilitate Recovery? *Schizophrenia Bulletin* 39, no. 5 (2013): 962–5.

Hopper, Kim. "Returning to the Community—Again." *Psychiatric Service* 53, no. 11 (2002): 1355.

———. "Rethinking Social Recovery in Schizophrenia: What a Capabilities Approach Might Offer." *Social Science & Medicine* 65, no. 5 (2007b): 868–79.

IMS Health Inc. "IMS National Sales Perspectives 2007". 2007. Accessed May 31, 2014. http://www.imshealth.com.

Insel, Thomas R. "Director's Blog: Transforming Diagnosis". In *NIMH Director's Blog*, edited by T. Insel, Vol. 2014. 2013. Accessed May 31,2014. http://www.nimh.nih.gov/about/director/2013/transforming-diagnosis.shtml.

———. "Disruptive Insights in Psychiatry: Transforming a Clinical Discipline." *The Journal of Clinical Investigation* 119, no. 4 (2009): 700–705.

Jablensky, Assen and Flavie Waters. "RDoC: A Roadmap to Pathogenesis?" *World Psychiatry* 13, no. 1 (2014): 43–44.

Janzen, John M. *The Quest for Therapy in Lower Zaire*. Berkeley: University of California Press, 1978.

Jenkins, Janis H. and Elizabeth Carpenter-Song. "Stigma Despite Recovery: Strategies for Living in the Aftermath of Psychosis." *Medical Anthropology Quarterly* 22, no. 4 (2008): 381–409.

Jenkins, Rachel Jenkins, Joseph Mbatia, Nicola Singleton, and Bethany White. "Prevalence of Psychotic Symptoms and Their Risk Factors in Urban Tanzania." *International Journal of Environmental Research and Public Health* 7, no. 6 (2010): 2514.

Johns, Louise C., James Y. Nazroo, Paul Bebbington, and Elizabeth Kuipers. "Occurrence of Hallucinatory Experiences in a Community Sample and Ethnic Variations." *The British Journal of Psychiatry* 180, no. 2 (2002): 174–8.

Kelleher, Ian, and Mary Cannon. "Psychotic-Like Experiences in the General Population: Characterizing a High-Risk Group for Psychosis." *Psychological Medicine* 41, no. 1 (2010): 1–6.

Kirkbride, James, Jeremy W. Coid, Craig Morgan, Paul Fearon, Paola Dazzan, Min Yang, Tuhina Lloyd, Glynn L. Harrison, Robin M. Murray, and Peter B. Jones. "Translating the Epidemiology of Psychosis into Public Mental Health: Evidence, Challenges and Future Prospects." *Journal of Public Mental Health* 9, no. 2 (2010): 4–14.

Kirmayer, Laurence J., and Ian Gold. "Re-Socializing Psychiatry: Critical Neuroscience and the Limits of Reductionism." In *Critical Neuroscience: A Handbook of the Social and Cultural Contexts of Neuroscience*, edited by J. S. Suparna Choudhury, 305–30. Oxford, UK: Wiley-Blackwell, 2012.

Kleinman, Arthur. *Rethinking Psychiatry: From Cultural Category to Personal Experience*. New York: The Free Press, 1988.

Leff, J., Williams, G., Huckvale, M., Arbuthnot, M., & Leff, A. P. "Avatar therapy for persecutory auditory hallucinations: what is it and how does it work?" *Psychosis*, 6, no. 2 (2014): 166-176.

Lende, Daniel H. and Greg Downey. *The Encultured Brain: An Introduction to Neuroanthropology*. Boston, MA: MIT Press, 2012.

Lewis, S. E. "Trauma and the making of flexible minds in the Tibetan exile community." *Ethos* 41, no. 3 (2013): 313-336.

Lloyd-Evans, B., E. Mayo-Wilson, B. Harrison, H. Istead, E. Brown, S. Pilling, S. Johnson, and T. Kendall. "A Systematic Review and Meta-Analysis of Randomised Controlled Trials of Peer Support for People with Severe Mental Illness." *BMC Psychiatry* 14, no. 1 (2014): 39.

Marrow, Jocelyn, and Tanya M. Luhrmann. "The Zone of Social Abandonment in Cultural Geography: On the Street in the United States, Inside the Family in India." *Culture, Medicine and Psychiatry* 46, no. 3 (2012): 495–513.

Martin, Emily. *Bipolar Expeditions: Mania and Depression in American Culture*. Princeton, NJ: Princeton University Press, 2007.

McGorry, P., M. Alvarez-Jimenez, and E. Killackey. "Antipsychotic Medication During the Critical Period Following Remission from First-Episode Psychosis: Less Is More." *JAMA Psychiatry* 70, no. 9 (2013): 898–900.

McGruder, Juli. "Madness in Zanzibar: An Exploration of Lived Experience." In *Schizophrenia, Culture, and Subjectivity: The Edge of Experience,* edited by J. H. Jenkins and R. J. Barrett, 255–81. Cambridge Studies in Medical Anthropology, Vol. 11. Cambridge: Cambridge University Press, 2004.

Metzl, Jonathan M. and Helena Hansen. "Structural Competency: Theorizing a New Medical Engagement with Stigma and Inequality." *Social Science & Medicine* 103 (2014): 126–33.

Miller, Greg. "Is Pharma Running Out of Brainy Ideas?" *Science* 329, no. 5991 (2010): 502–504.

Millon, T., P. P. Blaney, and R. Davis, eds. *Oxford Textbook of Psychopathology*. New York: Oxford University Press, 1999.

Moerman, Daniel E., and Wayne B. Jonas. "Deconstructing the Placebo Effect and Finding the Meaning Response." *Annals of Internal Medicine* 136 (2002): 471.

Morgan, Craig, Kwame McKenzie, and Paul Fearon, eds. *Society and Psychosis.* Cambridge: Cambridge University Press, 2008.

Myers, Neely. "Toward an Applied Neuroanthropology of Psychosis: The Interplay of Culture, Brains and Experience." *Annals of Anthropological Practice* 36, no. 1 (2012a): 113–30.

———. "Update: Schizophrenia across Cultures." *Current Psychiatry Reports* 13, no. 4 (2012b): 305–11.

Ndetei, D. M., L. Khasakhala, V. Mutiso, and A. W. Mbwayo. "Knowledge, Attitude and Practice (KAP) of Mental Illness among Staff in General Medical Facilities in Kenya: Practice and Policy Implications." *African Journal of Psychiatry (Johannesbg)* 14, no. 3 (2011): 225–35.

Newcomer, John W. "Antipsychotic Medications: Metabolic and Cardiovascular Risk." *Journal of Clincal Psychiatry* 68, no. 4 (2007): 1555–2101.

Newcomer, John W. and Charles H. Hennekens. "Severe Mental Illness and Risk of Cardiovascular Disease." *Journal of the American Medical Association* 298 (2007): 1794–6.

Ngoma, Mdimu, Martin Prince, and Anthony Mann. "Common Mental Disorders among Those Attending Primary Health Clinics and Traditional Healers in Urban Tanzania." *The British Journal of Psychiatry* 183, no. 4 (2003): 349–55.

Os, J. van, Linscott, R. J., Myin-Germeys, I., Delespaul, P., & Krabbendam, L. "A systematic review and meta-analysis of the psychosis continuum: evidence for a psychosis proneness-persistence-impairment model of psychotic disorder." *Psychological medicine*, 39 no. 2 (2009): 179-195.

Patel, Vikram. "Explanatory Models of Mental Illness in Sub-Saharan Africa." *Social Science and Medicine* 40, no. 9 (1995): 1291–8.

Pierre, Joseph. "A Mad World: A Diagnosis of Mental Illness Is More Common Than Ever—Did Psychiatrists Create the Problem, or Just Recognise It?" In *Aeon MAGAZINE,* Vol. 2014. Accessed May 31, 2014. http://aeon.co/magazine/being-human/have-psychiatrists-lost-perspective-on-mental-illness/: Aeon Media Ltd.

Plato. *Phaedrus.* 12 vols. Translated by H. N. Fowler. Volume 9. Cambridge, MA: Harvard University Press, 1925.

Robins, Eli and Samuel B. Guze. "Establishment of Diagnostic Validity in Psychiatric Illness: Its Application to Schizophrenia." *American Journal of Psychiatry* 126, no.7 (1970): 983–7.

Robins, Lee N. and Darrel A. Regier, eds. *Psychiatric Disorders in America: The Epidemiologic Catchement Area Study.* New York: The Free Press, 1991.

Romme, Marius, Sandra Escher, Jacqui Dillon, Dirck Corstens, and Mervyn Morris. *Living with Voices: 50 Stories of Recovery.* Gateshead, UK: Athaeneum Press, 2009.

Sartorius, Norman. "Short-Lived Campaigns Are Not Enough." *Nature* 468, no. 7321 (2010): 163–5.

Sartorius, Norman, A. Jablensky, A. Korten, G. Ernberg, M. Anker, J. E. Cooper and R. Day. "Early Manifestations and First Contact Incidence of Schizophrenia in Different Cultures." *Psychological Medicine* 16, no.4 (1986): 909–28.

Sato, Mitsumoto. "Renaming Schizophrenia: A Japanese Perspective." *World Psychiatry* 5, no. 1 (2006): 53–55.

Saxena, Saxena, Guillermo Paraje, Pratap Saharan, Ghassan Karam, and Ritu Sadana. "The 10/90 Divide in Mental Health Research: Trends over a 10-Year Period." *British Journal of Psychiatry* 188 (2006): 81–82.

Seligman, Rebecca. "The Unmaking and Making of Self: Embodied Suffering and Mind Body Healing in Brazilian Candomble." *Ethos* 38, no. 3 (2010): 297–320.

Shergill, Sukhwinder S., Robin M. Murray, and Philip K. McGuire. "Auditory Hallucinations: A Review of Psychological Treatments." *Schizophrenia Research* 32 (1998): 137–50.

Shorter, Edward. *A History of Psychiatry: From the Era of Asylum to the Age of Prozac.* New York: John Wiley & Sons, 1997.

Snyder, Sharon and David T. Mitchell. *Cultural Locations of Disability.* Chicago: University of Chicago Press, 2006.

Takahashi, Hidehiko, Takashi Ideno, Shigetaka Okubo, Hiroshi Matsui, Kazuhisa Takemura, Masato Matsuura, Motoichiro Kato, and Yoshiro Okubo. "Impact of Changing the Japanese Term for 'Schizophrenia' for Reasons of Stereotypical Beliefs of Schizophrenia in Japanese Youth." *Schizophrenia Research* 112, no. 1 (2009): 149–52.

Teplin, Linda A., Gary M. McClelland, Karen M. Abram, and Dana A. Weiner. "Crime Victimization in Adults with Severe Mental Illness: Comparison with the National Crime Victimization Survey." *Archives of General Psychiatry* 62, no. 8 (2005): 911–21.

Teuton, Joanna, Christopher Dowrick, and Richard P. Bentall. "How Healers Manage the Pluralistic Healing Context: The Perspective of Indigenous, Religious and Allopathic Healers in Relation to Psychosis in Uganda." *Social Science and Medicine* 65, no. 6 (2007): 1260–73.

Voosen, Paul. "A Revolution in Mental Health." *The Chronicle of Higher Education* (September 9, 2013).

Wakefield, Jerome C. "Wittgenstein's Nightmare: Why the RDoC Grid Needs A Conceptual Dimension." *World Psychiatry* 13, no. 1 (2014): 38–40.

Warner, Richard. *Recovery from Schizophrenia: Psychiatry and Political Economy.* London: Routledge, 1994.

Weinberger, Daniel R., and Terry E. Goldberg. "RDoCs Redux." *World Psychiatry* 13, no. 1 (2014): 36–38.

WHO (World Health Organization). *Policy Perspective on Medicines-Growing Needs and Potentials.* World Health Organization: Geneva, 2014.

———. *Mental Health Atlas.* Italy: World Health Organization, 2011.

Wunderink, Lex, Roeline M. Nieboer, Durk Wiersma, Sjoerd Sytema, and Fokko J. Nienhuis. "Recovery in Remitted First-Episode Psychosis at 7 Years of Follow-Up of An Early Dose Reduction/Discontinuation Or Maintenance Treatment Strategy: Long-Term Follow-Up of A 2-Year Randomized Clinical Trial." *JAMA Psychiatry* 70, no. 9 (2013): 913–20.

Yang, Lawrence H., Michael R. Phillips, Graciete Lo, Yuwen Chou, Xiaoli Zhang, and Kim Hopper. "Excessive Thinking" as Explanatory Model for Schizophrenia: Impacts on Stigma and "Moral" Status in Mainland China." *Schizophrenia Bulletin* 36, no. 4 (2009): 836–45.

10 The Lyme Wars

The Effects of Biocommunicability, Gender, and Epistemic Politics on Health Activation and Lyme Science

Georgia Davis and Mark Nichter

INTRODUCTION

Within the biomedical community, Lyme disease is considered a "well-defined, distinct clinical entity" (Baker 2009) with a widely accepted etiology and protocol for diagnosis and treatment (CDC 2013). Yet the disease remains one of the most contentious in recent history (Tonks 2007; Whelan 2007, 2010). On the one hand is an "establishment" group of credentialed doctors and researchers whose authority arises from their positions on the editorial boards of major medical journals and from the institutional backing of the powerful medical policy and advocacy group, the Infectious Diseases Society of America, and from the federal agency, the Centers for Disease Control and Prevention (CDC). Challenging this mainstream axis of medical-scientific expertise is a more loosely organized "alternative" network of patients, their friends and family members, and sympathetic doctors and scientists whose credibility is bolstered by professional organizations such as the Lyme Disease Association (Cohen 2004, 2007) and the International Lyme and Associated Diseases Society (ILADS 2014). This latter group has had some success challenging the "expert" science in scientific, legal, policy making, and more populist arenas. Several writers (for examples, see Stricker and Johnson 2014; Tonks 2007; Weintraub 2008), reflecting on the contentiousness between the two groups, have used the military metaphor the "Lyme Wars" to characterize the depth of the rancor and the fierce battles to sway scientists, patients, doctors, and policy makers to take sides.

The lingering contentiousness confounds those involved in the debate. Each group offers the explanation that the others' science must be corrupted, whereas its own remains pure. Viewing the Lyme debate through the lens of Hess's work on shifts in what it means to be a health citizen and perceptions of unfinished science makes it clear that such tensions are not surprising. Indeed, they are to be expected. According to Hess (Hess 2004), medicine is modernizing to make space—in a way we understand to be both literal and figurative—for an emerging scientific citizen. In the process, the old Enlightenment model of science, heavily critiqued by the field of Public Understanding of Science (Epstein 1996; Grosz 1994; Haraway 1997; Kroll-Smith and Floyd 1997), is losing its hegemonic power as objective and beyond social debate. Using the lens of epistemic politics, we review three scientific controversies related to Lyme diagnosis and we argue that the debate about Lyme disease is actually a debate about the proper role of society, and women in particular, in the production of medico-scientific knowledge. Our intent is not to make a case for whose science is right, but to see how differing epistemologies produce very different outcomes in terms of scientific inquiry and patient care.

THE "SUBURBAN DISEASE" IN AN ERA OF EPISTEMIC POLITICS

In 1975, an unnamed mother living in suburban Connecticut contacted her county health board to report that 12 children on her road had been diagnosed with juvenile rheumatoid arthritis, usually a rare condition. Within the same month, a second woman reported to the county that she, her family, and several neighbors had all been diagnosed with rheumatoid arthritis (Steere, Malawista et al. 1977). The latter mother, Judith Mensch, had been treated and sent home with aspirin. The former, Polly Murray, had been told by her doctor that she had psychological problems, and that her children—also sick—were mimicking her. Both women, based upon the number of people around them who had similar symptoms beyond joint pain and fatigue, refused to accept their doctor's diagnoses. Murray took the added step of using skills she had learned while working for the World Health Organization to conduct informal epidemiological work in her neighborhood (Weintraub 2008). When their doctors denied their patient-knowledge, both women appealed to the county to intervene. Eventually, the CDC sent in an epidemiological team to investigate what scientists were calling "Lyme arthritis," picking up on the label already assigned to the disease by area doctors and ignoring claims by Murray and Mensch that this was something else entirely.

It is now known that Murray and Mensch were right. Their disease was caused by a zoonotic bacterial infection of the *Borrelia burgdorferi* (*Bb*) spirochete, which is transmitted through the bite of a tick. Spirochetes, which are corkscrew-shaped and propel themselves by drilling into gelatinous tissues, are now known to cause other multi-systemic diseases—such as syphilis—and to produce multiple symptoms, including arthritis (Buhner 2005). It is also now known that *Bb* organisms were formed 100 million years ago, and have infected humans for at least 5,000 years (Keller et al. 2012). Modern medical accounts of Lyme-related rashes (erythema migrans, or EM) and arthritis dating back to the 1800s can be found in European literature (Matuschka et al. 1995), and doctors in the northeastern United States have been treating Lyme disease for many decades, colloquially referred to by names such as Montauk Knee (Horowitz 2013).

Despite a long history of making humans ill, Lyme disease only became a part of the national conversation due to the efforts of two middle-class, sub-urban women who, acting on behalf of themselves, their families, and their neighbors, alerted the government to a pathogen that scientists and public health officials had missed.

Notably, Murray and Mensch did exactly what was expected of good, female health citizens. They monitored their own and their family's health, and sought out medical expertise when confronted with illness. When their efforts were disregarded and they were further marginalized by their doctors (Weintraub 2008), they did not act irrationally. Rather, they went about doing something that, within the context of health citizenship, was very rational: they asked questions, gathered local data, compiled their findings, and contacted health boards about a public health concern in their area. In short, these two mothers became what we refer to as *activated health citizens*. Their activation was motivated when they personally experienced the tension between an older "doctor knows best" model of medicine where patients are passive and compliant, and a newer participatory model, where responsibility for health decision-making requires a proactive health consumer that adheres to a negotiated treatment plan. This emerging health consumer role is being taken up and performed by many other women who, like Murray and Mensch, hail from privileged socio-economic sections of society that have access to a wide range of information resources and an interest in science.

Despite their role in bringing attention to the unknown disease, Murray and Mensch remained unnamed in the reports on the phenomena. As Briggs and Hallin (2007) have noted, when the science is unclear or when there are gaps in medico-scientific knowledge, credentialed experts are assigned the role of filling in the holes, not lay publics. So it was in the case of Lyme. Government-backed scientists took charge, and a newly minted CDC epidemiologist, Allen Steere, was credited with discovering and naming the disease after Lyme, Connecticut, the location where he had been deployed (Steere et al. 1977). Treated as an emerging disease at a time when disease outbreaks around the globe threatened to disrupt the public's widespread faith that biomedical science would someday eliminate all infectious disease (Garrett 1994), Lyme disease became the focus of intensive research. This resulted in a succession of discoveries from the causative agent (Burgdorfer 1984), the vector (Oliver et al. 1993; Spielman 1985), the vector's ecology (Matuschka Fr 1986), and suitable therapies (Steere et al. 1980), to definitive diagnostic guidelines (Wormser et al. 2006). The field of public health congratulated itself on the quick containment of an emerging disease threat within America's own backyard. To this end, Halperin et al. wrote, "[T]wenty-five years after the description of Lyme disease we have come far; clinical features are well described, accurate tests support diagnosis, effective therapy is available, and there is an effective vaccine" (2013: 418).

The Lyme success story was short lived. The first problem to arise was patients, in mass, consulting doctors for what appeared to be a disease of the day, gaining press visibility. Concerns were voiced about the "health burden" this situation was creating for impacted states (Schwartz et al. 1989; Coyle et al. 1996), and the redirection of funds from vector control to treating inaccurate diagnoses of Lyme (Reid et al. 1998). Not surprisingly, many doctors, scientists, and health officials blamed the media for inciting fear and creating "Lyme anxiety" and "Lyme hysteria" (Aronowitz 1991). Markedly, the phenomena increasingly began being described in gendered terms, as a "suburban" disease (Barbour and Fish 1993; unknown 2001) associated with anxious women.

Activated female patients, in turn, pushed back, advocating for a more patient-centered model of medicine after being confronted by an evidence-based model that failed to address their lived health issues.[1] A Lyme movement emerged with women on the frontlines, vetting doctors who might become "Lyme-literate," locating scientists willing to collaborate with them, and gathering and sharing all manner of scientific knowledge. While it is beyond the scope of this chapter to interrogate the identity politics of the Lyme health movement, it is important to note that it was women who coined the term "Lymie" to signify their emerging health consumerist role as informed, domestic health care managers engaging in citizen science (Irwin 1995), true to the neoliberal principles of "taking responsibility."

THE SCIENCE OF LYME: CONTROVERSIES AND ALIGNMENTS

The scientific differences between Lyme debate participants are multiple. In this chapter, we focus on three areas of scientific disagreement related to the Lyme diagnosis. In each case, we first present the "mainstream" perspective, followed by "alternative" claims. We are fully aware that positioning the debate as an either/or reifies the problematic binary thinking that is at the heart of Lyme epistemic politics. Indeed, it may be argued that the debate has essentialized Lymies and mainstream voices alike, obscuring differences within camps. At the same time, the bifurcation of the Lyme debate into a mainstream and an alternative camp is a narrative that has certainly gained traction and is a common focus of discourse.[2] We use the two-sided narrative as a heuristic for understanding the ways in which people have aligned themselves and how such alignments have produced very different kinds of science.[3]

Signs of Lyme Disease

Symptoms are not typically identified as a major point of contention in the Lyme wars. We argue, however, that it is impossible to engage the Lyme debate without first understanding how some symptoms and not others came to be included as signs in the diagnosis of Lyme disease.

I. Mainstream

When the CDC-led investigative team first started cataloging the symptoms of Lyme disease, it noticed that most patients developed a distinctive bullseye-shaped rash (the EM) that subsided even without treatment. This led them to conclude that the disease was self-limiting (Steere et al. 1977). Over time, the EM rash became the hallmark of early Lyme infection (Wormser et al. 2006). They further observed that some Lyme patients developed swollen joints weeks after the EM rash cleared completely (Steere et al. 1980). They conjectured that joint swelling was most likely a post-infection immune response, a phenomenon seen in other infectious diseases (Steere 1993). Investigators also noted other symptoms associated with Lyme, ranging from extreme fatigue and flu-like symptoms to problems with short-term memory and cognition, and heart and neurological abnormalities that developed along with arthritis.

Whereas scientists took special interest in Lyme-related arthritis, and the manner in which *Bb* affected the human body, proactive patients sought explanations for other debilitating but more difficult-to-quantify symptoms, such as cognitive problems and profound fatigue (Aucott et al. 2013; Horowitz 2013; Johnson et al. 2014). Conflicting matters of concern (Latour 2005) created tension between scientists and patients, who had different opinions about treatment priorities. Scientists prioritized the resolution of rashes, arthritis, and pain and numbness in hands and feet, quantifiable symptoms that would resolve with antibiotics and time, as in other post-infectious conditions (Steere 2008). Patients, in contrast, wanted their debilitating fatigue and mental fog to resolve so they could get on with life (Johnson et al. 2014).

Cost of treatment for persistent and nebulous symptoms also played a role in diagnosis. Public health officials expressed concern about Lyme-related health expenditures, which were attributed to "Lyme anxiety" and the inability of doctors to distinguish Lyme anxiety and other nebulous diseases that tended to affect women, such as chronic fatigue syndrome (CFS) (Wormser and Shapiro 2009) and fibromyalgia (FMS) (Sigal 1994). For example, in a widely cited study (Dattwyler et al. 1988), the authors pointedly recommended against using "chronic fatigue" to diagnose Lyme. Doctors were advised that if a patient treated for Lyme continued to complain of nebulous symptoms, the recommended course of action was not to treat "chronic Lyme disease" (CLD), but to question the initial Lyme disease diagnosis, and to consider a diagnosis of fibromyalgia (Sigal 1994) or depression (Berman and Wenglin 1995) instead. When the American College of Physicians Lyme guidelines writing team finally met several years later, one member penned the following about the experience of sorting out Lyme symptoms from female syndromes:

> The consensus was that people with chronic symptoms, even those with serologic evidence of previous exposure to *Borrelia burgdorferi*, should be given a diagnosis of Lyme disease only if they have one of

a few well-defined late presentations, each of which contains one or more threshold conditions that is either a physician-discovered sign (for example, frank arthritis with observable and 'tapable' fluid) or an objective test result (such as cerebral spinal fluid findings consistent with aseptic meningitis). This decision did not simply follow from biological evidence that only persons who met these criteria had *B. burgdorferi* infection or its immunologic sequulae. We did not and do not have the technological means to reliably and directly apprehend the underlying pathologic processes that presumably cause the late symptoms of Lyme disease. (Aronowitz 2001: 807)

As noted by Aronowitz, the Lyme guidelines that ended up being produced were consensus-based, not strictly evidence-based, and served to rule out a Lyme diagnosis sought by troublesome patients in search of a legitimate diagnosis for vague sets of persisting complaints.[4]

Several researchers voiced the opinion that psychiatric disorders are the most likely cause of ongoing 'Lyme' symptoms, and suggested that the effects of somaticizing were considerably worse than the illness itself. "Assumption of the 'sick role,'" one study suggested, "leaves an invisible scar that may be the most devastating effect of 'chronic Lyme disease'" (Halperin et al. 2013). The overriding concern was women who really had CFS and FMS, but were unwilling to accept that there was little biomedicine could do to help them. Instead, it was presumed, they shopped around for a doctor willing to give them a Lyme label (Aronowitz 1991, Barbour and Fish 1993). This behavior was described as detrimental to society at large, because it occurred at taxpayer expense and skewed science, making Lyme surveillance numbers inaccurate (Reid et al. 1998; Wormser and Shapiro 2009).

II. Alternative

Whereas investigative scientists focused on a few observable signs to track the progression of Lyme disease and to distinguish it from female syndromes, some doctors treating Lyme used a much wider range of patient-reported criteria to diagnose and track the progression of the disease (Cameron et al. 2014). Richard Horowitz writes about his early experience treating Lyme patients in the late 1980s.

I wanted all of my patients to get better. Why did roughly 75 percent of the patients treated early on get better but 25 percent appeared to develop chronic symptoms? These patients presented with a strange litany of symptoms, such as fatigue, aches and pains that migrated around their bodies, tingling and numbness, memory and concentration problems, and a host of other unexplained symptoms. I asked my colleagues for input, but no one seemed to know the answers (Horowitz 2013: 10).

Horowitz, now a leading "Lyme-literate doctor" (LLMD) who travels the world educating doctors and public health officials about alternative protocols for the treatment of Lyme, was one of many clinicians who noted a wide range of patient-reported symptoms that occurred after a standard round of antibiotic treatment, many of which could not be easily quantified or explained (Buhner 2005; Makris 2011; McFadzean 2010).

In conjunction with their doctors, activated patients created more extensive lists of symptoms. As these individuals collectivized, they organized their symptom lists into a nosology that divided the disease into two phases: early and late infection. Their experience of Lyme disease ran counter to the mainstream definition and they began searching for doctors willing to work with patient expertise to develop treatment practices. This growing Lyme community then used their emerging nosology to train new LLMDs in how to respond to the disease.

Remarkably, activated patients not only played a role in producing knowledge about Lyme, but also in ferrying that knowledge between doctors, who may or may not speak to one another, and who may have different interpretations of patient-reported symptoms. Consider this comment by Carol, an activated Lyme patient in the northeastern United States. "I have actually connected doctors at conferences. They are all highly independent. Each has their own idea of what is at the root of chronic Lyme—is it autoimmune? Is it co-infection? Is it different serotypes of Lyme, etc.?—and how to treat it. Some think herbs are good. Others think they mask symptoms but only aggressive antibiotics work."

As scientists joined the movement, ensuing research sought scientific explanations to support the patient-reported nosology of a disease that develops in stages. In vitro studies, for example, revealed that *Bb* inhibits CD-57 cells and kills T- and B-cells, all of which are used by the immune system to fight disease. In early infection, while the body is still able to produce these cells, the germ load is low and patient symptoms are generally mild and usually curable (Buhner 2005; Makris 2011; Williams 2011). Research also found that once the bacteria has managed to compromise the host immune system, it can multiply and move out of the skin to infect other bodily systems. At this point, a patient's germ load is high and their symptoms increase in severity and kind (Burrascano 2008). The alternative Lyme camp refers to the surfacing of multi-system symptoms after a latent period as late disseminated infection. It is when patients begin to experience arthritis, along with cardiac and neurological dysfunctions. To diagnose a disseminated Lyme infection, LLMDs take into account a range of symptoms from fatigue to light and sound sensitivity, stiff neck, fevers, alternating sweats and chills, problems with memory and concentration, sleep disorders, shortness of breath, heart palpitations, migrating muscle aches, gastrointestinal disturbances, and psychiatric symptoms (Bean and Fein 2008; Blanc and Gebly 2007; Savely 2011). According to doctors endorsing chronic Lyme, it is not individual symptoms, but the wide constellation of severe symptoms that may wax and wane, shift over time, and migrate around the body that are indicative of an ongoing Lyme infection. This group attributes the changing symptom picture to spirochetes moving through the body, and changing bacterial loads related to the *Bb* life cycle (Burrascano 2008).

LLMDs have also sought to differentiate Lyme from other diseases. Their intent, however, is not to rule Lyme out, but to rule it *in*. In 1997, one research team compared post-treatment Lyme and CFS, finding that Lyme patients exhibited more overall cognitive impairment than CFS patients, and that they may have problems with verbal memory, verbal fluency, auditory attention, and finger tapping speed that CFS patients did not (Gaudino et al. 1997). Another study found that patients with Lyme often developed depression, even when they had no previous history of mental illness. They argued that depression is actually a symptom of Lyme disease (Hajek et al. 2002). Still others have linked Lyme disease to a range of unexplained neurological or psychiatric disorders found in previously healthy patients (Blanc and Gebly 2007). Some research has found Lyme spirochetes in a higher-than-expected rate of neuro-psych patients, suggesting Lyme disease—like its cousin, syphilis—may cause a range of psychiatric disorders (Hajek et al. 2006).

III. Discussion

Many of the symptoms Lyme patients report as most debilitating are difficult to measure. Furthermore, because a patient only complains about these problems once he/she is sick, the clinician has no comparable baseline from when the individual was healthy. Also, some symptoms may be different for women than men (Schwarzwalder et al. 2010). To use a range of patient-reported symptoms rather than a few objective signs, however, the expert must rely on a lay individual's subjective experiences, and his/her interpretation of those experiences. If, for example, a patient reports experiencing severe fatigue or depression, the clinician must trust the patient when he/she says he/she did not have these problems before being bitten by a tick, and that he/she is capable of assessing the progression and changing magnitude of his/her symptoms. Trust and the importance of feedback lies at the heart of the patient-centered care advocated by those in the alternative Lyme community.

The mainstream community, in contrast, only counts symptoms as valid if they can be observed and measured by trained experts, often using medical technologies. They also only include a narrow group of symptoms in the diagnostic guidelines. This fits with a managed care system that uses quantitative assessments, both conducted and interpreted by credentialed experts, to determine evidence-based practice across a variety of clinical settings.

The fight over which symptoms count is really a fight over who has the expertise to define Lyme disease. Is it the expert patient or the expert scientist? This very question about whose authority counts was one addressed by the panel that met to write the treatment guidelines and definition for Lyme disease. Members upheld the authority of trained experts when they excluded symptoms like fatigue and memory loss, which female patients were said to complain about the most.

In upholding medical authority, however, the panel also reproduced gendered assumptions about Lyme. Members reified the discursive link between growing health care expenditures, social anxiety, and women's bodies, causing women's bodies to come under further scrutiny. Soon women were not only blamed for the perceived public panic, they were also blamed for their ongoing symptoms (Hsu et al. 1993; Wormser and Shapiro 2009). Aronowitz partly spoke to this in his retrospective on the guidelines writing process:

> The critical appraisal of medical evidence could not be separated from knowledge of who would be the likely winners and losers if Lyme disease were defined one way or another. To no one's surprise, attempts such as this one to keep symptom clusters out of the Lyme disease definition have been controversial (Aronowitz 2001: 807).

Today, the guidelines remain largely intact despite several critical reviews (Johnson and Stricker 2008; Koopman and Cameron 2009; Stricker and Johnson 2010). The prevailing consensus within the wider biomedical community is that guidelines must be specific and narrow to exclude misdiagnoses. Although the mention of gender is conspicuously absent from the guidelines (Wormser et al. 2006), gender stereotypes are implicit. In contrast, the Lyme community credits the guidelines for forcing patients to activate; they have no choice if they are to regain their former health. "There is a reason so many Lyme sufferers seek out alternative treatments. It is not because they are insane, uneducated, overly hysterical, stupid, or gullible. It is because they are ill, they know they are ill, and because conventional medical treatment has not worked for them" (Buhner 2005: 7).

PTLDS/Chronic Lyme

Although early on the mainstream camp adopted the term chronic Lyme disease to describe post-treatment arthritis, it now rejects that label due to the term's "misuse" by the alternative camp to incorrectly signify ongoing infection (Sigal 2002). The mainstream now widely uses the label PTLDS, or Post-treatment Lyme Disease Syndrome, to classify people who have been diagnosed and treated for Lyme but who continue to suffer. In contrast, the alternative camp argues that people do not have a syndrome, they have an active infection caused by a complex bacteria that is sophisticated enough to evade efforts to eradicate it. The solution, until better drugs can be discovered, is to treat with antibiotics until symptoms resolve. The PTLDS/chronic Lyme debate is one of the most contentious in the Lyme wars.

I. Mainstream
Because investigative scientists noted a period of recovery in between the bullseye rash and the Lyme arthritis, they determined that the bacterial infection was short-lived. It was determined, in some unusual cases, that

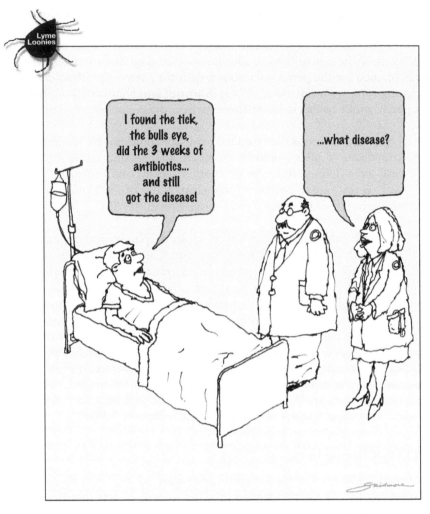

Figure 10.1   From the "Lyme Loonies" series by cartoonist David Skidmore. "Lyme Loonies" refers to an email written by outgoing National Institutes of Health Lyme program officer, Phillip Baker, in which he states, "I will certainly miss all of you people—the scientists—but not the Lyme loonies" (Mary Beth Pfeiffer, "Chronic Lyme: Is it Real," *Poughkeepsie Journal*, May 20, 2013). Members of the Lyme camp have taken up the term to highlight the degree of marginalization by those within federal health institutions.

the body's immune system will continue to fight the disease even after it is eradicated, causing an inflammatory illness—marked by arthritis—that can last six months or longer (Logigian et al. 1990). At first, the initial research team was ambivalent about the effectiveness of antibiotic treatments (Steere et al. 1977), but later, they began routinely prescribing antibiotics to treat Lyme disease based on clinical evidence that 7–10 days of antibiotic therapy led to the faster resolution of EM rashes, and significantly reduced the likelihood that patients would go on to develop arthritis (Steere et al. 1980). By 1998, researchers had discovered that after a second course of antibiotics, the "objective evidence of active disease, including arthritis, resolved in all patients over a 3-month period, with the exception of peripheral neuropathy, which resolved more slowly" (Dattwyler et al. 1988: 1442), and that the arthritis did not relapse in the eight-month follow-up period. From this, scientists concluded that because any other ongoing symptoms, such as fatigue, inflammation, headache, musculoskeletal pain, and neuropathy, were part of a post-infection inflammation response that should resolve itself in a matter of months, antibiotics would do more harm than good (Logigian et al. 1990; Sigal 1994; Steere 1993). In 2001, Klempner et al. (2001) conducted a pivotal study that is still cited as a justification for limiting antibiotic therapies for Lyme (Baker et al. 2010). Scientists observed the effects of an additional 90 days of antibiotics on post-treatment fatigue, musculoskeletal pain, and neurocognitive problems. Because researches noted no significant differences compared to the placebo group, they discontinued the study after only 107 of the 260 enrolled patients had been retreated, rather than continue to use potentially dangerous and costly therapies without evidence of treatment success (Shapiro 2014: 684). Today, the Lyme treatment guidelines state that patients be prescribed up to 28 days of oral or intravenous antibiotics, followed by another two to four weeks of antibacterial treatment for only those individuals whose *arthritis* symptoms have improved but not completely resolved (Wormser, Dattwyler et al. 2006).

The search, now, is not to understand Lyme disease—as that has already happened—but to find an explanation for why the immune system remembers a past infection (Steere 2008). One line of inquiry addresses what it is about the bacteria that could provoke an immune response. Several researchers have found evidence that dead organisms might leave behind highly inflammatory remnants (Norgard et al. 1995; Singh and Girschick 2006). Others have located the immune-related chemicals and pathways that are activated and could be targeted for therapies (Benhnia et al. 2005; Guerau-De-Arellano and Huber 2005). One group of researchers has found that people with PTLDS have elevated numbers of anti-neural antibodies, similar to patients with ALS and other neurological syndromes (Chandra et al. 2010). Still others have studied the possibility that ongoing symptoms could result from tissue damage caused by *Bb* during the active infection (Pachner and Steiner 2007). Scientists, however, remain unclear if it is damage to the tissues, pro-inflammatory proteins in the bacteria, the human immune system, or some combination thereof that causes the ongoing inflammation. This work continues.

Another line of inquiry, an offshoot of Lyme anxiety research, explored biopsychosocial mechanisms. This included the study that found a link between negative thinking, maladaptive coping styles, and prolonged illness (Satalino 2008). One study of post-infection fatigue to include Lyme fatigue found that the brain is biologically adapted to respond to illness, signaling the individual to withdraw in order to divert energy toward getting well. The author theorized that, in some patients, the brain dysfunctions for as-of-yet undetermined reasons, and the withdrawal signal continues even after an infection has cleared (James 2008).

II. Alternative

Lyme doctors who based their conclusions on patient-reported symptoms and not the diagnostic guidelines noted that "while on medication their problems all improved, but many quickly relapsed once the antibiotics were stopped" (Horowitz 2013: 10). This finding led many, like Horowitz, to conclude that symptoms were indicative of an active bacterial infection that could not necessarily be eradicated by antibiotics (Buhner 2005; Weintraub 2008). The alternative camp supports using open-ended courses of antibiotics until all symptoms are resolved. Depending on how long someone has been infected, that can take from weeks to months, and sometimes even years. These treating clinicians did not engage in clinical trials, nor did they collaborate with one another. In fact, it was only recently that they even published their findings. Instead, they treated more and more patients, who collectivized, organized, and distributed these doctors' findings within their growing Lyme network. As scientists were enrolled, they began to study the mechanisms that could allow the *Bb* bacteria to survive in a hostile environment.

This group does not discount the theory that the immune system may be over-responsive and that therapies targeted at calming the resulting inflammation may be helpful to Lyme patients. This group, however, maintains that this process is driven, at least in part, by the presence of live bacteria (Fallon et al. 1999). They cite studies in which scientists have been able to recover motile *Bb* spirochetes from mice (Hodzic et al. 2014), dogs (Straubinger et al. 1997), rhesus macaques (Embers et al. 2012), and humans after treatment with antibiotics (Georgilis et al. 1992).

Scientific inquiry has followed several different tracks. One seeks to understand how *Bb* can evade the human immune system, even when it is over-activated. According to this group, the immune response is modulated, meaning parts of it are activated—ostensibly to draw the body's "attention" away from the site of infection—while other parts that could be more deadly for the spirochete are deactivated (Diterich et al. 2003). Another theory advanced by this group is that spirochetes have the ability to bore deep into the body and its tissues, allowing *Borrelia* to hide out within host cells, and in hard-to-reach places (Burrascano 2008; Cameron et al. 2014). Another theory is that the bacteria can actually alter its outer surface, making it difficult for the body to produce antibodies that have the right shape to attach to and kill the invader (Diterich et al. 2003). Because *Bb* can evade detection—using whatever sophisticated mechanism(s) it has developed over the centuries—some patients' immune systems cannot mop up the residual bacteria that inevitably remain after treatment (Barthold et al. 2010).

Another line of research suggests that *Bb* cannot only withstand the human immune system, it has developed ways to shield itself from toxins, like antibiotics. Alan MacDonald was instrumental in recognizing that *Bb* may take on different shapes entirely, forming cysts, granules, and fragments (MacDonald 1988) that come back to life once the threat is removed, even after months of antibiotics. Along these same lines, another group of researchers is presently studying the ability of *Bb* to form biofilms. A biofilm is an interactive community of microbes that adhere to one another and coat themselves in a sticky substance (Horowitz 2013). This sticky coating, the theory goes, makes the bacteria more impervious to antibiotics (Sapi et al. 2011). Some of those studying atypical *Bb* forms have found that not only do antibiotics have different effects—and sometimes no effect at all on these various forms in vitro (Feng et al. 2014: 5)—but antibiotics may actually encourage *Bb* to take on these antibiotic-resistant shapes. "Our results are consistent with the idea that antibiotic treatment is effective only in the earliest stages of *Lyme borreliosis*. Antibiotics such as penicillin and its derivative doxycycline induce round body formation and quiescence of symptoms rather than cure" (Brorson et al. 2009: 18659).

III. Discussion

Initially, patients with ongoing symptoms were given another disease label. Those complaining of chronic Lyme symptoms were most likely to be classified as having FMS, CFS, or depression, conditions largely associated with women's bodies. This led patient-consumers who disagreed with these diagnoses to seek out doctors who would treat them based upon a wider variety and duration of symptoms. In time, this group adopted the chronic Lyme label to signify the ability of a complex bacteria to use sophisticated means to survive antibiotic therapy and the human immune system.

As chronic Lyme came to signify chronic infection, the mainstream abandoned the label and rejected any notion that Lyme could survive long durations of treatment (Halperin et al. 2013). Today, patients who have had a previous Lyme diagnosis and who continue to experience symptoms are likely to be diagnosed with Post-treatment Lyme Disease Syndrome. This signifies a shift in thinking from blaming somaticizing patients for their continuing illness, to recognizing that those who have been properly diagnosed and treated may still be "genuinely suffering" (Saunders 2014). This shift gives legitimacy to those who have followed expert advice and remained unwell, even though biomedical science can do little at this point to alleviate their symptoms. There is some evidence that the PTLDS label is also meant to appease patients who might otherwise activate, and join the Lyme movement, although a discourse analysis would be necessary to examine this claim further

Recognizing PTLDS amounts to an admission that medico-science does not have all the answers. Yet, this does not diminish the power of credentialed experts, and not patients, to fill in the gaps. Indeed, it is the nosology produced by the early, government-led research team that continues to guide mainstream thinking about Lyme disease. The counter-nosology, produced through patient-consumer partnerships with doctors, has driven the alternative science. Consequently, two very different modes of thinking are producing very different kinds of evidence about Lyme disease, even as only one has been given institutional authority.

Tests

Lyme testing protocol was established in 1994 during a conference in Dearborn, Michigan. The conference occurred at a time when there was heightened sensitivity about Lyme disease and anxiety amongst suburban women. The special meeting was meant to be a review of best practices for determining a *Bb* infection with the goal of standardizing the testing procedure and minimizing doctor subjectivity, thereby reducing high rates of misdiagnosis (Barbour 1989). The final report from that conference recommended that all patients be given not one, but two tests for Lyme disease. Furthermore, the Dearborn report narrowed the criteria for defining what could be considered a positive blot (ASTPHLD 1994). Although the tests have improved over the years with new technologies, the process and evidence used to determine a Lyme infection has remained constant. The alternative community, in contrast, believes that the two-step testing process advocated by the mainstream is deeply flawed.[5]

I. Mainstream

The rationale for the two-step testing process is that no single test is specific enough to distinguish Lyme from another disease it might mimic. The two tests both use sera drawn from a patient's blood. The sera is put into contact with *Bb* antigens in a culture and then tested to see if the antibodies in the sera sample bind to the antigens. The first test, usually an ELISA test, is widely used for detecting infectious diseases and measures the total number of antibodies in a sample. The test is known for being sensitive, in that it catches most cases of a given infection, but is not specific enough to always distinguish between infections. Consequently, the ELISA is known for returning too many false positives (Bazovska et al. 2001). To ensure that Lyme is distinguished from another condition with similar symptoms, patients who test positive or equivocal on an ELISA must also test positive on a western blot (Barbour 1989). The blot identifies specific antibody proteins and looks for patterns that suggest a *Bb* infection. Even though the western blot is more specific to Lyme, the mainstream recommends against using it alone because the test is only "semiquantitative." Individuals have to read the results and determine, based upon shading, if a particular protein antibody band is dark enough to be considered a positive (Wormser et al. 2006). Wide variations in the way different labs interpret the same test results have been noted (Bakken et al. 1992).[6]

There is one exception to the testing rule, for those instances when patients show up at their doctor's office with an evident bullseye rash. It became clear, around the time of the Dearborn conference, that antibody tests regularly return false negatives during the first month of infection (Hofmann 1996). One study found that the first-tier ELISA missed 41 percent of cases of patients who had the diagnostic EM rash (Stanek et al. 1999). This is the time when the bacteria have not disseminated past the initial infection site, and the immune system has not yet mounted a full response (Steere 2008). Because the rash is an early marker of Lyme disease, doctors can use the EM to diagnose an early case of Lyme without lab verification. Today, the mainstream community continues to call for caution in administering "Lyme tests:"(CDC 2005) "Considering the 2.7 million diagnostic assays for *B. burgdorferi* that are conducted annually in the United States, even a small proportion of false positive results could dwarf the number of reported cases" (Diuk-Wasser et al. 2012: 320).

II. Alternative

According to this group, available tests are useful but not reliable. Tests return both false positives and false negatives (Bazovska et al. 2001), and may actually miss between 55 and 80 percent of Lyme infections (Blanc et al. 2007; Burrascano 2008). This group offers up several explanations for the inaccuracy of the tests. Some have to do with problems with the test guidelines. For example, one logic is that the western blot uses the wrong set of protein bands; other bands, this camp argues, are more specific to Lyme disease (Ma et al. 1991). Most Lyme doctors and Lymies recommend the private lab IGENX, which interprets results using the bands favored by LLMDs. Patients who have received negative results elsewhere are asked to send samples to IGENX for a second opinion. Another critique levied at the process, but not necessarily at the tests themselves, is the decision to use only one strain of *Bb*, B31, (Burrascano 2008; Mervine 2013), even though research has shown that other strains are pathogenic (Clark et al. 2013).

Some Lymies venture the opinion that the *Bb* bacteria is much too evolved and complex to act in the same way as other bacteria, which makes tests that work for other pathogens less reliable when used to test for *Bb* (Nields and Kveton 1991; Blanc et al. 2007). This also makes it difficult to culture *Bb* (Sapi et al. 2013), a fastidious organism that does not survive or multiply to measurable quantities in most culture media (Clark 2004).

III. Discussion

Because the inclusion criteria for many Lyme clinical trials is a positive test result, the alternative camp has argued that the tests have produced the science, and not the other way around (Stricker and Johnson 2008). The result is that science, coupled with flawed policies, has discounted many bodies that are sick, and continue to get sicker due to lack of treatment for *Bb*. The mainstream has countered that the tests are nearly 100 percent accurate, and thus serve as the most precise way to determine if someone has been infected. This makes them a useful and objective tool for scientists and doctors who suspect Lyme (Johnson 2011).

Geography

According to the CDC, 95 percent of confirmed cases of Lyme disease occur in 14 states in the Northeast and Midwest, with a small cluster of cases in northern coastal California (CDC 2014). The risk of catching Lyme anywhere else in the United States is less than 1 percent (Johnson 2011). The alternative camp disagrees with the three-region hypothesis, believing that whereas the disease may not be as prevalent in non-endemic areas, it does exist and is all-too-frequently missed (Sherr 2006; Smith 2013).

I. Mainstream

By the late 1970s, researchers had identified two tick vectors, the *Ixodes dammini* tick in the Northeast and upper Midwest, and *Ixodes pacificus*, along the coast of northern California (Spielman 1985; Steere and Malawista 1979). Using physician referrals, letters, reports, and case studies published in the medical literature, Steere and Malawista determined that Lyme's range had three distinct foci: the Northeast, the Midwest, and northern California, foci that fit neatly with the ranges of the *I. pacificus* and *I. dammini* ticks. Thus, with the identification of three foci and two vectors, Lyme disease was given a geography.

In 1982, the Centers for Disease Control and Prevention began officially surveilling cases of Lyme disease (CDC 2014). Initially, most reports corresponded to the anticipated geography of Lyme disease. Every year, however, the number of diagnoses increased, until by 1988—during the height of "Lyme anxiety"—the reported geographic range extended across the United States, making Lyme the most frequently reported vector-borne disease in the country (Taylor 1991). Then, in 1993, the existence of *I. dammini* was discredited, and the *Ixodes scapularis* tick was identified as the vector (Oliver et al. 1993). The range of the *I. scapularis* tick was known to stretch "along the eastern coast from Massachusetts to Florida, the southern coast to Texas, inland in the Southeast, and in Wisconsin" (Steere and Malawista 1979: 731); yet, the geography of Lyme disease did not change to fit the expanding case reports or the range of the tick. CDC researchers at the time noted that variable reporting methods between states limited the usefulness of surveillance data "to monitor trends, not to represent the true incidence of disease" (Ciesielski et al. 1988: 287), while government-funded scientists cited behavioral differences between northern and southern ticks to explain why they expected to see low incidence rates in the South (Kerr 2012).

With the identification of three focal areas, and the dismissal of other *I. scapularis* habitats as risk areas, the mainstream reframed its guidelines.

The Northeast, Upper Midwest, and coastal northern California were no longer the sites of an emerging *epidemic*; they were *endemic* for Lyme. The rest of the United States, by comparison, became *nonendemic*. With the new geography, surveillance numbers also changed significantly and the resulting map came to represent the three focal area hypothesis. Scientists explained the change thusly, "Georgia reported hundreds of cases of Lyme disease until it was documented that there were few ticks bearing *B. burgdorferi* in this state" (Barbour and Fish 1993, 1610).

The geographically focused view of Lyme gained scientific legitimacy as it was taken up by researchers to study variables favorable to tick habitats in endemic areas (Kitron and Kazmierczak 1997; Killileaet al. 2008), to develop risk reduction measures (Frank et al. 1998), and to create geographic models of variable disease risk within endemic areas (Cortinas et al. 2002). Today, geography is cited as a useful tool for making sure health care expenditures go where they are needed, that doctors in endemic areas recognize the symptoms of Lyme disease, and that the public is given appropriate information to protect itself from risk (Diuk-Wasser et al. 2012). Notably, geography is also integral to a diagnosis. The guidelines recommend that doctors only test for Lyme disease when a patient lives in, or can prove a travel history to, an endemic area (CDC 2014). Patients who present with a bullseye rash but have only been in nonendemic areas, are not to be tested for Lyme, and reported cases of Lyme in most southern states are generally to be disregarded because of "the absence of infected host-seeking nymphal *I. scapularis* in this region" (Diuk-Wasser et al. 2012: 325).

II. Alternative

The alternative camp believes that one can catch Lyme disease almost anywhere in the United States. Rates may be lower in some areas, but that puts people at greater risk because of the likelihood that they will not be diagnosed. This group cites the early surveillance numbers in places like Texas (Rawlings et al. 1987), and doctors diagnosing but not reporting Lyme disease in places like Georgia (Boltri et al. 2002), as more indicative of the true prevalence of Lyme disease. They attribute the geographic mandate promoted by mainstream medicine as a product of political decision-making, not science (Smith 2013).

This camp often brings up the work of Ed Masters, a Missouri physician who diagnosed and reported cases of Lyme disease to the CDC in patients who had been bitten by the aggressive lone star, and not an *I. scapularis*, tick (Masters et al. 1998). Masters ended up in a fight with the CDC after CDC scientists reviewed his patient data and determined that the people Masters had treated were clinically different from patients with Lyme disease in the Northeast (Wormser et al. 2005). The CDC concluded that the patients had Southern Tick Associated Rash Illness, not Lyme, or quite possibly an allergic reaction to a tick bite (Dennis 2005). Masters refuted the findings, pointing to flaws in the CDC study, and refused to withhold antibiotic therapy from his patients (Masters 2006). According to the alternative camp, Masters was correct, and his work shows that even if southern *I. scapularis* ticks tend not to bite humans, other ticks do, and they may be infected with *Bb*.

This camp uses the Masters story to illustrate how the three-foci representation of Lyme disease has served to obscure other tick vectors and ecologies that affect *Bb* transmission. Members support a far broader geography for Lyme and back this claim up with research. In the mid-90s, James Oliver found that strains of *Borrelia* are much more varied in the South than in the North, indicating that more ticks could serve as competent vectors and that the enzootic cycle is more complex in the southern United States.[7] Epidemiologist and environmental health scientist Kerry Clark has found DNA sequences from *Bb* in both *I. scapularis* and *A. americanum* (e.g., lone star) ticks, showing that questing *I. scapularis* ticks do carry the bacteria that causes Lyme disease and that the lone star tick might indeed be a competent vector of Lyme disease (Clark 2004). More recently, Clark and colleagues studied patients in Georgia and Florida who presented with bullseye rashes and/or other Lyme symptoms (Clark et al. 2013). Using PCR and DNA sequences, the team found evidence of the other *Borrelia* strains in people sick with diseases, all of which these researchers say is Lyme. According to the authors, this study raises questions about the various *Borrelia* strains that might be causing human illness, including the *B. lonestari* found in lone star ticks.

III. Discussion

Researchers aligned with the alternative camp have adopted the terminology *Bb sensu lato* ("in the broad sense") to indicate the constellation of potentially disease-causing *Borrelia*, and to further signify a broader understanding of Lyme disease than is encapsulated in the mainstream guidelines and in the dominant geographic model. Contrarily, the mainstream has stuck to the *Bb sensu stricto* ("in the strict sense") label, insisting that evidence is needed to prove that other strains are pathogenic, as there are hundreds of types of *Borrelia*, but not all of them are infectious to humans.

It is also important to note an emerging line of research from the alternative camp that is not necessarily geographic, but which could change the requirement that exposure be a factor of geography. Because it is a related to syphilis, the alternative camp has long speculated that Lyme may be sexually transmitted. A group of researchers recently presented their work on finding viable spirochetes in seminal and vaginal fluid (Burke et al. 2014), leading to further questions about breast milk. It has not been proven that spirochetes in bodily fluids have the ability to infect nursing infants or sexual partners. It is likely researchers are pursuing that question now. Others in the Lyme community speculate that Lyme, and possibly its co-infections, could be transmitted through donated blood and organs, raising doubts about the security of the blood supply (Williams 2011). Such routes of transmission, fetal, sexual, and donor, are not proven, but they certainly have potential to disrupt the diagnostic model in which exposure and geography are synonymous.

FROM THEN TO NOW, THE ONGOING TRAJECTORY OF THE LYME WARS

Increasingly, health care decision-making falls to the individual (Beck 1994), who must locate or enroll providers who offer care that is deemed appropriate. Responsibility is further heightened for those who are expected to manage lifelong health conditions like diabetes (Schulze and Hu 2005), heart disease (Clarke and Binns 2006), or a genetic risk (Kenen 1996; Kenen et al. 2003). The responsible patient is tasked with keeping up with the expert science, weighing available evidence, and using calculations of risk to determine what measures to take to guard one's health (Crawford 2006). In many cases, the patient must choose between conflicting evidence (Briggs and Hallin 2007), sometimes while making incredibly difficult medical decisions (Rose 2001). Indeed, working through complicated science in order to promote good health has become a marker of health citizenship (Boero 2007; Crawford 2004), and increasingly, women are taking up this identity, assuming more responsibility especially with regard to the *care* of the family and familial risk (Mansfield 2012; Rapp 1999; Singh 2004). Lyme's women are indicative of this trend. They believed they were making informed, rational, and responsible decisions about their families' embodied health experiences, but their ability to assume the mantle of good health citizen was being impeded by political and economic factors, from policies that cut off antibiotics before all symptoms were resolved to a lack of access to alternative treatments and later affordable tests.

Concomitantly, the last four decades have seen a proliferation of evidence-based treatment guidelines (Upshur 2014). Medico-scientific experts, and not patients, sit on the panels that decide these guidelines and thus get to determine what facts count. The facts they privilege have widespread influence on clinical practice, insurance coverage, and the direction of research and funding (Asher 2010). Increasingly, activated Lyme patients, who have had embodied experiences that mismatch with these expertly crafted guidelines, want a say in the process and are prepared to shop around to find agreeable doctors and scientists in order to get one.

It is important to note that although individuals have become obligated to take on more responsibility, their authority remains limited. For example, patients are routinely instructed to stick to a doctor-ordered treatment plan (Pols 2014), even when that plan does not fit within their busy schedules or, in the case of Lyme, resolve the symptoms they want resolved. Not only is it unrealistic to expect all patients to follow their doctor's medico-scientific advice to the letter, tension results when patients take the added step of altering their care plan to fit their own lived needs. For Lyme's pioneering women, not only did they alter the treatment plan, they threw it out when it did not work for them, creating unease within the biomedical community and receiving a backlash from Lyme's frontline researchers.

Doctors are increasingly caught in the middle. In the face of diagnostic uncertainty, doctors may find themselves having to mediate between those who do the science, those who write the guidelines, those who pay the bills, those who want more individualized care, and those who suffer the effects of illness. The situation is exacerbated when punitive measures are attached to treatment guidelines (Boyer and Lutfey 2010). Such has been the case for Lyme. Some doctors have lost their medical licenses for treating with long-term antibiotics. Most LLMDs avoid problems with insurance companies by not taking insurance at all. Still other doctors express sympathy for Lyme patient suffering, but are hesitant to veer away from the norm. And still others refuse to hear Lymies' version of the science at all. It would take another paper to explore the many ways doctors have negotiated between parties, and why some have opted to align themselves with the alternative Lyme community knowing their choice may result in stigma and litigation. Suffice it to say that a range of responses has occurred, and whereas some doctors have chosen to take a side in the debate, many have not or will not until some definitive scientific evidence is provided one way or another.

Briggs and Hallin (2007), using an analytic they call biocommunicability, refer to the modern conception of medicine as the *patient-consumer model* in order to highlight the way notions about the neoliberal consumer who has the freedom to shop around have coincided with expectations that the individual will weigh expertly determined risk assessments to make deeply personal healthcare decisions. The patient-consumer model draws further attention to the assigned hierarchy of roles between scientists, doctors, policy makers, and patients. Many medico-scientific experts want to retain this model and their authority to determine what constitutes evidence, what outcomes matter, and what guidelines to use to determine best practices. This model, however, neglects to consider what happens when a patient is activated by an embodied illness experience that modern medicine cannot explain or fix (Kroll-Smith and Floyd 1997), and who wants a different role in the process. Nor does that model consider the way gendered relations are related to role assignments. Activated patients[8] attempted to assert their patient knowledge about Lyme disease. In return, suburban women were held accountable for the public response, and later blamed for causing illness. In response, these women did not retreat to their homes, engage in cognitive-behavioral therapy (see Hsu et al. 1993), or assume the identity of someone living with a mental disorder or female syndrome (see Reid et al. 1998). Instead, they countered by holding onto their good health citizen identity, while also publicly asserting a different model of care, one that is more centered on the patient. In so doing, these women also launched a health social movement that is growing in scope and size, as more women *and* men, patients *and* scientists, and kin *and* doctors, come on board to this way of thinking.

DISCUSSION

The early construction of Lyme along gendered and classed lines has become largely invisible, even as it continues to inform the science and the debate. Not only has the ongoing mainstream science of Lyme risk been centered on the suburbs (for continuing examples, see Barbour and Fish 1993; Mayer 1996; Frank et al. 1998; Ward and Brown 2004; Kilpatrick et al. 2014), the disease definition has been limited to include only symptoms that can be measured, and outcomes that can be rationalized. The female-driven, health-citizen-centered model of Lyme disease, in contrast, has produced a completely different geographical and clinical picture of the disease.

Those wishing to hold onto the more conventional, expert-driven system of medical science, not surprisingly, have sought various ways to minimize the threat (Douglas 1992), at first successfully dismissing activated patients as chronic—female—complainers, and then blaming their uneducated doctors for causing their confusion (Sigal 2002). However, as more professional doctors and scientists joined the movement, they challenged preconceived ideas about what a health activist should look like (Brown et al. 2004). More recently, mainstream Lyme scientists have shifted their position, admitting that old school medicine *was* more driven by profit motivations, dogmatism, and elitism. It made sense, then, for patients to be scornful and resistant. But medicine, this group insists, has progressed, becoming evidence based, and, consequently, more credible. And the science just does not justify expensive and extended therapies for Lyme disease (Auwaerter et al. 2011).

It would seem from these comments that activated Lyme patients have remained stuck in a past way of thinking. Our evidence indicates otherwise. It has also been suggested that that they are working to subvert expert medicine. This is not at all their intent. Their ultimate goal has not been to dismantle the system of expertise; it has been about making the system work better for them. As Warren and Manderson note in their chapter on Parkinson's, diagnostic uncertainty creates lived uncertainty for those suffering from the disease. Similarly, as Lyme parents and sufferers experienced uncertainty through treatments that did not address their most troubling symptoms and technologies that failed to diagnose them, they found themselves confronting medical professionals and raising doubts about the efficacy of the existing scientific knowledge. When their efforts were dismissed, they activated and collectivized, at first seeking relief for their symptoms and, later, corrections to a system that they perceived had worked against them. To this day, Lyme patients serve as exemplars of activated health consumers, responding to uncertainty by working to improve access to a particular kind of patient-centered care.

In each scientific controversy, it is possible to see how Lymies have not retreated to the fringes. Instead, they have *increasingly* collaborated with doctors and scientists to advance a future in which activated health citizens can point to undone science (Hess 2009), pose new research questions (Akrich et al. 2013), and legitimize symptoms (Fair 2009) alongside biomedical professionals. The tension Lymies face from being caught between challenging a system while also relying upon it, is one that researchers studying health social movements have noted elsewhere (Brown et al. 2004). It is also one that feminist scholars have examined, particularly in the case of breast cancer, where women who have struggled to resist the patriarchal system of biomedicine have come to depend upon it to make them well (Kaufert 1998). Likewise, Lyme's original activist women looked to the system for answers, showing a deep faith in the progress of science and medicine, values that are decidedly white, middle class . . . and gendered (Klawiter 1994).

Because of their successes, Lymies have been able to shift their gaze to include other diseases. Prominent AIDS activists have become involved in the Lyme health movement (Bernstein 2014) and increasingly, Lyme scientists are searching for links between Lyme and largely unexplained diseases such as Alzheimer's (MacDonald 1988), multiple sclerosis (Marshall 1988), autism (Bransfield et al. 2008), and mental illness (Hajek et al. 2002; Hajek et al. 2006). Lymies have begun to share science with these other communities and have encouraged individuals within them to question their diagnoses and, because of the overlapping symptom clusters, to even consider being tested for a Lyme infection. In the face of these new challenges, the mainstream has adjusted its message, linking the Lyme health movement to a wider, "anti-science" movement—to include those campaigning against vaccines—wanting to "subvert evidence-based medicine and peer-reviewed science" (Auwaerter et al. 2011: 713). This is a message that acknowledges the breadth and successes of the Lyme movement even as it seeks to diminish its power.

Four decades after it began, the Lyme Wars have not been won. Indeed, one reason is that it is not a war at all, despite being widely characterized as such. The story of Lyme is not that of a two-sided fight between experts and activists, nor are there clear and stable boundaries between the opposing camps. Rather, the story of Lyme is about the emergence of a disease, simultaneous to the emergence of citizen science in an advanced neoliberal society (Hess 2004). As Hess tells us, such emergences necessarily lead to points of tension. Differently placed people do not universally shift their way of thinking, taking up new epistemologies at the same time and in the same ways. Tensions erupt in different times and places, and between differently placed actors.

Lyme is also the story of women who—despite overwhelming pressure to the contrary—asserted their right to take control of their own and their families' illnesses. Along the way, they reframed their responsibility to maintain their health as a right to intercede when the medical system failed to help. They interpreted medicine's failures as giving them the right, and the responsibility, to push doctors, scientists, and policy makers to address undone science. In so doing, these women did not intend to subvert medical science. They activated so that their broken bodies could become useful again, as instruments in the search for a scientific solution to end Lyme suffering. Their goal, a goal toward which they have made considerable progress, was to open space for new conversations, new science, and new models of care.

NOTES

1 Our genealogy of Lyme is not meant to exclude men. Men are being diagnosed with Lyme (CDC (2014). Lyme Disease Data, Centers for Disease Control.), and men are taking part in the Lyme health movement (Edlow, J. A. (2003). *Bull's-Eye: Unraveling the Medical Mystery of Lyme Disease*. New Haven, Yale University Press, Rosner, B. (2009) "Lyme Disease: Real Disease or Medical Myth?" *Townsend Letter*, 51-.). Women, in contrast, have long been the *face* of Lyme disease.

2 We note that the terms "mainstream" and "alternative" are additionally problematic; we use them intentionally to highlight the way knowledge has been constructed as bifurcated and hierarchical.

3 These are not the only controversies. For example, much work remains to be done on conflicts over the Lyme vaccine.

4 There was clearly a gender subtext implicit in the guidelines. Researchers questioned why chronic Lyme was more prevalent in women than men, even though more men were diagnosed and treated for early Lyme. One study of 105 women with FMS or CLD found that all participants reported higher levels of self-blame, neuroticism, perceived stress, self-distraction, and difficulty identifying feelings than the healthy controls (Hassett, A. L., D.C. Radvanski, S. Buyske, S.V. Savage, M. Gara, J.I. Escobar and L.H. Sigal (2008). "Role of Psychiatric Comorbidity in Chronic Lyme Disease." *Arthritis Care and Research* 59(12): 1742–1749.) Hassett et al. compared patients who complained of suffering from CLD with patients who had been diagnosed and treated successfully for Lyme. They found that those who considered themselves to be chronic Lyme sufferers were mostly women and were significantly more likely to suffer from depression and anxiety.

5 While the alternative camp has circumnavigated the standardized testing process by developing new tests and by treating patients based on their reported symptoms, the mainstream has used institutional enforcement mechanisms in an attempt to prevent such activities (FDA 2014). This is an emerging point of contention and will be the focus of future papers.

6 Despite the two-step process, which backers say is 99 percent specific for Lyme disease (Johnson, B. (2011). Laboratory Diagnostic Testing for *Borellia Burgdorferi* Infection. *Lyme Disease: An Evidence-Based Approach*. J. J. Halperin, CAB International.), the mainstream still voices trepidation about false

positive results, a concern that arose in late 80s and early 90s at the height of "Lyme anxiety." Credentialed researchers expressed concern that "the growing use of Lyme disease serological testing may or may not be an appropriate response to the rising incidence of this illness, but it seems that the growth in the use of the diagnostic test may be greater than the rising incidence of the disease" (Schwartz, B.S., M.D. Goldstein, J.C. Ribeiro, T.L. Schulze and S.I. Shahied (1989). "Antibody Testing in Lyme Disease a Comparison of Results in Four Laboratories." *JAMA* 262(24): 3431–3434.). This caused some to question the amount governments and insurance companies were paying to cover potentially unnecessary lab work (Dattwyler, R.J., D.J. Volkman, B.J. Luft, J.J. Halperin, J. Thomas and M.G. Golightly (1988). "Seronegative Lyme Disease." *New England Journal of Medicine* 319(22): 1441–1446, Steere, A.C. (1993). "Seronegative Lyme Disease." *The Journal of the American Medical Association* 270(11): 1369–1369.) and to speculate that with large numbers of (putatively female) people seeking Lyme tests, "the ratio of persons with false-positive reactions to those who have actual *B. burgdorferi* infections will predictably rise" (Barbour, A.G. (1989). "The Diagnosis of Lyme Disease—Rewards and Perils." *Annals of Internal Medicine* 110(7): 501–502.).

7   Clark was able to isolate *Bb* from a variety of mice, rats, and ticks in South Carolina. He noted that not all of the ticks were species that bite humans, but that they serve as important reservoirs for keeping the infection circulating within the local animal and arthropod population. His study further pointed to the complexity of the zoonotic transmission cycle in the South. This complexity, rather than negating the existence of Lyme disease in the South, he argued, signals that the Lyme bacteria are endemic to the region. (Clark, K.L., B. Leydet and S. Hartman (2013). "Lyme borreliosis in Human Patients in Florida and Georgia, USA." *International Journal of Medical Sciences* 10(7): 915–931.).

8   Only anecdotal reports exist as to the gendered composition of early activated Lyme patients; therefore, it is not possible to state with authority that this group was dominated by women. This is an area that could use further study.

BIBLIOGRAPHY

Akrich, Madeline, Orla O'Donovan, and Vololona Rabeharisoa. "The Entanglement of Scientific and Political Claims: Towards a New Form of Patient Activism." In *CSI Working Papers Series*. Centre de Sociologie de L'Innovation Mines ParisTech, 2013.

Aronowitz, Robert A. "When Do Symptoms Become a Disease?" [In No Linguistic Content]. *Annals of Internal Medicine* 134, no. 9 Part 2 (2001): 803–808.

———. "Lyme Disease: The Social Construction of a New Disease and Its Social Consequences." *The Milbank Quarterly* 69, no. 1 (1991): 79–112.

Asher, Tammy L. "Unprecedented Antitrust Investigation into the Lyme Disease Treatment Guidelines Development Process." [In English]. *Gonzaga Law Review* 46, no. 1 (2010): 117–145.

ASTPHLD. "Proceedings of the Second National Conference on the Serological Diagnosis of Lyme Disease." The Association of State and Territorial Public Health Laboratory Directors and The Centers for Disease Control: Dearborn, MI, 1994.

Aucott, J.N., A.W. Rebman, L.A. Crowder, and K.B. Kortte. "Post-Treatment Lyme Disease Syndrome Symptomatology and the Impact on Life Functioning: Is

There Something Here?" [In English]. *Quality of Life Research* 22, no. 1 (2013): 75–84.

Auwaerter, Paul G., Johan S. Bakken, Raymond J. Dattwyler, J. Stephen Dumler, John J. Halperin, Edward McSweegan, Robert B. Nadelman, et al. "Antiscience and Ethical Concerns Associated with Advocacy of Lyme Disease." *The Lancet Infectious Diseases* 11, no. 9 (2011): 713–19.

Baker, Carol J., William A. Charini, Paul H. Duray, Paul M. Lantos, Gerald Medoff, Manuel H. Moro, David M. Mushatt, Jeffrey Parsonett, and John Sanders. "Final Report of the Lyme Disease Review Panel." 65: Infectious Diseases Society of America, 2010.

Baker, Philip. "Lyme Disease Review Panel Hearing." Paper presented at the Infectious Diseases Society of America, 2009.

Bakken, L. L., K. L. Case, S. M. Callister, N. J. Bourdeau, and R. F. Schell. "Performance of 45 Laboratories Participating in a Proficiency Testing Program for Lyme Disease Serology." *JAMA* 268, no. 7 (1992): 891–5.

Barbour, Alan G. "The Diagnosis of Lyme Disease—Rewards and Perils." *Annals of Internal Medicine* 110, no. 7 (1989): 501–502.

Barbour, Alan G. and Durland Fish. "The Biological and Social Phenomenon of Lyme Disease." *American Association of the Advancement of Science* 260, no. 5114 (1993): 1610–16.

Barthold, S. W., E. Hodzic, D. M. Imai, S. Feng, X. Yang, and B. J. Luft. "Ineffectiveness of Tigecycline against Persistent Borrelia Burgdorferi." [In English]. *Antimicrobial Agents and Chemotherapy* 54, no. 2 (2010): 9.

Bazovska, S., M. Kondas, M. Simkovicova, E. Kmety, and P. Traubner. "Significance of Specific Antibody Determination in Lyme Borreliosis Diagnosis." [In English]. *Bratisl Lek Listy* 102, no. 10 (2001): 454–57.

Bean, Constance, and Lesley Ann Fein. *Beating Lyme: Understanding and Treating This Complex and Often Misdiagnosed Disease*. New York: AMACOM, 2008.

Beck, Ulrich. "The Reinvention of Politics: Towards a Theory of Reflexive Modernization." In *Reflexive Modernization: Politics, Tradition and Aesthetics in the Modern Social Order*. Stanford: Stanford University Press, 1994.

Benhnia, Mrei, D. Wroblewski, M. N. Akhtar, R. A. Patel, W. Lavezzi, S. C. Gangloff, S. M. Goyert, et al. "Signaling through Cd14 Attenuates the Inflammatory Response to Borrelia Burgdorferi, the Agent of Lyme Disease." *Journal of Immunology* 174, no. 3 (2005): 1539–48.

Bernstein, Jessica. "From Aids to Lyme: Will We Let History Repeat Itself?" *Truthout* (2014): 1–37.

Blanc, F. and GEBLY. "Neurologic and Psychiatric Manifestations of Lyme Disease." *Medecine Et Maladies Infectieuses* 37, no. 7–8 (2007): 435–45.

Blanc, F., B. Jaulhac, M. Fleury, J. de Seze, S. J. de Martino, V. Remy, G. Blaison, et al. "Relevance of the Antibody Index to Diagnose Lyme Neuroborreliosis among Seropositive Patients." *Neurology* 69, no. 10 (2007): 953–58.

Boero, Natalie. "All the News That's Fat to Print: The American 'Obesity Epidemic' and the Media." *Qualitative Sociology* 30 (2007): 41–60.

Boltri, John M., Robert B. Hash, and Robert L. Vogel. "Patterns of Lyme Disease Diagnosis and Treatment by Family Physicians in a Southeastern State." *Journal of Community Health* 27, no. 6 (2002): 395–402.

Boyer, Carol, and Karen Lutfey. "Examining Critical Health Issues Within and Beyond the Clinical Encounter: Patient-Provider Relationships and Help-Seeking Behavior." *Jourrnal of Health and Social Behavior* 51, no. 1 (2010): 80.

Bransfield, Robert C., Jeffrey S. Wulfman, William T. Harvey, and Anju I. Usman. "The Association between Tick-Borne Infections, Lyme Borreliosis and Autism Spectrum Disorders." *Medical Hypotheses* 70, no. 5 (2008): 967–74.

Briggs, Charles L., and Daniel C. Hallin. "The Neoliberal Subject and Its Contradictions in News Coverage of Health Issues." *Social Text 93*, no. 25 (2007): 43–65.

Brorson, O., S. H. Brorson, J. Scythes, J. MacAllister, L. Margulis, and A. Wier. "Destruction of Spirochete Borrelia Burgdorferi Round-Body Propagules (Rbs) by the Antibiotic Tigecycline." [In English]. *Proc. Natl. Acad. Sci. U. S. A. Proceedings of the National Academy of Sciences of the United States of America* 106, no. 44 (2009): 18656–661.

Brown, P., S. Zavestoski, S. McCormick, B. Mayer, R. Morello-Frosch, and R. Altman. "Embodied Health Movements: New Approaches to Social Movements in Health." *Sociology of Health and Illness* 26, no. 1 (2004): 50–80.

Buhner, Stephen Harrod. *Healing Lyme: Natural Prevention and Treatment of Lyme Borreliosis and Its Coinfections*. Randolph: Raven Press, 2005.

Burgdorfer, W. "Discovery of the Lyme Disease Spirochete and Its Relation to Tick Vectors." [In English]. *The Yale journal of Biology and Medicine* 57, no. 4 (1984): 515–20.

Burgdorfer, W., R. S. Lane, A. G. Barbour, R. A. Gresbrink, and J. R. Anderson. "The Western Black-Legged Tick, Ixodes Pacificus: A Vector of Borrelia Burgdorferi." *The American Journal of Tropical Medicine and Hygiene* 34, no. 5 (1985): 925.

Burke, Jennie, Augustin Franco, Yean Wang, Peter Mayne, Eva Sapi, Cheryl Bandoski, Hilary Schlinger, and Raphael Stricker. "Lyme Disease May Be Sexually Transmitted." In *Western Regional Meeting of the American Federation for Medical Research*, 280–81. Carmel, CA: The Journal of Investigative Medicine, 2014.

Burrascano, Joseph. *Advanced Topics in Lyme Disease: Diagnostic Hints and Treatment Guidelines for Lyme and Other Tick Borne Illnesses*. Burrascano. 2008.

Cameron, Daniel J., Lorraine B. Johnson, and Elizabeth L. Maloney. "Evidence Assessments and Guideline Recommendations in Lyme Disease: The Clinical Management of Known Tick Bites, Erythema Migrans Rashes and Persistent Disease." *Expert Review of Anti-infective Therapy* 12, no. 9 (2014): 1103–35.

CDC (Centers for Disease Control and Prevention). "Concerns Regarding a New Culture Method for *Borrelia Burgdorferi* Not Approved for the Diagnosis of Lyme Disease." *Morbidity and Mortality Weekly Report* 333 (2014): 333.

———. "Lyme Disease Data and Statistics." Accessed September 25, 2014. http://www.cdc.gov/lyme/stats/index.html.

———. "Lyme Disease Diagnosis and Testing." Accessed January 29, 2014. http://www.cdc.gov/lyme/diagnosistesting/index.html.

———. "Lyme Disease." Accessed January 3, 2014. http://www.cdc.gov/lyme/index.html.

———. "Notice to Readers: Caution Regarding Testing for Lyme Disease." *Morbidity and Mortality Weekly Report* 125 (2005): 125.

Chandra, Abhishek, Gary P. Wormser, Mark S. Klempner, Richard P. Trevino, Mary K. Crow, Norman Latov, and Armin Alaedini. "Anti-Neural Antibody Reactivity in Patients with a History of Lyme Borreliosis and Persistent Symptoms." *Brain, Behavior, and Immunity* (in press).

Ciesielski, Carol A., Lauri E. Markowitz, Rose Horsley, Allen W. Hightower, Harold Russell, and Claire V. Broome. "The Geographic Distribution of Lyme Disease in the United States." *Annals of the New York Academy of Sciences* 539, no. 1 (1988): 283–88.

Clark, Kerry L. "Borrelia Species in Host-Seeking Ticks and Small Mammals in Northern Florida." [In English]. *Journal of clinical microbiology* 42, no. 11 (2004): 5076.

Clark, Kerry L., Brian Leydet, and Shirley Hartman. "Lyme Borreliosis in Human Patients in Florida and Georgia, USA." *International Journal of Medical Sciences* 10, no. 7 (2013): 915–31.

Clarke, Juanne Nancarrow, and Jeannine Binns. "The Portrayal of Heart Disease in Mass Print Magazines, 1991–2001." [In English]. *Health Communication* 19, no. 1 (2006): 39–48.

Clover, J. R., and R. S. Lane. "Evidence Implicating Nymphal Ixodes Pacificus (Acari: Ixodidae) in the Epidemiology of Lyme Disease in California." *The American Journal of Tropical Medicine and Hygiene* 53, no. 3 (1995): 237–40.

Cohen, Marcus A. *Lyme Disease Update: Science, Policy & Law*. Jackson, NJ: Lyme Disease Association, 2004.

Cortinas, M. Roberto, Marta A. Guerra, Carl Jones, and Uriel Kitron. "Detection, Characterization, and Prediction of Tick-Borne Disease Foci." *International Journal of Medical Microbiology* 291, no. 33 (2002): 11–20.

Coyle, Bonnie S., G. Thomas Strickland, Yale Y. Liang, César Peña, Robert McCarter, and Ebenezer Israel. "The Public Health Impact of Lyme Disease in Maryland." *The Journal of Infectious Diseases* 173, no. 5 (1996): 1260–62.

Crawford, Robert. "Health as a Meaningful Social Practice." *Health: An Interdisciplinary Journal for the Social Study of Health, Illness and Medicine* 10, no. 4 (2006): 401–20.

———. "Risk Ritual and the Management of Control and Anxiety in Medical Culture." *Health: An Interdisciplinary Journal for the Social Study of Health, Illness and Medicine* 8, no. 4 (2004): 505–28.

Dattwyler, Raymond J., David J. Volkman, Benjamin J. Luft, John J. Halperin, Josephine Thomas, and Marc G. Golightly. "Seronegative Lyme Disease." *New England Journal of Medicine* 319, no. 22 (1988): 1441–46.

Dennis, David T. "Rash Decisions: Lyme Disease, or Not?" *Clinical Infectious Diseases* 41, no. 7 (2005): 966–68.

Diterich, I., C. Rauter, C. J. Kirschning, and T. Hartung. "Borrelia Burgdorferi-Induced Tolerance as a Model of Persistence Via Immunosuppression." [In English]. *Infection and Immunity* 71, no. 7 (2003): 9.

Diuk-Wasser, Maria A., Anne Gatewood Hoen, Paul Cislo, Robert Brinkerhoff, Sarah A. Hamer, Michelle Rowland, Roberto Cortinas, et al. "Human Risk of Infection with Borrelia Burgdorferi, the Lyme Disease Agent, in Eastern United States." *The American Journal of Tropical Medicine and Hygiene* 86, no. 2 (2012): 320–27.

Douglas, Mary. *Risk and Blame: Essays in Cultural Theory*. London: Routledge, 1992.

Edlow, Jonathan A. *Bull's-Eye: Unraveling the Medical Mystery of Lyme Disease*. New Haven: Yale University Press, 2003.

Embers, Monica E., Sephen W. Barthold, Juan T. Borda, Lisa Bowers, Lara Doyle, Emir Hodzic, Mary B. Jacobs, et al. "Persistence of *Borrelia Burgdoferi* in Rhesus Macaques Following Antibiotic Treatment of Disseminated Infection." *PLoS One* 7, no. 1 (2012).

Epstein, S. "Impure Science: Aids, Activism, and the Politics of Knowledge." [In English]. *Medicine and Society* (1996): 1–466.

Fair, Brian. "Morgellons: Contested Illness, Diagnostic Compromise and Medicalisation." *Sociology of Health and Illness* 32, no. 4 (2009): 597–612.

Fallon, Brian A., Felice Tager, Lesley Fein, Kenneth Liegner, John Keilp, Nicola Weiss, and Michael Liebowitz. "Repeated Antibiotic Treatment in Chronic Lyme Disease." *Journal of Spirochetal and Tick-Borne Diseases* 6 (1999): 10.

FDA. "FDA Takes Steps to Help Ensure the Reliability of Certain Diagnostic Tests." news release, 2014, http://www.fda.gov/NewsEvents/Newsroom/PressAnnouncements/ucm407321.htm.

Feng, Jie, Ting Wang, Wanliang Shi, Shuo Zhang, David Sullivan, Paul G. Auwaerter, and Ying Zhang. "Identification of Novel Activity against *Borrelia Burdorgferi* Persisters Using an FDA Approved Drug Library." *Emerging Microbes and Infections* 3 (2014): 8.

Frank, Denise H., Durland Fish, and Fred H. Moy. "Landscape Features Associated with Lyme Disease Risk in a Suburban Residential Environment." [In English]. *Landscape Ecology* 13, no. 1 (1998): 27–36.

Garrett, Laurie. *The Coming Plague: Newly Emerging Diseases in a World out of Balance*. New York: Farrar, Straus and Giroux, 1994.

Gaudino, E. A., P. K. Coyle, and L. B. Krupp. "Post-Lyme Syndrome and Chronic Fatigue Syndrome: Neuropsychiatric Similarities and Differences." *Archives of Neurology* 54, no. 11 (1997): 1372–76.

Georgilis, K., M. Peacocke, and M. S. Klempner. "Fibroblasts Protect the Lyme Disease Spirochete, Borrelia Burgdorferi, from Ceftriaxone in Vitro." *Journal of Infectious Diseases* 166, no. 2 (1992): 440–44.

Grosz, Elizabeth. "Refiguring Bodies." Chap. 1 in *Volatile Bodies: Toward a Corporeal Feminism*, 3–24. Bloomington: Indiana University Press, 1994.

Guerau-De-Arellano, M., and B. T. Huber. "Chemokines and Toll-Like Receptors in Lyme Disease Pathogenesis." *Trends in Molecular Medicine* 11, no. 3 (2005): 114–20.

Hajek, T., J. Libiger, D. Janovska, P. Hajek, M. Alda, and C. Hoschl. "Clinical and Demographic Characteristics of Psychiatric Patients Seropositive for Borrelia Burgdorferi." *European Psychiatry* 21, no. 2 (2006): 118–22.

Hajek, T., B. Paskova, D. Janovska, R. Bahbouh, P. Hajek, J. Ligiber, and C. Hoschl. "Higher Prevalence of Antibodies to Borrelia Burgdorferi in Psychiatric Patients Than in Healthy Subjects." *American Journal of Psychiatry* 159, no. 2 (2002): 297–301.

Halperin, John J., Philip Baker, and Gary P. Wormser. "Common Misconceptions about Lyme Disease." [In English]. *The American Journal of Medicine* 126, no. 3 (2013): 1–7.

———. "The Reply." *The American Journal of Medicine* 126, no. 8 (2013): e11–e12.

Haraway, Donna. "The Persistence of Vision." In *Writing on the Body: Female Embodiment and Feminist Theory*, edited by Katie Conboy, Nadia Medina and Sarah Stanbury, 384. New York: Columbia University Press, 1997.

Hassett, A. L., D. C. Radvanski, S. Buyske, S. V. Savage, M. Gara, J. I. Escobar, and L. H. Sigal. "Role of Psychiatric Comorbidity in Chronic Lyme Disease." [In English]. *Arthritis Rheum* 59, no. 12 (2008): 1742–49.

Hess, David J. "The Potentials and Limitations of Civil Society Research: Getting Undone Science Done." *Sociological Inquiry* 79, no. 3 (2009): 306–27.

———. "Medical Modernisation, Scientific Research Fields and the Epistemic Politics of Health Social Movements." [In English]. *Sociology of Health and Illness* 26, no. 6 (2004): 695–709.

Hodzic, E., S. Feng, and S. W. Barthold. "Resurgence of Persisting Non-Cultivable *Borrelia Burdorferi* Following Antibiotic Treatment in Mice." *PLoS One* 9, no. 1 (2014).

Hofmann, H. "Lyme Borreliosis—Problems of Serological Diagnosis." *Infection* 24, no. 6 (1996): 470–72.

Horowitz, Richard I. *Why Can't I Get Better? Solving the Mystery of Lyme and Chronic Disease*. New York: St. Martin's Press, 2013.

Hsu, Vivien M., Sondra J. Patella, and Leonard H. Sigal. " 'Chronic Lyme Disease' as the Incorrect Diagnosis in Patients with Fibromyalgia." *Arthritis & Rheumatism* 36, no. 11 (1993): 1493–500.

ILADS. "International Lyme and Associated Diseases Society." Accessed January 29, 2014. http://www.ilads.org/.

James, Jones F. "An Extended Concept of Altered Self: Chronic Fatigue and Post-Infection Syndrome." *Psychoneuroendocrinology* 33 (2008): 119–29.

Johnson, Barbara. "Laboratory Diagnostic Testing for *Borellia Burgdorferi* Infection." In *Lyme Disease: An Evidence-Based Approach*, edited by J. J. Halperin, 73–88. Cambrigde, MA: CAB International, 2011.

Johnson, Lorraine, and Dr. Raphael Stricker. "Attorney General Forces Infectious Diseases Society of America to Redo Lyme Guidelines Due to Flawed Development Process." *Journal of Medical Ethics* 35 (2008): 283–88.

Johnson, Lorraine, Spencer Wilcox, Jennifer Mankoff, and Raphael B. Stricker. "Severity of Chronic Lyme Disease Compared to Other Chronic Conditions: A Quality of Life Survey." *PeerJ* 2 (2014): 21.

Kaufert, P. A. "Women, Resistance, and the Breast Cancer Movement." [In English]. *Cambridge Studies in Medical Anthropology* no. 5 (1998): 287–309.

Keller, Andreas, Angela Graefen, Markus Ball, Mark Matzas, Valesca Boisguerin, Frank Maixner, Petra Leidinger, et al. "New Insights into the Tyrolean Iceman's Origin and Phenotype as Inferred by Whole-Genome Sequencing." *Nature Communication* 3 (2012): 698.

Kenen, Regina H. "The at-Risk Health Status and Technology: A Diagnostic Invitation and the "Gift" of Knowing." *Social Science & Medicine* 42, no. 11 (1996): 1545–53.

Kenen, Regina H., Audrey Ardern-Jones, and Rosalind Eeles. "Living with Chronic Risk: Healthy Women with a Family History of Breast/Ovarian Cancer." *Health, Risk and Society* 5, no. 3 (2003): 315–31.

Kerr, Kaetlyn T. "A Northern Vs. Southern United States Comparison of Host Infestation by the Lyme Borreliosis Vector, Ixodes Scapularis." M.S., Hofstra University, 2012.

Killilea, Mary E., Andrea Swei, Robert S. Lane, Cheryl J. Briggs, and Richard S. Ostfeld. "Spatial Dynamics of Lyme Disease: A Review." *EcoHealth* 5 (2008): 167–95.

Kilpatrick, Howard J., Andrew M. Labonte, and Kirby C. Stafford. "The Relationship between Deer Density, Tick Abundance, and Human Cases of Lyme Disease in a Residential Community." *Journal of Medical Entomology* 51, no. 4 (2014): 777–84.

Kitron, Uriel, and James J. Kazmierczak. "Spatial Analysis of the Distribution of Lyme Disease in Wisconsin." *American Journal of Epidemiology* 145, no. 6 (1997): 558–66.

Klawiter, Maren. "Racing for the Cure, Walking Women, and Toxic Touring: Mapping Cultures of Action within the Bay Area Terrain of Breast Cancer." *Social Problems* 46, no. 1 (1994): 104–26.

Klempner, Mark S., Linden T. Hu, Janine Evans, Christopher H. Schmid, Gary M. Johnson, Richard P. Trevino, DeLona Norton, et al. "Two Controlled Trials of Antibiotic Treatment in Patients with Persistent Symptoms and a History of Lyme Disease." *New England Journal of Medicine* 345, no. 2 (2001): 8.

Koopman, Cheryl, and Daniel Cameron. "Critique of IDSA Constraints on Lyme Research." *Lyme Times*, 2009, 43–46.

Kroll-Smith, J. Stephen, and H. Hugh Floyd. *Bodies in Protest : Environmental Illness and the Struggle over Medical Knowledge* [In English]. New York: New York University Press, 1997.

Latour, Bruno. "From Realpolitik to Dingpolitik or How to Make Things Public." In *Making Things Public—Atmosphers of Democracy*, edited by Bruno Latour and Peter Weibel. Karlsruhe: MIT Press and ZKM, 2005.

Logigian, E. L., R. F. Kaplan, and A. C. Steere. "Chronic Neurologic Manifestations of Lyme Disease." *The New England Journal of Medicine* 323 (1990): 1438–44.

Ma, Bingnan, Beyat Christen, Danton Leung, and Carmen Vigo-Pelfrey. "Serodiagnosis of Lyme Borreliosis by Western Immunoblot: Reactivity of Various

Significant Antibodies against *Borellia Burdgorferi.*" *Journal of Clinical Microbiology* 30, no. 370–76 (1991): 370–376.

MacDonald, Alan B. "Concurrent Neocortical Borreliosis and Alzheimer's Disease: Demonstration of a Spirochetal Cyst Form" *Annals of the New York Academy of Sciences*, no. 539 (1988):468-470.

Makris, Katina. *Out of the Woods: Healing Lyme Disease—Body, Mind and Spirit.* Santa Rosa, CA: Elite Books, 2011.

Mansfield, Becky. "Gendered Biopolitics of Public Health: Regulation and Discipline in Seafood Consumption Advisories." *Environment and Planning D: Society and Space* 30 (2012): 588–602.

Marshall, Vincent. "Multiple Sclerosis Is a Chronic Central Nervous System Infection by a Spirochetal Agent." *Medical Hypotheses* 25, no. 2 (1988): 89–92.

Masters, Edwin J. "Lyme-Like Illness Currently Deserves Lyme-Like Treatment [with Reply]." *Clinical Infectious Diseases* 42, no. 4 (2006): 580–82.

Masters, Edwin J., Scott Granter, Paul Duray, and Paul Cordes. "Physician-Diagnosed Erythema Migrans and Erythema Migrans-Like Rashes Following Lone Star Tick Bites." *Archives of Dermatology* 134, no. 8 (1998): 955–60.

Matuschka, F., A. Ohlenbusch, H. Eiffert, D. Richter, and Spielman A. "Antiquity of the Lyme-Disease Spirochaete in Europe." [In English]. *Lancet* 346, no. 8986 (1995): 1367.

Matuschka Fr, Spielman A. "The Emergence of Lyme Disease in a Changing Environment in North America and Central Europe." [In English]. *Experimental & Applied Acarology* 2, no. 4 (1986): 337–53.

Mayer, Jonathan D. "Geography, Ecology and Emerging Infectious Diseases." *Social Science & Medicine* 50 (1996): 937–52.

McFadzean, Nicola. *The Lyme Diet.* San Diego, CA: Legacy Line Publishing, 2010.

Mervine, Phyllis. "Advocates Accuse CDC of Harming Patients." *The Lyme Times*, 2013, 23–25.

Nields, Jenifer A., and John F. Kveton. "Tullio Phenomenon and Seronegative Lyme Borreliosis." [In English]. *The Lancet* 338, no. 8759 (1991): 128–9.

Norgard, M. V., B. S. Riley, J. A. Richardson, and J. D. Radolf. "Dermal Inflammation Elicited by Synthetic Analogs of Treponema-Pallidum and Borrelia-Burgdorferi Lipoproteins." *Infection and Immunity* 63, no. 4 (1995): 1507–15.

Oliver, J. H., M. R. Owsley, H. J. Hutcheson, A. M. James, C. S. Chen, W. S. Irby, E. M. Dotson, and D. K. McLain. "Conspecificity of the Ticks Ixodes-Scapularis and Ixodes-Dammini (Acari, Ixodidae)." [In English]. *Journal of Medical Entomology* 30, no. 1 (1993): 54–63.

Pachner, Andrew R., and Israel Steiner. "Lyme Neuroborreliosis: Infection, Immunity, and Inflammation." *The Lancet Neurology* 6, no. 6 (2007): 544–52.

Pols, Jeannette. "Knowing Patients: Turning Patient Knowledge into Science." *Science, Technology, and Human Values* 39, no. 1 (2014): 73–97.

Rapp, Rayna. *Testing Women, Testing the Fetus: The Social Impact of Amniocentesis in America.* London: Routledge, 1999.

Rawlings, J. A., P. V. Fournier, and G. J. Teltow. "Isolation of Borrelia Spirochetes from Patients in Texas." *Journal of Clinical Microbiology* 25, no. 7 (1987): 1148–50.

Reid, M. Carrington, Robert T. Schoen, Janine Evans, Jennifer C. Rosenberg, and Ralph I. Horwitz. "The Consequences of Overdiagnosis and Overtreatment of Lyme Disease: An Observational Study." *Annals of Internal Medicine* 128, no. 5 (1998): 354–62.

Rose, Nikolas. "The Politics of Life Itself." [In English]. *Theory, Culture and Society* 18, no. 6 (2001): 1–30.

Sapi, Eva, Navroop Kaur, Samuel Anyanwu, David F Luecke, Seema Patel, Michael Rossi, and Raphael B. Stricker. "Evaluation of in-Vitro Antibiotic Susceptibility of Different Morphological Forms of Borrelia Burgdorferi." *Infection and Drug Resistance* 4 (2011): 97–113.

Sapi, Eva, Namrata Pabbati, Akshita Datar, Ellen M. Davies, Amy Rattelle, and Bruce A. Kuo. "Improved Culture Conditions for the Growth and Detection of Borrelia from Human Serum." *Journal of Medical Sciences* 10, no. 4 (2013): 362.

Satalino, Anna. "Personality Traits, Perceived Stress, and Coping Styles in Patients with Chronic Lyme Disease and Fibromyalgia." Ph.D., Walden University, 2008.

Saunders, Russell. *Predator Doctors Take Advantage of Patients with 'Chronic Lyme' Scam.* Tech-and-Health. The Daily Beast, 2014.

Savely, Ginger. "Lyme Disease: A Diagnostic Dilemma." Tucson, Arizona, 2011.

Schulze, Matthias B., and Frank B. Hu. "Primary Prevention of Diabetes: What Can Be Done and How Much Can Be Prevented?" *Annual Review of Public Health* 26 (2005): 445–67.

Schwartz, B. S., M. D. Goldstein, J. C. Ribeiro, T. L. Schulze, and S. I. Shahied. "Antibody Testing in Lyme Disease a Comparison of Results in Four Laboratories." *JAMA* 262, no. 24 (1989): 3431–34.

Schwarzwalder, Alison, Michael F. Schneider, Alison Lydecker, and John N. Aucott. "Sex Differences in the Clinical and Serologic Presentation of Early Lyme Disease: Results from a Retrospective Review." [In English]. *Gender Medicine* 7, no. 4 (2010): 10.

Shapiro, Eugene D. "Lyme Disease." *New England Journal of Medicine* 371, no. 7 (2014): 683–84.

Sherr, Virginia T. " 'Bell's Palsy of the Gut' and Other Gi Manisfestations of Lyme and Associated Disease." *The Human Side of Lyme: Research & Writings of Virginia T. Sherr, MD* (2006). http://www.lymenet.de/literatur/vtsherr_gut.htm.

Sigal, Leonard H. "Misconceptions about Lyme Disease: Confusions Hiding Behind Ill-Chosen Terminology." *Annals of Internal Medicine* 136, no. 5 (2002): 413.

———. "Persisting Complaints Attributed to Chronic Lyme Disease: Possible Mechanisms and Implications for Management." *The American Journal of Medicine* 96 (1994): 365–74.

Singh, Ilina. "Doing Their Jobs: Mothering with Ritalin in a Culture of Mother-Blame." *Social Science & Medicine* 59 (2004): 1193–1205.

Singh, S. K., and H. J. Girschick. "Toll-Like Receptors in Borrelia Burgdorferi-Induced Inflammation." *Clinical Microbiology and Infection* 12, no. 8 (2006): 705–17.

Smith, Pat. "LDA President Rebuts CDC's Arguments." *The Lyme Times*, 2013, 3–4.

Spielman, A. "Ecology of Ixodes Dammini-Borne Human Basesiosis and Lyme Disease." *Annual Review of Entomology* 30, no. 1 (1985): 439–60.

Stanek, G., F. Breier, G. Menzinger, B. Schaar, M. Hafner, and H. Partsch. "Erythema Migrans and Serodiagnosis by Enzyme Immunoassay and Immunoblot with Three Borrelia Species." [In English]. *Wien Klin Wochenschr* 111, no. 22–23 (1999): 951–56.

Steere, Allen C. "Reply to Stricker and Johnson." *Clinical Infectious Diseases* no. 47 (2008): 2.

———. "Seronegative Lyme Disease." *The Journal of the American Medical Association* 270, no. 11 (1993): 1369.

Steere, Allen C., and S. E. Malawista. "Cases of Lyme Disease in the United States: Locations Correlated with Distribution of Ixodes Dammini." *Annals of Internal Medicine* 91, no. 5 (1979): 730.

Steere, Allen C., S. E. Malawista, J. H. Newman, P. N. Spieler, and N. H. Bartenhagen. "Antibiotic Therapy in Lyme Disease." *Annals of Internal Medicine* 93, no. 1 (1980): 1.

Steere, Allen C., S. E. Malawista, D. R. Snydman, R. E. Shope, W. A. Andiman, M. R. Ross, and F. M. Steele. "Lyme Arthritis: An Epidemic of Oligoarticular Arthritis in Children and Adults in Three Connecticut Communities." [In English]. *Arthritis and Rheumatism* 20, no. 1 (1977): 7–17.

Straubinger, Reinhard K., Brian A. Summers, Yung-Fu Chang, and Max J. G. Appel. "Persistence of Borrelia Burgdorferi in Experimentally Infected Dogs after Antibiotic Treatment." [In English]. *Journal of Clinical Microbiology* 35, no. 1 (1997): 6.

Stricker, Raphael B., and Lorraine Johnson. "Lyme Disease: Call for a "Manhattan Project" to Combat the Epidemic." *PLoS Pathogens* 10, no. 1 (2014): 3.

———. "The Lyme Disease Chronicles, Continued: Chronic Lyme Disease: In Defense of the Patient Enterprise." *The Federation of American Societies for Experimental Biology* 24 (2010): 4632–3.

———. "Serologic Tests for Lyme Disease: More Smoke and Mirrors." *Clinical Infectious Diseases* 47, no. 8 (2008): 1111–12.

Taylor, George C. "Lyme Disease: An Overview of Its Public Health Significance." *Journal of Environmental Health* 54, no. 1 (1991): 24–27.

Tonks, Alison. "Lyme Wars." *Infectious Diseases* 355 (2007): 910–12.

unknown. "Special Report: Lyme Disease, a Suburban Menace." *Nutrition Health Review* 81 (2001): 9.

Upshur, Ross E. G. "Do Clinical Guidelines Still Make Sense? No." *The Annals of Family Medicine* 12, no. 3 (2014): 202–3.

Ward, Sarah E., and Robert D. Brown. "A Framework for Incorporating the Prevention of Lyme Disease Transmission into the Landscape Planning and Design Process." *Landscape and Urban Planning* 66 (2004): 91–106.

Weintraub, Pamela. *Cure Unknown: Inside the Lyme Epidemic*. New York: St. Martin's Griffin, 2008.

Whelan, David. "Lyme Inc." *Forbes* 179, no. 5 (2007): 96–97.

Williams, Mara. *Nature's Dirty Needle: What You Need to Know About Chronic Lyme Disease and How to Get the Help to Feel Better*. San Francisco, CA: Bush Street Press, 2011.

Wormser, Gary P. and Eugene D. Shapiro. "Implications of Gender in Chronic Lyme Disease." [In English]. *Journal of Women's Health* 18, no. 6 (2009): 831–34.

Wormser, Gary P., Raymond J. Dattwyler, Eugene D. Shapiro, John J. Halperin, Allen C. Steere, Mark S. Klempner, Peter J. Krause, et al. "The Clinical Assessment, Treatment, and Prevention of Lyme Disease, Human Granulocytic Anaplasmosis, and Babesiosis: Clinical Practice Guidelines by the Infectious Diseases Society of America." *Clinical Infectious Diseases* 43, no. 9 (2006): 1089–134.

Wormser, Gary P., Edwin Masters, John Nowakowski, Donna McKenna, Diane Holmgren, Katherine Ma, Lauren Ihde, L. Frank Cavaliere, and Robert B. Nadelman. "Prospective Clinical Evaluation of Patients from Missouri and New York with Erythema Migrans—Like Skin Lesions." *Clinical Infectious Diseases* 41, no. 7 (2005): 958–65.

Afterword
Diagnosis: To Tell Apart

Atwood D. Gaines

In biomedicine, "diagnosis" literally means, "to tell apart." It comes from the Latin, derived from the Greek. In Greek, gnosis means "knowledge." That is, by distinguishing one entity from some other entity, we come to "know" it. It is thus unlike the French interrogative, "Qu'est que c'est ça?" "What is it that it is?" In other words, diagnosis distinguishes an entity from others rather than purely identifying the entity of clinical concern in and of itself.

Diagnosis is thus relational; it is also contextual not only in social and cultural terms, but also in nosological terms, the latter because a diagnoses in particular instances must draw from the array of extant possibilities. Such possibilities vary from time to time and context to context. As such, diagnoses carry temporally shifting meanings in all of the various medical specialties of biomedicine. For example, take the case of the OB/GYN diagnosis of menopause, which may not have previously existed as a diagnosis in some countries such as Japan (Lock 1993); however, it is being adopted now. So while problems associated with it could not have been diagnosed in that context 10 or 20 years ago, such a diagnosis of problems associated with menopause could be diagnosed now. Likewise, in my work at the inception of the anthropology of biomedicine in two psychiatric hospitals in the San Francisco Bay Area, the diagnosis of borderline personality disorder (in the *DSM-III*, 1980) was not uncommon in one, but was nonexistent in the other (Gaines 1979). Thus, as Davis and Nichter (this volume) show, physicians cannot make diagnoses of things they do not know about. Diagnoses have social implications and potential negative social and psychological consequences as well, as Hardon and Smith-Morris (this volume) argue.

The "proper" diagnosis also relates to therapies; certain diagnoses suggest particular therapies in all fields of biomedicine. In psychiatry today, a variety of pharmaceutical agents are available and these are usually, although not always, prescribed for specific conditions. There are "off label" uses, as many have noted, for many psychopharmaceuticals, as there are for other agents used elsewhere in biomedicine. In many cases, the agents can have very negative consequences, even if they are alleviating some of the target symptoms.

To be sure, as Crane (this volume) shows, a diagnosis can also be a reason for NOT treating certain people in whom alleged poor adherence would promote treatment-resistant strains of a disorder (in her case, HIV). And, paradoxically, persons may seek to achieve an otherwise highly stigmatized disease diagnosis, such as TB in Georgian prisons, as several scholars, including Paul Farmer (and Koch, this volume), have noted.

While social scientists and patients have been calling for a focus on experience and subjectivity in mental and other illnesses for some time, certain voices in psychiatry and elsewhere have called for ignoring such "ephemeral" things. Instead, they have called for an exclusive focus on Insel's (2013) call for a clinical neuroscience that has departed from the traditional model of psychiatric diagnosis, which is based on self-reported symptom checklists, and replaced this with data on neural systems and their dysregulation, which is asserted to create the manifest symptoms of mental illness. Such identification of these ultimate (for now) sources of illness can then be targeted for intervention to correct or prevent illness.

With comments such as this, we see that the issue in diagnosis is often one of ontology (Hacking 2002) and, perhaps, not epistemology (see Potter, this volume). This clinical neuroscience appears to be but a refinement on the shift in psychiatry away from the psychological (and psychoanalytic) to biology; only now, the biology is neurology. Purporting to be atheoretical and descriptive, the formulators of the American Psychiatry Association's *Diagnostic and Statistical Manual, Third Edition (1980,* 1987) asserted that they were moving away from explanation to a more positivist stance (in the correct sense of the term), that is, as a non-causal, non-explanatory position. In fact, the *DSM-III* was intended to advance other biological theories of disease by eliminating others (Gaines 1992a; Young 1991). We note that the key problem of any psychology is the demarcation between the normal and the abnormal (Devereux 1978).

That which is abnormal psychology becomes psychiatry's (or psychoanalysis's) objects of concern and, in other illth domains, a medical concern or something in the patient's head (e.g., Lyme disease in the case discussed by Davis and Nicther, this volume). The boundary between the normal and the abnormal is always shifting in any area of medicine, viz., the radical shift from medically defined normal cholesterol levels to the now defined pathological levels in the last ten or so years in the U.S.

While the cultural construction and meaning of psychiatric diagnosis is easier to see than in corporally focused biomedicine (Gaines 1992a; Nuckols 1992), the same cultural processes may be seen at work in both, for medical science, and all other sciences, are both science and culture (Pickering 1992) and, as Young (1995) says, science, while its highest form, is also cultural. Much of the changes in biomedical diagnosis reflect attempts, as with Insel (2013) (see Myers, this volume) to put diagnosis in a 'firm' biological basis, or, these days, a firm biogenetic or neurological basis. As we move further down the biotic line, can atomic or molecular neuropsychiatry be far behind?

This move to deeper and deeper levels of biology seeks to remove the often obvious cultural involvement with diagnosis and, hence, with treatment (or non-treatment). Hence, we have the cultural biases of "race" and gender reappearing in forms of the "advanced" and "more scientific" diagnostic practices, especially those said to be based in biology and genetics and the putative "new racial medicine" (Gaines 1992b; Hunt and Kreiner 2013; Lock 2008). Such a trajectory only adds to the problems with biomedicine that are carried with it to other lands as a panacea for global health (see Gaines 2011).

The present studies show clearly the multivocal meaning of diagnosis and the seeking of diagnoses in a variety of settings. Diagnosis is a contested and contentious set of practices that must engage the object of the practices. However, another level, consonant with the formulation of a synthetic, millennial medical anthropology (Gaines 2011; Gaines and Whitehouse 2006), is the engagement of the theory of diagnosis in particular specialties rather than the practice thereof. The former can greatly illuminate the latter. This work remains for us to develop as we step through the diagnostic door (see Smith-Morris, this volume), although we must be mindful that the color, shape, and location of the door(s) rapidly change, as does that which is to be encountered on the other side.

REFERENCES CITED

American Psychiatric Association. *Diagnostic and Statistical Manual IV (DSM IV)*. Washington, DC: American Psychiatric Association, 1990.
_____. *Diagnostic and Statistical Manual III-Revised (DSM III-R)*. Washington, DC: American Psychiatric Association, 1987.
_____. *Diagnostic and Statistical Manual III (DSM III)*. Washington, DC: American Psychiatric Association, 1980.
Devereux, George. "Normal and Abnormal: The Key Problem in Psychiatric Anthropology." In *Ethnopsychoanalysis: Psychoanalysis and Anthropology as Complementary Frames of Reference*, edited by George Devereux, 3–71. Berkeley: University of California Press, 1978.
Gaines, Atwood D. "Millennial Medical Anthropology: from There to Here and Beyond or, the Problem of Global Health." *Culture, Medicine and Psychiatry* 34, no. 1 (2011): 83–89.
———. "From DSM I to III-R, Voices of Self, Mastery and the Other: A Cultural Constructivist Reading of U.S. Psychiatric Classification." *Social Science and Medicine* 35, no. 1 (1992a): 3–24.
_____. "Medical/Psychiatric Knowledge in France and the United States: Culture and Sickness in History and Biology." In *Ethnopsychiatry: the Cultural Construction of Professional and Folk Psychiatries*, edited by Atwood D. Gaines, 171–201. Albany, NY: State University of New York Press, 1992b.
_____. "Definitions and Diagnoses: Cultural Implications of Psychiatric Help-Seeking and Psychiatrists' Definitions of the Situation in Psychiatric Emergencies." *Culture, Medicine and Psychiatry* 3, no. 4 (1979): 381–418.
Gaines, Atwood D. and Peter J. Whitehouse. "Building a Mystery: Alzheimer Disease, Mild Cognitive Impairment and Beyond." *Journal of Philosophy, Psychiatry and Psychology* 13, no. 1 (2006): 61–74.

Hacking, Ian. *Historical Ontology*. Cambridge, MA: Harvard University Press, 2002.

Hunt, Linda M. and Meta J. Kreiner. "Pharmacogenetics in Primary Care: The Promise of Personalized Medicine and the Reality of Racial Profiling." *Culture, Medicine, and Psychiatry* 37, no. 1 (2013): 226–35.

Insel, Thomas R. "Director's Blog: Transforming Diagnosis." In *NIMH Director's Blog*, Edited by T. Insel, Vol. 2014, 2013, Accessed February 1, 2015. http://www.nimh.nih.gov/about/director/2013/transforming-diagnosis.shtml.

Lock, Margaret. "Biosociality and Susceptibility Genes: A Cautionary Tale." In *Biosocialities, Genetics and the Social Sciences*, edited by Sarah Gibbon and Carlos Novas, 56–78. London: Routledge, 2008.

_____. *Encounters with Aging: Mythologies of Menopause in Japan and North America*. Berkeley, CA: University of California Press, 1993.

Nuckolls, Charles, Editor. "The Cultural Construction of Psychiatric Categories." *Social Science and Medicine Special Issue* 35, no. 1 (1992).

Pickering, Andrew, Editor. *Science as Practice and Culture*. Chicago: University of Chicago Press, 1992.

Young, Allan. *A Harmony of Illusions: Inventing Post-Traumatic Stress Disorder*. Princeton: Princeton University Press, 1995.

_____. "Emil Kraepelin and the Origins of American Psychiatric Diagnosis." In *Anthropologies of Medicine*, edited by Beatrix Pfleiderer and Gilles Bibeau, 175–181. Wiesbaden, Germany: Vieweg und Sohn Verlag, 1991.

Contributors

EDITOR

Carolyn Smith-Morris is an Associate Professor and Director of the Health & Society Program in the Department of Anthropology at Southern Methodist University in Dallas, TX. Her work focuses on chronic disease and the health impacts of culture change in colonized and migrating groups. She is engaged in several research programs that work among migrating Mexican workers, with poor African Americans in Dallas, and for the Gila River Indian Community of Southern Arizona, a tribe that suffers from the highest recorded rates of type 2 diabetes in the world. She co-edited *Chronic Conditions, Fluid States: Chronicity and the Anthropology of Illness* with Lenore Manderson (2010, Rutgers University Press), and she published *Diabetes Among the Pima: Stories of Survival* in 2006 (University of Arizona Press).

AUTHORS

Johanna Crane is an Assistant Professor at the University of Washington Bothell. She is a medical anthropologist whose research and teaching focuses on questions of inequality in relation to medicine, science, and technology. Her most recent research documents the power dynamics that underlie global health research and practice. Her book *Scrambling for Africa: AIDS, Expertise, and the Rise of American Global Health Science* (Cornell University Press, 2013) uses ethnographic fieldwork conducted in the U.S. and Uganda to track how Africa has moved from being largely excluded from advancements in HIV medicine to a key locus of knowledge production in global health and HIV research. Dr. Crane earned her PhD from the UCSF/UC Berkeley Joint Program in Medical Anthropology in 2007, and her MA in anthropology from San Francisco State University in 1999.

Georgia Davis is a PhD candidate at the University of Arizona School of Geography and Development, and holds a postgraduate certificate in medical anthropology. Her work brings together her interest in health and her extensive training in broadcast journalism. Most recently, she worked for the public television affiliate in Tucson, Arizona, producing a weekly news magazine show featuring stories about science, medicine, and health. Prior to entering the PhD program, she spent 12 years in Florida working as a network radio bureau chief, political reporter, and public television news director.

Atwood D. Gaines is Professor of Anthropology, Bioethics, Nursing, and Psychiatry, and part of the Program Faculty Women's and Gender Studies at CWRU and its schools of medicine and nursing. His MA, CPhil and PhD, all in cultural anthropology, were earned at UC Berkeley. His MPH was received from UC Berkeley's School of Public Health. He also holds a certificate in (biomedical) ethics from Case's law school. He is editor-in-chief of the journal, *Culture, Medicine, and Psychiatry* and series Editor-in-Chief for the *Millennial Medical Anthropology* and the *Cultural Studies of Science and Medicine*, both with Springer. His books include Ethnopsychiatry (1992) and two volumes edited with Robert Hahn called Physicians of Western Medicine (1982, 1985), which initiated the cultural studies of biomedicine (i.e., the anthropology of biomedicine). He has published nearly 90 articles in journals and books in medical anthropology (on the subjects of anthropology of biomedicine, ethnopsychiatry, dementia (especially Alzheimer's disease), aging, and bioethics) and in the anthropology of religion, social identity, cultural studies of science, American studies, and Europeanist anthropology. His work on dementia with Peter Whitehouse, MD, PhD, has contributed to the deconstruction of Alzheimer's as a disease. Other key contributions include the cultural interpretation of U.S. psychiatric classifications (1991) and the cultural construction and variation of depression (with Paul Farmer). Dr. Gaines is a contributing author of the Cultural Formulation Appendix for the American Psychiatric Association's *Diagnostic and Statistical Manual, Fourth Edition (DSM-IV)* (2000).

Anita Hardon has been trained as a medical biologist and medical anthropologist (PhD). Her research career has taken shape around multi-site anthropological studies of global health technologies. Over the course of these research programs, she has provided intensive guidance to young researchers (many from Africa and Asia), engaging them in the joint writing of books and special issues of journals. At present she is the Scientific Director at the Amsterdam Institute for Social Science Research, and a Professor in Anthropology of Care and Health. She co-directs the global health research priority area of the University of Amsterdam. Anita Hardon is the co-author of the *Social Lives of Medicines* (2002). She publishes regularly in a wide number of journals, including *Social Science and Medicine*, Medical Anthropology and Culture Health and Sexuality. Recently, she edited a special issue on secrecy as an embodied practice (2012). She is currently conducted a study on the chemical lives of young people called Chemical Youth, which was awarded an ERC advanced grant.

Erin Koch is an Associate Professor of Anthropology at the University of Kentucky. Her research in medical anthropology and science and technology studies focuses on global health, biomedical standardization, infectious disease, and humanitarianism. She has conducted research in Georgia about contemporary tuberculosis control and about the health effects of protracted displacement and humanitarian interventions among ethnic Georgians displaced by civil war in the early 1990s.

Lenore Manderson, PhD, is Professor of Public Health and Medical Anthropology in the School of Public Health at the University of the Witwatersrand (South Africa), a visiting professor of anthropology at the Institute for the Study of Environment and Society at Brown (USA), and Adjunct Professor in Anthropology at Monash University. She is a medical anthropologist, but she has also contributed to sociology, the social history of medicine, and public health, undertaking field research and training across these disciplines primarily in Malaysia, Thailand, the Philippines, China, Ghana, and South Africa. Her recent books include *Surface tensions: surgery, bodily boundaries and the social self* (2011), *Technologies of sexuality, identity and sexual health* (ed., 2012), and *Disclosure in health and illness* (ed. With Mark Davis, 2014). She is editor of the international journal *Medical Anthropology*. Lenore is a Fellow of the Academy of Social Sciences of Australia (1995) and the World Academy of Art and Science (2004).

Neely Myers received her PhD in 2009 in comparative human development from the University of Chicago. She is a sociocultural anthropologist who specializes in the study of culture, madness, and disability. In 2014, she joined the Department of Anthropology at Southern Methodist University. Dr. Myers has conducted over a decade of ethnographic fieldwork among people with symptoms of serious mental illness in the United States and, more recently, in Tanzania. Her work has been supported by a three-year National Institutes of Health (NIH) postdoctoral fellowship through the University of Virginia and Georgetown University, the Nathan Kline Institute's NIH-funded Center to Study Recovery in Social Contexts, and the George Washington University's Elliott School of International Affairs Institute for Global and International Studies. Recent projects include a preliminary investigation of women, mental health, and mental illness in Tanzania, as well as a recently funded (NIH) project on how young people with early psychosis, primarily African Americans, make decisions about early treatment. Her forthcoming book (2015) is *Mad Dreamers: Madness, Moral Agency, and Recovery*, from Vanderbilt University Press.

Mark Nichter is a Regents' Professor and the coordinator of the medical anthropology graduate training program at the University of Arizona. He received a BA in philosophy and psychology at George Washington University (1971), a PhD in social anthropology from the University of Edinburgh (1977), a MPH in international health from the Johns Hopkins School of Public Health (1978), and postdoctoral training in clinically applied anthropology from the University of Hawaii (1980–83). He holds joint appointments in the Department of Family and Community Medicine and the College of Public Health at the University of Arizona. Dr. Nichter has over 30 years of experience conducting health-related research in Asia, Africa, and North America. His most recent research has focused on neglected and emerging diseases, tobacco, and pharmaceutical practice. Dr. Nichter is the author of over 130 articles and book chapters in a wide variety of health-related fields and four books, including *Global Health: Why Cultural Perceptions, Social Representations, and Biopolitics Matter* (2008).

Nancy Nyquist Potter is Professor of Philosophy at the University of Louisville. She teaches and writes about ethical theory and practice and her current focus is in philosophy and psychiatry. She has published extensively in this area. Her books include *How Can I Be Trusted? A Virtue Theory of Trustworthiness* (Rowman-Littlefield, 2002), the edited volume *Trauma, Truth, and Reconciliation: Healing Damaged Relationships* (Oxford University Press, 2006), and *Mapping the Edges and the In-Between: A Critical Analysis of Borderline Personality Disorder* (Oxford University Press, 2009). She is part of the health care team at the University of Louisville's Emergency Psychiatry Department. Her most recent book project is *The Virtue of Defiance and Psychiatric Engagement: Psychiatry and Norms for Compliant Behavior* (to be published by Oxford University Press).

Fabiola Rohden received a PhD in social anthropology at the Federal University of Rio de Janeiro (2000). She is an Associate Professor and coordinator of the Center for Research in Anthropology of the Body and Health at the Department of Anthropology at the Federal University of Rio Grande do Sul. She is also an associate researcher at the Latin American Center on Sexuality and Human Rights and a researcher for the National Council of Science and Technology. She is engaged in research on gender, sexuality, the anthropology of science, and the history of gynecology, and has published a series of articles on gender relations, the anthropology of the body, and sexuality, gender, and science. She is the author of the books *A science of difference: sex and gender in women's medicine* (Fiocruz, 2001; 2009), *Deceptive nature: contraception, abortion and infanticide in the early twentieth century* (Fiocruz, 2003), and *Living sciences: anthropology of science in perspective*, a volume she edited with Claudia Fonseca and Paula Machado (Terceiro Nome, 2012)

Lisbeth Sachs is a medical anthropologist with experience as professor/researcher in the Department of Communication Studies at Linköping University and as a researcher in the Department of International Health Care Research at Karolinska Institute, Stockholm. She is a scientific advisor at the Skaraborg Institute in Skövde, and affiliated as senior research advisor with the Osher Center for Integrative Medicine, at Karolinska Institute. She is a member of the Council for Culture at the Karolinska Institute and is a member of the board of the Hagströmer Medico-Historical Library.

Narelle Warren, PhD, is a lecturer in the anthropology program at the School of Social Sciences at Monash University. Her current research focuses on understanding the relationship between the lived experience of neurological conditions, biomedical representations of the brain, and temporality, from both the perspectives of people living with such conditions and their informal caregivers. She works in Australia and Southeast Asia, where she is undertaking ethnographic research into community factors and recovery from stroke in rural Malaysia. Much of her work to date has been concerned with understanding how people's experiences of chronic conditions vary by gender, age, geographical location, and culture, and what mechanisms underlie these experiences. She is the co-editor, along with Lenore Manderson, of *Reframing Quality of Life and Physical Disability* (2013).

Index

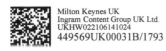